Cutting-Edge Concepts in Knee Surgery

Cutting-Edge Concepts in Knee Surgery

Guest Editor

Dhong Won Lee

MDPI

Basel • Beijing • Wuhan • Barcelona • Belgrade • Novi Sad • Cluj • Manchester

Guest Editor
Dhong Won Lee
Orthopaedic Surgery
Konkuk University Medical
Center, Konkuk University
Seoul
Republic of Korea

Editorial Office
MDPI AG
Grosspeteranlage 5
4052 Basel, Switzerland

This is a reprint of the Special Issue, published open access by the journal *Medicina* (ISSN 1648-9144), freely accessible at: https://www.mdpi.com/journal/medicina/special_issues/PJLO484LS9.

For citation purposes, cite each article independently as indicated on the article page online and as indicated below:

Lastname, A.A.; Lastname, B.B. Article Title. *Journal Name* **Year**, *Volume Number*, Page Range.

ISBN 978-3-7258-6564-2 (Hbk)
ISBN 978-3-7258-6565-9 (PDF)
https://doi.org/10.3390/books978-3-7258-6565-9

Contents

About the Editor

Dhong Won Lee

Dhong Won Lee is a Professor in the Department of Orthopaedic Surgery at Konkuk University Medical Center in Seoul, Republic of Korea, where he specializes in knee surgery and sports medicine. His clinical practice is focused on joint preservation procedures, including ligament reconstruction, meniscal surgery, cartilage restoration, alignment correction, and arthroplasty, with a strong emphasis on evidence-based surgical decision making.

His research interests encompass meniscal allograft transplantation, cartilage repair strategies, biomechanical factors influencing knee alignment, and the assessment of clinical and functional outcomes following joint-preserving surgery. He has authored and co-authored numerous peer-reviewed publications in international journals and is actively involved in academic activities as a reviewer and Guest Editor.

Through the integration of clinical expertise and academic research, Professor Lee aims to advance the understanding of knee pathology and to contribute to improved long-term functional outcomes and surgical precision for patients with complex knee disorders.

Preface

Knee surgery has undergone rapid evolution over the past few decades, driven by advances in biomechanics, imaging technology, biologic treatments, and an increasing emphasis on joint preservation. As patients remain active longer and expectations for functional recovery continue to rise, surgeons are challenged to adopt strategies that balance symptom relief with long-term joint health. This Reprint, "*Cutting-Edge Concepts in Knee Surgery*", brings together a series of high-quality contributions that address key clinical and scientific questions in contemporary knee surgery. The included articles cover a broad spectrum of topics, ranging from ligament reconstruction and meniscal surgery to cartilage repair, alignment correction, and arthroplasty, reflecting the multidisciplinary nature of modern knee care. The Guest Editor hopes that this Reprint will serve not only as a practical reference for daily clinical decision making but also as a platform to stimulate further discussion and research aimed at improving outcomes for patients with complex knee disorders.

Dhong Won Lee
Guest Editor

medicina

MDPI

Review

Usefulness of 3-Dimensional Computed Tomography Assessment of Femoral Tunnel after Anterior Cruciate Ligament Reconstruction

Min-Jeong Kim [1], Sung-Gyu Moon [2], Ji-Hee Kang [2] and Dhong-Won Lee [3,*]

1 Department of Radiology, Incheon Sarang Hospital, Incheon 22135, Republic of Korea; ish1283@saranghospital.com
2 Department of Radiology, KonKuk University Medical Center, Konkuk University School of Medicine, Seoul 05030, Republic of Korea; sgmoon@kuh.ac.kr (S.-G.M.); 20200184@kuh.ac.kr (J.-H.K.)
3 Department of Orthopaedic Surgery, KonKuk University Medical Center, Konkuk University School of Medicine, Seoul 05030, Republic of Korea
* Correspondence: osdoctorknee@kuh.ac.kr

Abstract: Positioning of the femoral tunnel during anterior cruciate ligament (ACL) reconstruction is the most crucial factor for successful procedure. Owing to the inter-individual variability in the intra-articular anatomy, it can be challenging to obtain precise tunnel placement and ensure consistent results. Currently, the three-dimensional (3D) reconstruction of computed tomography (CT) scans is considered the best method for determining whether femoral tunnels are positioned correctly. Postoperative 3D-CT feedback can improve the accuracy of femoral tunnel placement. Precise tunnel formation obtained through feedback has a positive effect on graft maturation, graft failure, and clinical outcomes after surgery. However, even if femoral tunnel placement on 3D CT is appropriate, we should recognize that acute graft bending negatively affects surgical results. This review aimed to discuss the implementation of 3D-CT evaluation for predicting postoperative outcomes following ACL re-construction. Reviewing research that has performed 3D CT evaluations after ACL reconstruction can provide clinically significant evidence of the formation of ideal tunnels following anatomic ACL reconstruction.

Keywords: anterior cruciate ligament anatomy; anterior cruciate ligament reconstruction; 3-dimensional computed tomography; tunnel position; femoral tunnel; quadrant method

1. Introduction

An anterior cruciate ligament (ACL) injury is a common sports-related knee injury that can cause knee instability and secondary meniscal damage [1]. The goal of ACL reconstruction is to restore the knee to a state that is anatomically, biomechanically, and functionally similar to normal [1]. Several factors are involved in achieving the best surgical outcomes, including the choice of graft, method of graft fixation, and postoperative rehabilitation exercises [2]. However, the positioning of the femoral and tibial tunnels during ACL reconstruction is the most crucial factor for successful procedure [3–7]. In particular, small changes in the femoral tunnel position can have large effects on the graft-length pattern during knee flexion and extension [8,9]. In other words, this can have significant implications not only for graft maturation and failure but also for knee biomechanics. Much research has been conducted on tunnel positioning during ACL reconstruction, and surgical techniques have evolved based on the evidence for establishing the position of the femoral tunnel [10–18].

Owing to inter-individual variability in the intra-articular anatomy, such as the bony ridges of the femoral condyle, it can be challenging to obtain precise tunnel placement and ensure consistent results, even when guided by intra-articular landmarks during reconstruction surgery. This concept of anatomical ligament reconstruction has led to an increase in the use of imaging to validate tunnel placement during and after surgery [10–21]. A consensus on the anatomical centers of the femur and tibia is crucial for practical and clinically efficient use of imaging to confirm tunnel placement [22].

The accuracy of imaging in depicting tunnel placement has been validated in cadaver studies using radiographs, computed tomography (CT) scan, and magnetic resonance imaging (MRI) [23]. Currently, three-dimensional (3D) reconstruction of CT scans is considered the best method to determine whether the femoral and tibial tunnels are positioned correctly [23,24].

This narrative review aims to present the formation of ideal femoral tunnels and to discuss the implementation of 3D-CT evaluation for predicting postoperative outcomes following ACL reconstruction based on the current literature.

2. Femoral Tunnel Assessments

2.1. Cadaveric Anatomy

Several studies assessed the femoral footprint of the native ACL in cadaveric specimens [25–31]. These studies used the Bernard and Hertel grid, known as the quadrant method, as described by Bernard et al. [32] to represent the ACL center. The center of the ACL footprint was determined in the high to low direction and deep to shallow direction and presented as the percentage of the distance from the roof of the intercondylar notch and the posterior edge of the lateral femoral condyle (Figure 1). The centers of anteromedial (AM) bundle and posterolateral (PL) bundles are summarized in Table 1.

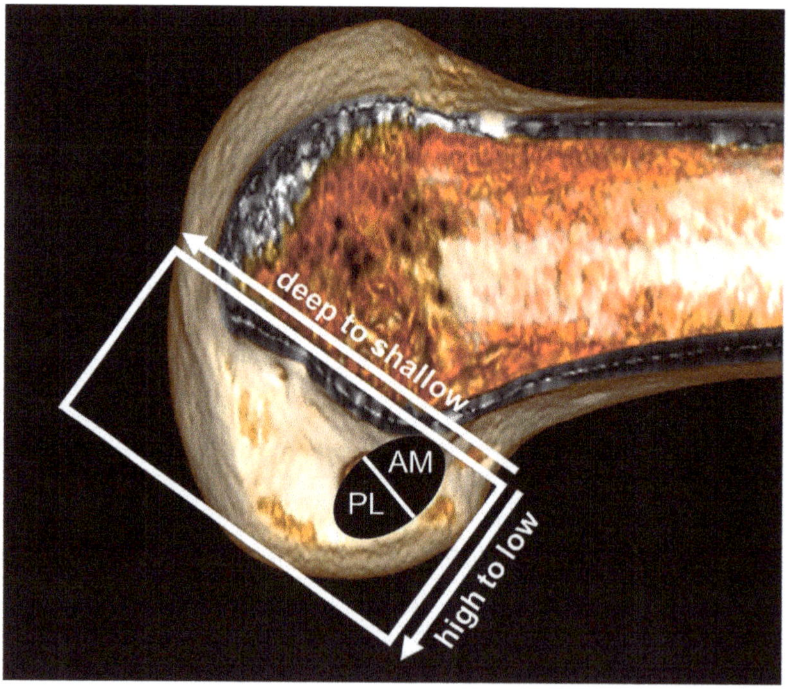

Figure 1. Femoral tunnel placement by the quadrant method. AM—anteromedial; PL—posterolateral.

Table 1. Anatomic Center of ACL Femoral Footprint.

Study	Whole Bundle		Anteromedial Bundle		Posterolateral Bundle	
	High to Low (%)	Deep to Shallow (%)	High to Low (%)	Deep to Shallow (%)	High to Low (%)	Deep to Shallow (%)
Colombet et al. [25]	36.5	29.4	25.3	26.4	47.6	32.3
Forsythe et al. [31]	44.3	28.4	33.2	21.7	55.3	35.1
Lee et al. [26]	41.0	37.3	25.6	33.9	56.4	40.6
Lorenz et al. [29]	33.5	24.0	22.0	21.0	45.0	27.0
Luites et al. [27]	28.5	25.5	10.0	23.0	47.0	28.0
Musahl et al. [30]	26.6	26.3	Not applicable	Not applicable	Not applicable	Not applicable
Tsukada et al. [28]	30.0	30.4	17.8	25.9	41.1	34.8

Piefer et al. [33] systematically reviewed the anatomic center of the ACL femoral footprint. After analyzing eight items, the mean whole bundle center was 35.2% for the high to low direction and 28.5% for the deep to shallow direction. The mean centers of the AM bunle and PL bundle were 23.1% and 48.8% in the high to low direction and 21.5% and 32% in the deep to shallow direction, respectively. Parkar et al. [22] conducted a systematic review of the literature on the anatomic center of the ACL. In their systematic review, 218 knees demonstrated that the weighted mean and the weighted median of the femoral center were 35% and 34% for the high to low direction and 29% and 26% for the deep to shallow direction, respectively. The weighted 5th and 95th percentiles for high to low direction were 28% and 43%, and for deep to shallow direction were 24% and 37%, respectively. They suggested the use of the 5th and 95th percentiles when evaluating postoperative femoral placement to be 'in or out of the anatomic range.' These systematic reviews of anatomy studies have clinical relevance for orthopedic surgeons who believe that anatomical ACL reconstruction results in improved outcomes.

2.2. Postoperative 3D CT-Based Study

Intra-articular anatomy is influenced by inter-individual variability, and in anatomical studies, structures such as the lateral intercondylar ridge or bifurcate ridge of the femoral condyle have been described to exhibit variations among individuals [34–36]. Moreover, in cases of chronic rupture or re-rupture, these intra-articular structures are often not clearly visible, making it challenging for surgeons to determine whether the femoral tunnel has been accurately positioned during the operation [37]. Therefore, using only intra-articular landmarks may result in significant variations in femoral tunnel placement. To overcome this problem, many authors are trying to use intraoperative fluoroscopy or ACL computer-assisted surgery, but this is still at a challenging stage, and further verification studies are needed [38,39].

The usefulness of feedback after ACL reconstruction using 3D-CT has been reported in several studies [10,38,40]. Inderhaug et al. [38] switched from a transtibial to a trans-AM portal technique for ACL reconstruction, and they compared the femoral tunnel positions between the trans-AM portal technique without postoperative 3D-CT feedback (AM 1) and the trans-AM portal technique after 3D-CT feedback (AM 2). Mean femoral tunnel placements in high to low direction were 8%, 26%, and 29% in transtibial group, AM 1, and AM 2, and for deep to shallow direction were 32%, 43%, and 27% in transtibial group, AM 1, and AM 2, respectively. The femoral tunnel placement gradually approached the ideal femoral tunnel center (34% in high to low direction and 27% in deep to shallow direction) described by Bird et al. [19] in all groups over time. In particular, AM 2 showed a significant improvement in the distance from the ideal femoral tunnel center over time throughout the feedback period compared to AMI 1 (p = 0.001) (Figure 2). Changing from the transtibial to the trans-AM portal technique and postoperative 3D-CT feedback were critical points in the improvement of femoral tunnel placement (Figures 2 and 3). It is important to perform repeated surgeries to increase the accuracy of femoral tunnel placement; however, radiological feedback is equally important. Sirleo et al. [10] performed

ACL reconstruction using the outside-in technique in a series of 60 consecutive patients, providing 3D-CT feedback within 48 h after each surgery. Subsequently, they divided the patients into three groups of 20 patients each according to the order of surgery (three consecutive series) and compared the femoral tunnel placement among these groups. The ideal femoral tunnel placement was 35.2% in high to low direction and 28.5% in deep to shallow direction, reported by Piefer et al. [33]. They confirmed progressive improvement in femoral tunnel placement from the first to the second series, and from the second to the third series. Both the accuracy and precision of the femoral tunnel placement increased from the first to the third series. They concluded that postoperative 3D-CT feedback was effective in the learning process to improve accuracy (+52.4%) and precision (+55.7%) of femoral tunnel placement to perform appropriate anatomic ACL reconstruction.

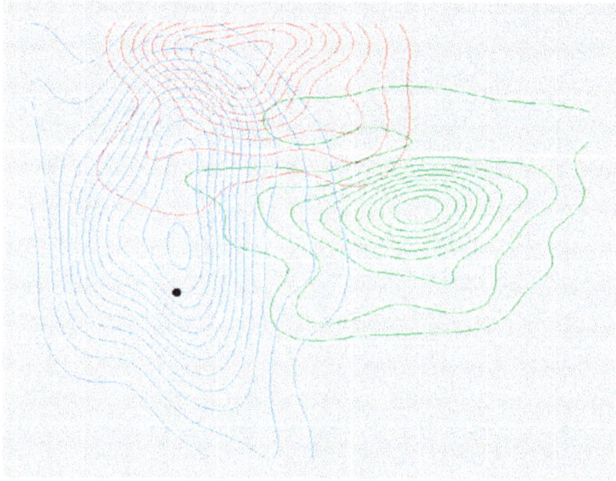

Figure 2. Contour plot of the spread of the femoral tunnels in transtibial group, trans-AM portal technique without feedback (AM 1) and trans-AM portal technique after feedback (AM 2) groups (red transtibial group, green AM 1 group, blue AM 2 group). Black dot means an ideal femoral tunnel center (34% in high to low direction and 27% in deep to shallow direction) described by Bird et al. [19]. (Reprinted with permission from Springer [38]).

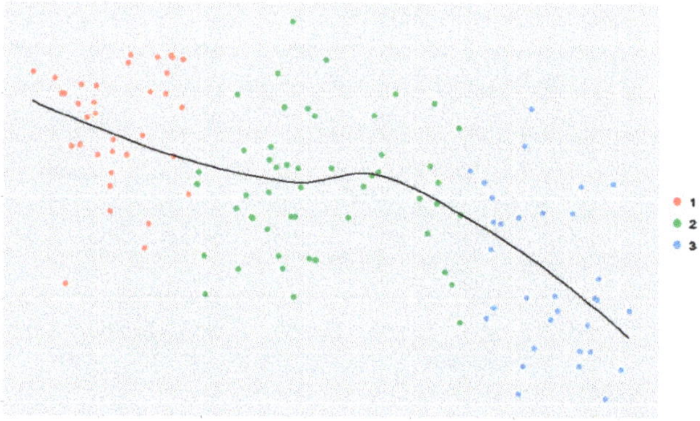

Figure 3. Relative distance (*Y*-axis indicates relative distance from ideal femoral tunnel center in absolute value) from femoral tunnel to ideal femoral tunnel center as a function of time (*X*-axis indicates time from first to last surgery). *Red (1) transtibial group, green (2) trans-AM portal technique without feedback, blue (3) trans-AM portal technique after feedback.* (Reprinted with permission from Springer [38]).

2.3. Clinical Relevance of Postoperative 3D CT

Parkinson et al. [41] demonstrated that shallow nonanatomic femoral tunnel placement was significant predictor of graft failure (hazard ratio 4.3; 95% CI, 1.6–11.6; p = 0.004). Among 97 patients assessed using postoperative 3D-CT, failure rates were 30% for shallow nonanatomic placement and 21% for deep anatomic placement. Shallow femoral tunnel placement is the most common cause of ACL reconstruction failure [42–44]. They recommended postoperative 3D-CT to ensure appropriate femoral tunnel placement and to decrease the risk of non-anatomic femoral tunnel positioning and failure. Mhaskar et al. [40] analyzed 60 ACL reconstructions and categorized femoral tunnel placement into type I (well-placed), type II (slightly malpositioned), and type III (grossly malpositioned) according to postoperative 3D-Ct. There were 32 type I, 28 type II, and no type III tunnels. There were significant differences in postoperative Lysholm score and International Knee Documentation Committee (IKDC) score between type I and II tunnels (62.2 ± 16.2 vs. 48.5 ± 17.2, p = 0.002, and 62.5 ± 14.3 vs. 52.7 ± 15.1, p = 0.012, respectively).

Some authors reported that femoral tunnel placement on 3D-CT can influence graft inclination and maturation on MRI. Lee et al. [45] reported that a total of 60 patients who underwent anatomical ACL reconstruction using flexible reamer system showed femoral tunnel located at 24.1 ± 5.9% in high to low direction and at mean 29.7 ± 4.4% in deep to shallow direction on postoperative 3D-CT. They aimed to target the femoral tunnel position slightly toward the AM bundle rather than the center of the entire bundle and received 3D-CT feedback after each procedure. As a result, all patients had a comparable sagittal and coronal graft inclination to them of the native ACL (52.4 ± 4.6° and 69.2 ± 4.7°, respectively). Femoral tunnels created at anatomical positions on 3D-CT ultimately result in a graft inclination similar to that of the normal ACL, and this similarity in graft inclination can have implications for clinical outcomes and graft laxity [46,47]. Lee et al. [48] proved that positioning the femoral tunnel near the AM bundle and center led to better graft signal intensity on postoperative MRI (one year after anatomic ACL reconstruction) than positioning the femoral tunnel near the PL bundle, although there were no differences in clinical outcomes or knee laxity. MRI signal intensity reflects graft maturation [16,48,49]. In their study, the mean femoral tunnel placements were 20.3%, 33.76%, and 47.56% in high to low direction in AM bundle positioned group, center positioned group, and PL bundle positioned groups, respectively. Regarding deep to shallow direction, mean femoral tunnel placements were 21.67%, 25.95%, and 30.23% in AM bundle positioned group, center positioned group, and PL bundle positioned groups, respectively. They assumed that the AM bundle and center positions led to less graft excursion during knee flexion and extension than the PL bundle position.

Even when similar femoral tunnel positions are observed on 3D-CT, the graft bending angle varies between femoral drilling techniques. Because the graft bending angle can influence graft stress, it is necessary in the future to analyze not only the tunnel position but also the graft bending angle for receiving feedback. Lee et al. [16] compared the femoral tunnel placement, the graft bending angle at the femoral tunnel on 3D-CT, and the signal/noise quotient (SNQ) on MRI between single-bundle ACL reconstruction using modified transtibial and outside-in techniques. Femoral tunnel placement for the high to low direction were 39.8 ± 2.4% and 40.9 ± 1.9% (p = 0.087), and deep to shallow direction were 31.3 ± 2.9% and 33.2 ± 2.5% (p = 0.517) in modified transtibial group and outside-in group, respectively. However, the femoral graft bending angle was reduced in the modified transtibial group, and SNQ at the femoral intraosseous and proximal grafts on MRI were lower in the modified transtibial group than in the outside-in group (p < 0.01). These results showed that an acute femoral graft bending angle could negatively affect graft maturation, even though the femoral tunnel was positioned anatomically. Niki et al. [21] compared the femoral tunnel placement and graft bending angle on 3D-CT between double-bundle ACL reconstruction using outside-in and trans-AM portal techniques. There were no significant differences in femoral tunnel placement between the two groups. Femoral tunnel placement for the high to low direction were 19.8 ± 6.2% (AM bundle) and 47.9 ± 8.5% (PL bundle) in the outside-in group, and 22.9 ± 8.0% (AM bundle) and 48.6 ± 8.8% (PL bundle) in the trans-AM portal group. The deep-to-shallow directions were 18.4 ± 5.6% (AM bundle) and 22.5 ± 6.0% (PL bundle) in the outside-in group, and 21.0 ± 5.5% (AM bundle) and 24.6 ± 4.8% (PL bundle) in the trans-AM portal group. However, the graft bending angles of the AM bundle and PL bundle were greater in the outside-in group ($p < 0.001$). These results can help surgeons choose a technique that shows an obtuse graft bending angle while creating a femoral tunnel in an appropriate position.

The 3D-CT can provide surgeons with useful information for revision ACL reconstruction. During revision ACL reconstruction, accurate determination of the position of the femoral tunnel created is essential for planning whether revision surgery should be performed in a one- or two-stage manner. In this context, 3D-CT serves as a tool to accurately assess femoral tunnel placement. Magnussen et al. [50] developed a femoral tunnel classification according to 3D-CT, which yielded a moderate to substantial inter- and intra-observer reliability (kappa coefficient of 0.57 and 0.67, respectively) (Table 2). They suggested that type I should consider a re-using tunnel, type 2 should consider a two-stage procedure when there is a possibility of tunnel convergence, and type 3 should consider a new tunnel without concern of convergence.

Table 2. Classification system for previous tunnel placement according to 3D-CT.

Femoral Tunnel Type		Location Relative to the Lateral Intercondylar Ridge
I	Well positioned	Inferior and posterior
II-Vertical II-Anterior II-Both	Slightly malpositioned	Overlapping
III	Significantly malpositioned	Entirely vertical and/or anterior

3. Authors' Suggestions

Because it is important to create a femoral tunnel at the anatomical footprint for successful ACL reconstruction, surgeons must accurately identify the anatomical femoral footprint as identified in various cadaveric experiments. However, owing to the large individual variations in bony landmarks, it is often difficult to evaluate whether the femoral tunnel is created in the desired position when operated in a limited arthroscopic field of view. If a surgeon does not recognize that the femoral tunnel placement is incorrect and performs the same surgery, the surgeon is likely to make the same mistake. To avoid such errors, radiological feedback is required. In order to receive feedback on the target point you chose during surgery, it is better to review it within 48 to 72 h after the surgery.

In addition, it is important for surgeons to know the results of the surgery and explain them to the patient.

4. Conclusions

Postoperative 3D-CT feedback, which is considered the best method for determining whether femoral tunnels are positioned correctly, is effective in improving the accuracy of femoral tunnel placement. Precise tunnel formation obtained through feedback may have a positive effect on graft maturation, graft failure, and clinical outcomes after surgery.

5. Future Directions

Even if femoral tunnel placement on 3D-CT is appropriate, we should recognize that acute graft bending negatively affects surgical results. Therefore, in the future, it will be necessary to utilize 3D-CT to analyze femoral tunnel placement as well as various factors such as the graft bending angle and graft contact area. This will enable the receipt of feedback that will facilitate the selection of appropriate surgical techniques.

Author Contributions: Conceptualization, D.-W.L.; investigation, M.-J.K. and J.-H.K.; resources, S.-G.M.; writing—original draft preparation, M.-J.K. and J.-H.K.; writing—review and editing, D.-W.L. and S.-G.M.; supervision, D.-W.L. All authors have read and agreed to the published version of the manuscript.

Funding: This research received no external funding.

Institutional Review Board Statement: Not applicable.

Informed Consent Statement: Not applicable.

Data Availability Statement: All relevant data generated or analyzed during this study are included in this published article.

Conflicts of Interest: The authors declare no conflict of interest.

References

1. Louboutin, H.; Debarge, R.; Richou, J.; Selmi, T.A.S.; Donell, S.T.; Neyret, P.; Dubrana, F. Osteoarthritis in patients with anterior cruciate ligament rupture: A review of risk factors. *Knee* **2009**, *16*, 239–244. [CrossRef] [PubMed]
2. Tuca, M.; Valderrama, I.; Eriksson, K.; Tapasvi, S. Current trends in anterior cruciate ligament surgery. A worldwide benchmark study. *J. ISAKOS* **2023**, *8*, 2–10. [CrossRef] [PubMed]
3. Moran, T.E.; Ignozzi, A.J.; Werner, B.C. Comparing the Use of Flexible and Rigid Reaming Systems Through an Anteromedial Portal for Femoral Tunnel Creation During Anterior Cruciate Ligament Reconstruction: A Systematic Review. *Orthop. J. Sports Med.* **2021**, *9*, 23259671211035741. [CrossRef] [PubMed]
4. Vijayan, S.; Kyalakond, H.; Kulkarni, M.S.; Aroor, M.N.; Shetty, S.; Bhat, V.; Rao, S.K. Clinical outcome of anterior cruciate ligament reconstruction with modified transtibial and anteromedial portal. *Musculoskelet. Surg.* **2021**, *107*, 37–45. [CrossRef]
5. Fernandes, T.L.; Moreira, H.H.; Andrade, R.; Sasaki, S.U.; Bernardo, W.M.; Pedrinelli, A.; Espregueira-Mendes, J.; Hernandez, A.J. Clinical Outcome Evaluation of Anatomic Anterior Cruciate Ligament Reconstruction With Tunnel Positioning Using Gold Standard Techniques: A Systematic Review and Meta-analysis. *Orthop. J. Sports Med.* **2021**, *9*, 23259671211013327. [CrossRef]
6. Wang, H.; Fleischli, J.E.; Zheng, N.N. Transtibial versus anteromedial portal technique in single-bundle anterior cruciate ligament reconstruction: Outcomes of knee joint kinematics during walking. *Am. J. Sports Med.* **2013**, *41*, 1847–1856. [CrossRef]
7. Fox, M.A.; Engler, I.D.; Zsidai, B.T.; Hughes, J.D.; Musahl, V. Anatomic anterior cruciate ligament reconstruction: Freddie Fu's paradigm. *J. ISAKOS* **2023**, *8*, 15–22. [CrossRef]
8. Musahl, V.; Plakseychuk, A.; VanScyoc, A.; Sasaki, T.; Debski, R.E.; Mcmahon, P.J.; Fu, F.H. Varying femoral tunnels between the anatomical footprint and isometric positions: Effect on kinematics of the anterior cruciate ligament-reconstructed knee. *Am. J. Sports Med.* **2005**, *33*, 712–718. [CrossRef]
9. Zantop, T.; Diermann, N.; Schumacher, T.; Schanz, S.; Fu, F.H.; Petersen, W. Anatomical and nonanatomical double-bundle anterior cruciate ligament reconstruction: Importance of femoral tunnel location on knee kinematics. *Am. J. Sports Med.* **2008**, *36*, 678–685. [CrossRef]
10. Sirleo, L.; Innocenti, M.; Innocenti, M.; Civinini, R.; Carulli, C.; Matassi, F. Post-operative 3D CT feedback improves accuracy and precision in the learning curve of anatomic ACL femoral tunnel placement. *Knee Surg. Sports Traumatol. Arthrosc.* **2018**, *26*, 468–477. [CrossRef]
11. Vermersch, T.; Lustig, S.; Reynaud, O.; Debette, C.; Servien, E.; Neyret, P. CT assessment of femoral tunnel placement after partial ACL reconstruction. *Orthop. Traumatol. Surg. Res.* **2016**, *102*, 197–202. [CrossRef] [PubMed]
12. Tomihara, T.; Hashimoto, Y.; Taniuchi, M.; Shimada, N. Relationship between femoral tunnel location and graft bending angle in outside-in and transportal technique for ACL double bundle reconstruction in 3D-CT study. *Arch. Orthop. Trauma Surg.* **2015**, *135*, 839–846. [CrossRef] [PubMed]
13. Vadlamudi, A.; Kale, A.; Sharma, J.; Patil, V.; Pai, M. Comparison of Inside-Out and Outside-In Methods of Femoral Tunnel Preparation in Anterior Cruciate Ligament (ACL) Reconstruction Using 3D-CT. *Cureus* **2022**, *14*, e23367. [CrossRef] [PubMed]
14. Seo, Y.J.; Song, S.Y.; Im, W.Y.; Kim, Y.S.; Jang, S.W. Effects of flexible reamer on the femoral tunnel characteristics in anterior cruciate ligament reconstruction. *Medicine* **2021**, *100*, e27833. [CrossRef] [PubMed]
15. Yoon, K.H.; Kim, J.H.; Kwon, Y.B.; Kim, E.J.; Lee, S.H.; Kim, S.G. A two-portal technique using a flexible reamer system is a safe and effective method for transportal anterior cruciate ligament reconstruction. *Arch. Orthop. Trauma Surg.* **2020**, *140*, 383–390. [CrossRef]
16. Lee, D.W.; Kim, J.G.; Lee, J.H.; Park, J.H.; Kim, D.H. Comparison of Modified Transtibial and Outside-In Techniques in Anatomic Single-Bundle Anterior Cruciate Ligament Reconstruction. *Arthroscopy* **2018**, *34*, 2857–2870. [CrossRef]
17. Kim, J.G.; Wang, J.H.; Lim, H.C.; Ahn, J.H. Femoral graft bending angle and femoral tunnel geometry of transportal and outside-in techniques in anterior cruciate ligament reconstruction: An in vivo 3-dimensional computed tomography analysis. *Arthroscopy* **2012**, *28*, 1682–1694. [CrossRef]
18. Youm, Y.S.; Cho, S.D.; Eo, J.; Lee, K.J.; Jung, K.H.; Cha, J.R. 3D CT analysis of femoral and tibial tunnel positions after modified transtibial single bundle ACL reconstruction with varus and internal rotation of the tibia. *Knee* **2013**, *20*, 272–276. [CrossRef]

19. Bird, J.H.; Carmont, M.R.; Dhillon, M.; Smith, N.; Brown, C.; Thompson, P.; Spalding, T. Validation of a new technique to determine midbundle femoral tunnel position in anterior cruciate ligament reconstruction using 3-dimensional computed tomography analysis. *Arthroscopy* **2011**, *27*, 1259–1267. [CrossRef]
20. de Abreu-e-Silva, G.M.; Baumfeld, D.S.; Bueno, E.L.; Pfeilsticker, R.M.; de Andrade, M.A.; Nunes, T.A. Clinical and three-dimensional computed tomographic comparison between ACL transportal versus ACL transtibial single-bundle reconstructions with hamstrings. *Knee* **2014**, *21*, 1203–1209. [CrossRef]
21. Niki, Y.; Nagai, K.; Harato, K.; Suda, Y.; Nakamura, M.; Matsumoto, M. Effects of femoral bone tunnel characteristics on graft-bending angle in double-bundle anterior cruciate ligament reconstruction: A comparison of the outside-in and transportal techniques. *Knee Surg. Sports Traumatol. Arthrosc.* **2017**, *25*, 1191–1198. [CrossRef] [PubMed]
22. Parkar, A.P.; Adriaensen, M.; Vindfeld, S.; Solheim, E. The Anatomic Centers of the Femoral and Tibial Insertions of the Anterior Cruciate Ligament: A Systematic Review of Imaging and Cadaveric Studies Reporting Normal Center Locations. *Am. J. Sports Med.* **2017**, *45*, 2180–2188. [CrossRef] [PubMed]
23. Parkar, A.P.; Adriaensen, M.E.; Fischer-Bredenbeck, C.; Inderhaug, E.; Strand, T.; Assmus, J.; Solheim, E. Measurements of tunnel placements after anterior cruciate ligament reconstruction—A comparison between CT, radiographs and MRI. *Knee* **2015**, *22*, 574–579. [CrossRef]
24. Parkar, A.P.; Adriaensen, M.E.; Strand, T.; Inderhaug, E.; Harlem, T.; Solheim, E. How to read post-operative radiographs and CT scans after single-bundle anterior cruciate ligament reconstruction. *Skeletal. Radiol.* **2013**, *42*, 1489–1500. [CrossRef] [PubMed]
25. Colombet, P.; Robinson, J.; Christel, P.; Franceschi, J.-P.; Djian, P.; Bellier, G.; Sbihi, A. Morphology of anterior cruciate ligament attachments for anatomic reconstruction: A cadaveric dissection and radiographic study. *Arthroscopy* **2006**, *22*, 984–992. [CrossRef] [PubMed]
26. Lee, J.K.; Lee, S.; Seong, S.C.; Lee, M.C. Anatomy of the anterior cruciate ligament insertion sites: Comparison of plain radiography and three-dimensional computed tomographic imaging to anatomic dissection. *Knee Surg. Sports Traumatol. Arthrosc.* **2015**, *23*, 2297–2305. [CrossRef] [PubMed]
27. Luites, J.W.; Wymenga, A.B.; Blankevoort, L.; Kooloos, J.G. Description of the attachment geometry of the anteromedial and posterolateral bundles of the ACL from arthroscopic perspective for anatomical tunnel placement. *Knee Surg. Sports Traumatol. Arthrosc.* **2007**, *15*, 1422–1431. [CrossRef]
28. Tsukada, H.; Ishibashi, Y.; Tsuda, E.; Fukuda, A.; Toh, S. Anatomical analysis of the anterior cruciate ligament femoral and tibial footprints. *J. Orthop. Sci.* **2008**, *13*, 122–129. [CrossRef]
29. Lorenz, S.; Elser, F.; Mitterer, M.; Obst, T.; Imhoff, A.B. Radiologic evaluation of the insertion sites of the 2 functional bundles of the anterior cruciate ligament using 3-dimensional computed tomography. *Am. J. Sports Med.* **2009**, *37*, 2368–2376. [CrossRef]
30. Musahl, V.; Burkart, A.; Debski, R.E.; Van Scyoc, A.; Fu, F.H.; Woo, S.L. Anterior cruciate ligament tunnel placement: Comparison of insertion site anatomy with the guidelines of a computer-assisted surgical system. *Arthroscopy* **2003**, *19*, 154–160. [CrossRef]
31. Forsythe, B.; Kopf, S.; Wong, A.K.; Martins, C.A.; Anderst, W.; Tashman, S.; Fu, F.H. The location of femoral and tibial tunnels in anatomic double-bundle anterior cruciate ligament reconstruction analyzed by three-dimensional computed tomography models. *J. Bone Jt. Surg. Am.* **2010**, *92*, 1418–1426. [CrossRef]
32. Bernard, M.; Hertel, P.; Hornung, H.; Cierpinski, T. Femoral insertion of the ACL. Radiographic quadrant method. *Am. J. Knee Surg.* **1997**, *10*, 14–21, discussion 21–12. [PubMed]
33. Piefer, J.W.; Pflugner, T.R.; Hwang, M.D.; Lubowitz, J.H. Anterior cruciate ligament femoral footprint anatomy: Systematic review of the 21st century literature. *Arthroscopy* **2012**, *28*, 872–881. [CrossRef]
34. Ferretti, M.; Ekdahl, M.; Shen, W.; Fu, F.H. Osseous landmarks of the femoral attachment of the anterior cruciate ligament: An anatomic study. *Arthroscopy* **2007**, *23*, 1218–1225. [CrossRef] [PubMed]
35. Tsukada, S.; Fujishiro, H.; Watanabe, K.; Nimura, A.; Mochizuki, T.; Mahakkanukrauh, P.; Yasuda, K.; Akita, K. Anatomic variations of the lateral intercondylar ridge: Relationship to the anterior margin of the anterior cruciate ligament. *Am. J. Sports Med.* **2014**, *42*, 1110–1117. [CrossRef] [PubMed]
36. van Eck, C.F.; Martins, C.A.; Vyas, S.M.; Celentano, U.; van Dijk, C.N.; Fu, F.H. Femoral intercondylar notch shape and dimensions in ACL-injured patients. *Knee Surg. Sports Traumatol. Arthrosc.* **2010**, *18*, 1257–1262. [CrossRef] [PubMed]
37. Brown, C.H., Jr.; Spalding, T.; Robb, C. Medial portal technique for single-bundle anatomical anterior cruciate ligament (ACL) reconstruction. *Int. Orthop.* **2013**, *37*, 253–269. [CrossRef]
38. Inderhaug, E.; Larsen, A.; Strand, T.; Waaler, P.A.; Solheim, E. The effect of feedback from post-operative 3D CT on placement of femoral tunnels in single-bundle anatomic ACL reconstruction. *Knee Surg. Sports Traumatol. Arthrosc.* **2016**, *24*, 154–160. [CrossRef]
39. Meuffels, D.E.; Reijman, M.; Verhaar, J.A. Computer-assisted surgery is not more accurate or precise than conventional arthroscopic ACL reconstruction: A prospective randomized clinical trial. *J. Bone Jt. Surg. Am.* **2012**, *94*, 1538–1545. [CrossRef]
40. Mhaskar, V.A.; Jain, Y.; Soni, P.; Fiske, R.; Maheshwari, J. How Important is the Tunnel Position in Outcomes Post-ACL Reconstruction: A 3D CT-Based Study. *Indian J. Orthop.* **2022**, *56*, 312–318. [CrossRef]
41. Parkinson, B.; Robb, C.; Thomas, M.; Thompson, P.; Spalding, T. Factors That Predict Failure in Anatomic Single-Bundle Anterior Cruciate Ligament Reconstruction. *Am. J. Sports Med.* **2017**, *45*, 1529–1536. [CrossRef] [PubMed]
42. Hosseini, A.; Lodhia, P.; Van de Velde, S.K.; Asnis, P.D.; Zarins, B.; Gill, T.J.; Li, G. Tunnel position and graft orientation in failed anterior cruciate ligament reconstruction: A clinical and imaging analysis. *Int. Orthop.* **2012**, *36*, 845–852. [CrossRef] [PubMed]

43. Marchant, B.G.; Noyes, F.R.; Barber-Westin, S.D.; Fleckenstein, C. Prevalence of nonanatomical graft placement in a series of failed anterior cruciate ligament reconstructions. *Am. J. Sports Med.* **2010**, *38*, 1987–1996. [CrossRef] [PubMed]
44. Trojani, C.; Sbihi, A.; Djian, P.; Potel, J.-F.; Hulet, C.; Jouve, F.; Bussière, C.; Ehkirch, F.-P.; Burdin, G.; Dubrana, F.; et al. Causes for failure of ACL reconstruction and influence of meniscectomies after revision. *Knee Surg. Sports Traumatol. Arthrosc.* **2011**, *19*, 196–201. [CrossRef] [PubMed]
45. Lee, D.W.; Lee, D.H.; Moon, S.G.; Kang, J.H.; Woo, Y.J.; Kim, W.J. Femoral Tunnel Geometry and Graft Inclination Angles in Anterior Cruciate Ligament Reconstruction Using a Flexible Reamer System. *Medicina* **2023**, *59*, 1031. [CrossRef] [PubMed]
46. Hagiwara, K.; Terauchi, M.; Hatayama, K.; Yanagisawa, S.; Ohsawa, T.; Kimura, M. Sagittal Inclination Angle of Graft Is Associated With Knee Stability After Anatomic Anterior Cruciate Ligament Reconstruction. *Arthroscopy* **2021**, *37*, 2533–2541. [CrossRef] [PubMed]
47. Snoj, Z.; Zupanc, O.; Strazar, K.; Salapura, V. A descriptive study of potential effect of anterior tibial translation, femoral tunnel and anterior cruciate ligament graft inclination on clinical outcome and degenerative changes. *Int. Orthop.* **2017**, *41*, 789–796. [CrossRef]
48. Lee, S.M.; Yoon, K.H.; Lee, S.H.; Hur, D. The Relationship Between ACL Femoral Tunnel Position and Postoperative MRI Signal Intensity. *J. Bone Jt. Surg. Am.* **2017**, *99*, 379–387. [CrossRef]
49. Ahn, J.H.; Jeong, H.J.; Lee, Y.S.; Park, J.H.; Lee, J.H.; Ko, T.S. Graft bending angle is correlated with femoral intraosseous graft signal intensity in anterior cruciate ligament reconstruction using the outside-in technique. *Knee* **2016**, *23*, 666–673. [CrossRef]
50. Magnussen, R.A.; Debieux, P.; Benjamin, B.; Lustig, S.; Demey, G.; Servien, E.; Neyret, P. A CT-based classification of prior ACL femoral tunnel location for planning revision ACL surgery. *Knee Surg. Sports Traumatol. Arthrosc.* **2012**, *20*, 1298–1306. [CrossRef]

medicina

MDPI

Article

Femoral Tunnel Geometry and Graft Inclination Angles in Anterior Cruciate Ligament Reconstruction Using a Flexible Reamer System

Dhong-Won Lee [1,*], Dong-Hwan Lee [1], Sung-Gyu Moon [2], Ji-Hee Kang [2], Young-Je Woo [1] and Woo-Jong Kim [3]

1. Department of Orthopaedic Surgery, Konkuk University Medical Center, Konkuk University School of Medicine, Seoul 05029, Republic of Korea
2. Department of Radiology, Konkuk University Medical Center, Konkuk University School of Medicine, Seoul 05029, Republic of Korea
3. Department of Orthopaedic Surgery, Soonchunhyang University Hospital Cheonan, Cheonan 31538, Republic of Korea

* Correspondence: osdoctorknee@kuh.ac.kr

Abstract: *Background and Objectives*: The aim of this study is to investigate the femoral tunnel geometry (femoral tunsnel location, femoral graft bending angle, and femoral tunnel length) on three-dimensional (3D) computed tomography (CT) and graft inclination on magnetic resonance imaging (MRI) after anatomic anterior cruciate ligament (ACL) reconstruction using a flexible reamer system. *Materials and Methods*: A total of 60 patients who underwent anatomical ACL reconstruction (ACLR) using a flexible reamer system were retrospectively reviewed. One day after the ACLR procedure was performed, all patients underwent three-dimensional computed tomography (3D-CT) and magnetic resonance imaging (MRI). The femoral tunnel location, femoral graft bending angle, femoral tunnel length, and graft inclination were assessed. *Results*: In the 3D-CTs, the femoral tunnel was located at 29.7 ± 4.4% in the posterior to anterior (deep to shallow) direction and at 24.1 ± 5.9% in the proximal to distal (high to low) direction. The mean femoral graft bending angle was 113.9 ± 5.7°, and the mean femoral tunnel length was 35.2 ± 3.1 mm. Posterior wall breakage was observed in five patients (8.3%). In the MRIs, the mean coronal graft inclination was 69.2 ± 4.7°, and the mean sagittal graft inclination was 52.4 ± 4.6°. The results of this study demonstrated that a comparable femoral graft bending angle and longer femoral tunnel length were observed compared with the reported outcomes from previous studies that used the rigid reamer system. *Conclusions*: ACLR using a flexible reamer system allowed for an anatomic femoral tunnel location and a comparable graft inclination to that of the native ACL. In addition, it achieved a tolerable femoral graft bending angle and femoral tunnel length.

Keywords: anterior cruciate ligament reconstruction; anteromedial portal; flexible reamer; femoral tunnel

1. Introduction

Of the various surgical methods used for anatomical anterior cruciate ligament (ACL) reconstruction (ACLR), femoral drilling methods that are independent of the tibial tunnel have garnered attention [1–3]. The recent purpose of anatomical reconstruction is not only to achieve anatomical neo-ACL reconstruction but also to preserve the residual ACL where possible [4,5]. The transportal technique, the representative independent femoral drilling method, has potential risks, such as iatrogenic femoral cartilage injury, short femoral tunnel, posterior wall breakage, and peroneal nerve injury [6,7]. To overcome such potential risks, hyperflexion of the knee needs to be maintained during femoral drilling, in which the surgical field is blocked by hyperflexion [8,9]. Nonetheless, hyperflexion is needed because a guide pin and reamer are rigid [8].

A flexible reamer system was developed to overcome the limitation of the transportal technique that uses the existing rigid reamer system. Because the femoral drilling in this system is performed without more than 120° of knee hyperflexion, securing the surgical field, a relatively long femoral tunnel can be generated [10]. This can reduce the incidence of posterior wall breakage and avoid the risk of peroneal nerve injury. Previous cadaver studies reported that a significantly longer femoral tunnel could be achieved with a flexible guide pin than with a rigid guide pin [11,12]. A recently published systemic review reported that a clinical application of a flexible guide pin resulted in a longer and more anteverted femoral tunnel than a rigid guide pin [13]. In an attempt to overcome the inherent limitations of the transportal technique, the retrograde drilling method was introduced [14]. However, it is known that it has not yet been successful in reducing the incidence of acute graft bending [15,16]. As a result, the authors chose to use the transportal technique with a flexible reamer.

Because the postoperative outcomes of ACLR are affected by not only the graft length within the tunnel but also the femoral graft bending angle and graft inclination angle, merely securing a long femoral tunnel is not sufficient to obtain a desirable outcome. It is known that the femoral graft bending angle affects graft stress within the femoral tunnel, leading to tunnel widening or graft failure when an acute graft bending angle is formed [17–19]. Although it is unclear if the maintenance of inclination in the native ACL during ACLR would help obtain functionally beneficial clinical outcomes, it has been reported that a larger graft inclination is associated with graft laxity [20,21].

However, there has not been a comprehensive analytical study on femoral tunnel geometry and graft inclination after ACLR using a flexible reamer system. Therefore, the aim of the current study as a case series is to investigate the femoral tunnel geometry (femoral tunnel location, femoral graft bending angle, and femoral tunnel length) on three-dimensional (3D) computed tomography (CT) and graft inclination on magnetic resonance imaging (MRI) after anatomic ACLR using a flexible reamer system. It was hypothesized that ACLR using a flexible reamer system would result in an anatomical femoral tunnel location and an average femoral tunnel length of 35 mm or more while maintaining a tolerable graft bending angle. In addition, it was hypothesized that it would provide a relatively native graft inclination.

2. Materials and Methods

2.1. Patients

The medical records, 3D CT images, and MRI scans of 65 patients who underwent anatomical ACLR using a flexible reamer system at our institute from September 2021 to June 2022 were retrospectively reviewed. The inclusion criteria were primary ACLR; single-bundle reconstruction; the use of a soft-tissue graft; and availability to attend 3D CT and MRI evaluations. The exclusion criteria were selective bundle reconstruction, multiple-ligament injury, and revision ACLR. Among the 65 patients, 5 were excluded due to revision ACLR ($n = 3$), multiligament injury for which combined ligament reconstruction was performed ($n = 1$), and no follow-up MRI ($n = 1$). Finally, 60 patients were enrolled in this study. This retrospective investigation was conducted following approval from the Ethics Committee of Konkuk University Medical Center (KUMC 2023-01-001).

2.2. Surgical Techniques

All procedures were performed by a single experienced surgeon (DWL) using a flexible reamer system (VersiTomic, Stryker; Kalamazoo, MI, USA). In all patients, soft-tissue grafts (a hamstring autograft or hamstring autograft + tibialis allograft) were used, the diameters of which were 8–9 mm. The diameters of the femoral and tibial tunnels were equal to the diameter of the graft.

Three portals were created using a 30° arthroscope [22]. The anterolateral (AL) portal was established at the level of the patellar inferior pole as close as possible to the lateral border of the patellar tendon as a viewing portal. The anteromedial (AM) portal was established at the level of the patellar inferior pole as close as possible to the medial border of the patellar tendon as a viewing portal or working portal. This was in a slightly higher position than conventional to avoid the "sword fighting phenomenon." The accessory anteromedial portal (AAM) was located inferior and medial to the AM portal, just above the anterior horn of the medial meniscus. Care was taken to avoid chondral damage of the medial femoral condyle. This allows the ACL femoral attachment to be viewed through the AM portal while instruments are inserted through this AAM portal.

The ACL femoral attachment was removed to identify the bony landmarks (lateral intercondylar ridge and bifurcate ridge) while preserving the remnant tissue substantially using electrocautery (ArthroCare, Smith & Nephew; Austin, TX, USA). While visualizing through the AL portal, the center of the femoral tunnel was marked inferior to the lateral intercondylar ridge and just behind the bifurcate ridge using a microfracture awl through the AAM portal, with the knee in 90° of flexion (Figure 1A). The tunnel center was determined using an arthroscopic bendable ruler (Smith & Nephew Endoscopy, Andover, MA, USA), ensuring that the posterior wall remained 2–3 mm. A 45° curved drill guide was introduced through the AAM portal to the center of the femoral tunnel with superolateral trajectory viewing through the AL portal. A flexible guide pin was inserted through the curved drill guide and drilled with the knee in 100° of flexion (Figure 1B). After the curved drill guide was removed, a flexible reamer of 4.5 mm diameter was drilled out through the far cortex to pass through a suspensory fixation device (Figure 1C). A flexible reamer of a diameter equal to that of the prepared graft was drilled at the same knee flexion angles (Figure 1D). The femoral tunnel was confirmed via the AM portal (Figure 1E). An ACL guide (Linvatec; Largo, FL, USA) was used to establish the tibial tunnel at an angle of 47.5°. The ACL guide tip was located just anteromedial to the center of the ACL bundles. A rigid reamer of a diameter equal to that of the prepared graft was drilled to protect the remnant ACL bundles. The prepared graft was passed from the tibial tunnel to the femoral tunnel. If the femoral tunnel length was 35 mm or longer, EndoButton (Smith & Nephew; Andover, MA, USA) with 15 mm tape was used for fixing. In contrast, if it was shorter than 35 mm, UltraButton (Smith & Nephew; Andover, MA, USA) was used for femoral fixation to maintain the 20 mm or longer graft length within the tunnel. The tibial side was dually fixed using a bioabsorbable interference screw (Matryx, ConMed Linvatec; Largo, FL, USA) and an additional cortical screw or staple with the knee in 20° of flexion. The diameter of the interference screw was equal to that of the tibial tunnel. Finally, the reconstructed ACL graft containing the original remnant ACL tissue was evaluated (Figure 1F).

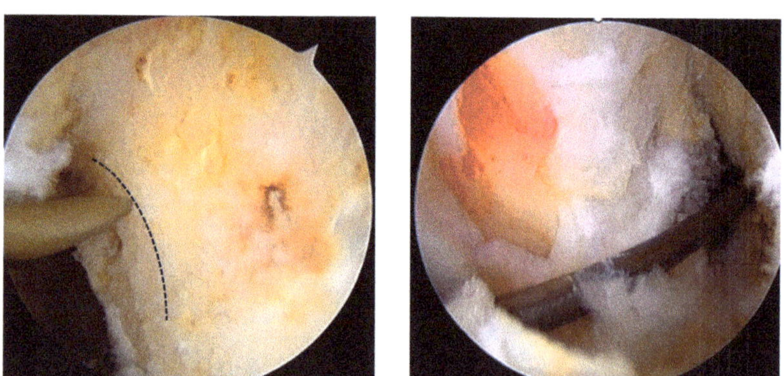

(A) **(B)**

Figure 1. *Cont.*

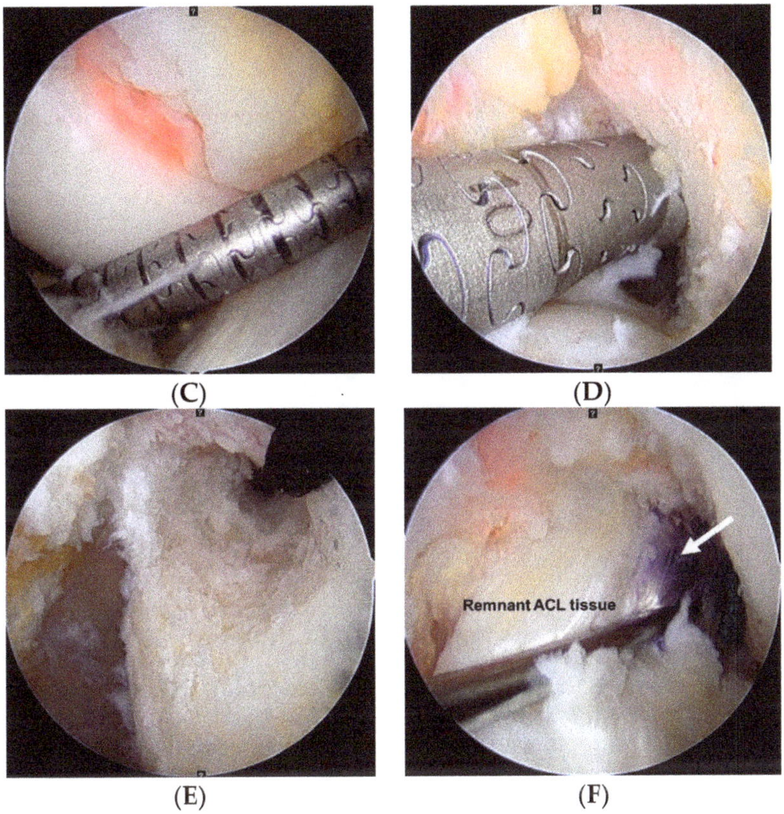

Figure 1. Anterior cruciate ligament (ACL) reconstruction of the left knee. (**A**) Anatomic center of the femoral tunnel is marked inferior to the lateral intercondylar ridge and just behind the bifurcate ridge (dotted line) using a microfracture awl through the accessory anteromedial (AM) portal, with the knee in 90° of flexion. (**B**) A flexible guide pin is inserted and drilled with the knee in 100° of flexion. (**C**) A flexible reamer of 4.5 mm diameter is drilled out through the far cortex to pass through a suspensory fixation device. (**D**) A flexible reamer of a diameter equal to that of the prepared graft is drilled. (**E**) The femoral tunnel is confirmed via the AM portal. (**F**) After tibial fixation, the reconstructed ACL graft containing the remnant tissue is evaluated.

2.3. *Three-Dimensional CT Evaluation*

One day after the ACLR procedure was performed, all patients underwent 3D CT scans (LightSpeed VCT XT, GE Medical Systems; Milwaukee, WI, USA). During the examination, the knee was extended as fully as possible.

To assess the femoral tunnel location, a true medial view of the lateral femoral condyle with the image of the medial femoral condyle erased at the center of the intercondylar notch was obtained. The quadrant methods used previously by Bernard et al. [23] and Forsythe et al. [24] facilitated the analysis of the femoral tunnel location (Figure 2). The tunnel location was determined in the proximal to distal (deep–shallow) and anterior to posterior (high–low) directions and presented as the percentage of the distance from the posterior edge of the lateral femoral condyle to the roof of the intercondylar notch. The measurements were performed on a picture archiving and communication system (PACS) workstation (Centricity RA 1000, GE Healthcare; Chicago, IL, USA).

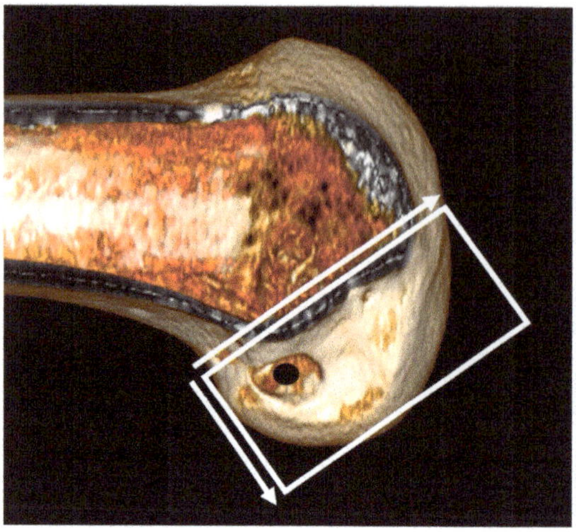

Figure 2. The femoral tunnel location is determined in the proximal to distal and anterior to posterior directions and presented as the percentage of the distance from the posterior edge of the lateral femoral condyle to the roof of the intercondylar notch.

The 3D CT scans were imported into 3D software (AW Sever 3.2 PACS system, GE Healthcare; Chicago, IL, USA) for the assessments of the femoral graft bending angle and femoral tunnel length. The femoral graft bending angle was defined as the angle formed by the longitudinal axis of the femoral tunnel and the line connecting the intra-articular aperture of the tibial tunnel and the intra-articular aperture of the femoral tunnel (Figure 3). The femoral tunnel length was defined as the distance between the center of the extra-articular aperture of the femoral tunnel and the center of the intra-articular aperture of the femoral tunnel in a plane where the entire femoral tunnel could be viewed (Figure 4). Posterior wall breakage of the femoral tunnel was also checked.

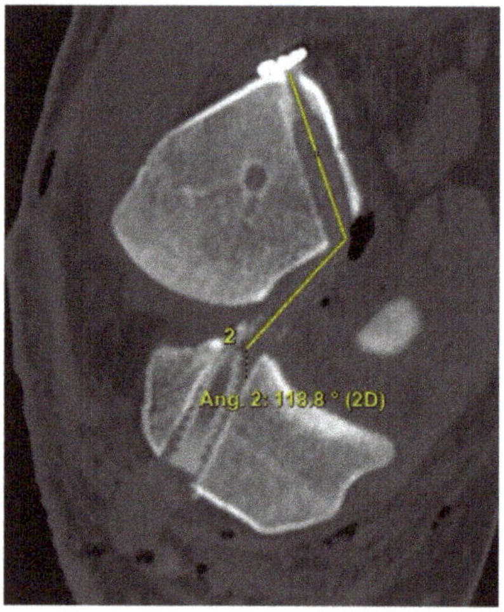

Figure 3. The femoral graft bending angle is defined as the angle formed by the longitudinal axis of the femoral tunnel and the line connecting the intra-articular aperture of the tibial tunnel and the intra-articular aperture of the femoral tunnel.

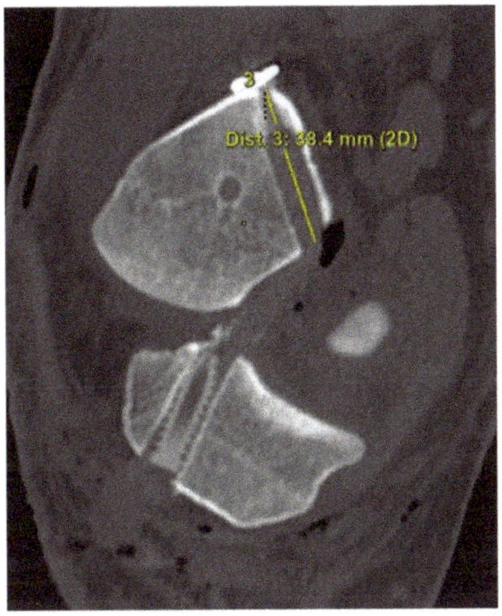

Figure 4. The femoral tunnel length is defined as the distance between the center of the extra-articular aperture of the femoral tunnel and the center of the intra-articular aperture of the femoral tunnel.

2.4. MRI Evaluation

One day after ACLR, all patients underwent MRI with a 3.0-T system apparatus (Signa HD, GE Healthcare; Milwaukee, WI, USA) to evaluate for graft inclination. The graft inclination on the coronal plane was defined as the angle between the medial margin of the ACL graft through more than one slice and a line parallel to the tibial plateau at the level of the middle of the medial collateral ligament (Figure 5A). Because the entire ACL graft is unable to be visualized on one slice, if the medial margin of the ACL graft is marked and scrolled while watching the monitor, a line can be clearly drawn. The graft inclination on the sagittal plane was defined as the angle between the anterior margin of the ACL graft and a line perpendicular to the long axis of the tibia at the level of the Blumensaat line (Figure 5B).

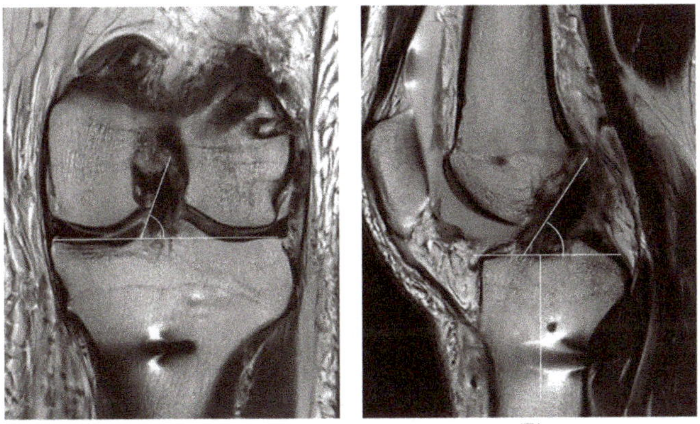

(**A**) (**B**)

Figure 5. The coronal graft inclination (**A**) is defined as the angle between the medial margin of the anterior cruciate ligament (ACL) graft and a line parallel to the tibial plateau at the level of the middle of the medial collateral ligament. The sagittal graft inclination (**B**) is defined as the angle between the anterior margin of the ACL graft and a line perpendicular to the long axis of the tibia at the level of the Blumensaat line.

2.5. Statistical Analysis

The statistical analysis was performed using SPSS software (IBM SPSS Statistics 21, IBM Corp.; Somers, NY, USA). Intrarater reliability was assessed using the intraclass correlation coefficient (ICC) with the following classifications: excellent (>0.9), good (0.75–0.9), moderate (0.5–0.75), and poor (<0.5). Interrater reliability between the examiners was assessed using kappa (k) values and classified as excellent (0.81–1.00), substantial (0.61–0.80), moderate (0.41–0.60), fair (0.21–0.40), or slight (0–0.20) [25]. All radiological measurements were independently performed by one experienced radiologist and one experienced orthopedic surgeon (SGM and DWL). Each investigator evaluated all images two times in intervals of 6 weeks and was blinded to the other investigator's evaluation. The average data of two measures were used for the analysis.

3. Results

The basic demographics of enrolled patients are summarized in Table 1. The kappa values for intraobserver and interobserver agreements for the measurements were all >0.81 (Table 2).

Table 1. Demographic data.

	$N = 60$
Age, y	28.4 ± 9.9
Sex, *n*, Male/Female	37/23
Body Mass Index, kg/m^2	23.2 ± 5.3
Side, *n*, Right/Left	29/31

Table 2. Reliability of each radiological measurement.

	Tunnel Location		FGBA	Tunnel Length	Graft Inclination	
	Posterior to Anterior	Proximal to Distal			Coronal	Sagittal
Examiner 1	0.91	0.89	0.89	0.97	0.91	0.94
Examiner 2	0.89	0.87	0.86	0.94	0.89	0.90
Interexaminer	0.86	0.84	0.85	0.96	0.89	0.91

FGBA, femoral graft bending angle.

Regarding the femoral tunnel location, it was located at 29.7 ± 4.4% in the posterior to anterior (deep to shallow) direction and at 24.1 ± 5.9% in the proximal to distal (high to low) direction. The mean femoral graft bending angle was 113.9 ± 5.7°, and the mean femoral tunnel length was 35.2 ± 3.1 mm (Table 3). There were no cases of a femoral tunnel length <30 mm because the guide pin was redirected for those <30 mm while making the knee joint flexion to approximately 110°. Posterior wall breakage was observed in five patients (8.3%). In the MRIs, the mean coronal graft inclination was 69.2 ± 4.7°, and the mean sagittal graft inclination was 52.4 ± 4.6° (Table 3). The mean posterior tibial slope 241 was 7.9 ± 3.5, and there was no posterior tibial slope of more than 12°.

Table 3. Femoral tunnel geometry and graft inclination.

	$N = 60$
Femoral tunnel location, %	
Proximal to distal (deep–shallow)	28.8 ± 4.7
Anterior to posterior (high–low)	24.1 ± 5.9
Femoral graft bending angle, °	113.9 ± 5.7
Femoral tunnel length, mm	35.2 ± 3.1
Graft inclination, °	
Coronal inclination	69.2 ± 4.7
Sagittal inclination	52.4 ± 4.6

There were no cases of iatrogenic chondral damage of the medial femoral condyle during the procedure. The mean operative time was 72.4 ± 12.1 min.

The results of this study were compared with those of previous studies in which an anatomical single-bundle ACLR using a flexible reamer system or rigid reamer system was performed (Table 4).

Table 4. Current findings and previously reported femoral tunnel geometry in anatomical single-bundle anterior cruciate ligament reconstruction.

Study	Cases, n	Technique	Femoral Tunnel Location, %		Femoral Graft Bending Angle, °	Femoral Tunnel Length, mm	Posterior Wall Breakage, *n* (%)
			Deep–Shallow	High–Low			
Current study	60	TP (3 portals)/FR	28.8 ± 4.7	24.1 ± 5.9	113.9 ± 5.7	35.2 ± 3.1	5 (8.3)
Yoon et al. [26]	30	TP (2 portals)/FR	29.6 ± 5.5	20.1 ± 6.7	108.4 ± 6.9	32.8 ± 4.5	2 (6.6)
Seo et al. [27]	14	TP (3 portals)/FR	28.0 ± 6.3	23.7 ± 5.8	109.8 ± 9.4	36.7 ± 2.9	N/A
	14	TP (3 portals)/RR	32.1 ± 4.3	21.5 ± 5.2	118.1 ± 7.2	32.9 ± 9.0	
Park et al. [28]	21	TP (3 portals)/RR	26.7 ± 4.5	32.1 ± 8.0	107.9 ± 10.0	29.6 ± 3.9	7 (33.3)
	30	OI/RR	31.3 ± 6.0	27.6 ± 10.1	101.3 ± 8.2	33.0 ± 3.5	1 (3.3)

TP, transportal; FR, flexible reamer; RR, rigid reamer; OI, outside–in; N/A, Not Available.

4. Discussion

The most substantial findings of the current study were that the flexible reamer system allowed for an anatomic femoral tunnel location and a comparable graft inclination to those of the native ACL. In addition, our results demonstrate that a comparable femoral graft bending angle and longer femoral tunnel length were observed compared with the reported outcomes from previous studies that used the rigid reamer system (Table 4).

Parkar et al. [29] published a systematic review of normal ACL center locations. In this systematic review, 218 knees demonstrated that the weighted 5th and 95th percentiles for the deep–shallow direction were 24% and 37%, respectively, and they were 28% and 43%, respectively, for the high–low direction. Piefer et al. [30] conducted a systematic review of the ACL femoral footprint anatomy. In their systematic review, the center of AM bundle ranged from 15% to 26.4% for the deep–shallow direction and 14.2% to 25.3% for the high–low direction. The center of the ACL footprint ranged from 23.5% to 43.1% for the deep–shallow direction and 27.5% to 44.25% for the high–low direction. In the present study, the center of the femoral tunnel was 28.8 ± 4.7% for the deep–shallow direction and 24.1 ± 5.9% for the high–low direction, and this femoral tunnel location was slightly closer to the AM bundle than the anatomical center of the ACL footprint. This indicates that the tunnel was well generated at the intended position because we targeted not the center between the AM bundle and the PL bundle but rather the region just posterior to the bifurcate ridge when marking the center of the femoral tunnel. To create a relatively consistent position of the femoral tunnel, we determined the tunnel center location using an arthroscopic bendable ruler (Smith & Nephew Endoscopy, Andover, MA, USA), ensuring that the posterior wall remained 2–3 mm.

In terms of graft inclination, Jamsher et al. [31] applied and compared four drilling techniques (the transportal technique using a flexible reamer system, the transportal technique using a rigid reamer system, outside–in retrograde drilling technique, and the transtibial drilling technique) for ACLR and demonstrated that the transportal technique using a flexible reamer system and outside–in retrograde drilling technique had outcomes more similar to those of sagittal and coronal inclinations than the transportal technique using a rigid reamer system and transtibial technique. In the study, the inclinations of the native ACL in the sagittal plane and coronal plane were 49.3 ± 4.2° and 73.6 ± 3.4°, respectively, and the graft inclination in ACLR with the transportal technique using a flexible reamer system in the sagittal plane and coronal plane were 49.9 ± 5.0° and 69.3 ± 4.5°, respectively. Other studies also reported that the sagittal inclination of the native ACL was 51–52° [20,32]. Snoj et al. [21] reported 52.2 ± 4.4° for the sagittal inclination of native ACL and 65.2 ± 6.6° for coronal inclination. Thus, the sagittal and coronal inclinations in our study were as close as within a 5° difference as those from inclinations of the native ACL reported by previous studies. Because a femoral offset guide was not used when applying the flexible reamer system, we were able to easily adjust the vertical position of the femur tunnel, which seemed to affect the outcome positively [31]. Although the effect of graft inclination on the clinical outcomes of ACLR has yet to be revealed, some report that it could have effects as considerable as the femoral tunnel location. Snoj et al. [21] demonstrated that there were significant correlations between anterior tibial translation and the sagittal ($p = 0.01$) and coronal ($p < 0.01$) inclinations. Hagiwara et al. [20] reported that the lateral sagittal inclination ranged from 45.8° to 65.4° after ACLR and that a larger graft inclination was significantly correlated with graft laxity.

Regarding the femoral graft bending angle, there are contradictory reports between the rigid reamer system and the flexible reamer system. Seo et al. [27] reported that the mean angles with the application of a flexible reamer system and a rigid reamer system for single-bundle ACLR were 109.8° and 118.1°, respectively, demonstrating a more acute outcome for the flexible reamer system. In contrast, Kim et al. [33] applied a flexible reamer system for double-bundle ACLR, resulting in 115.5° for a mean graft bending angle of AM bundle, which is less acute than that when a rigid reamer system was applied (108.4°). When applying a flexible reamer, Yoon et al. [26] made a tunnel in the lateral femoral condyle in a less perpendicular trajectory using a standard AM portal rather than an accessory AM portal. In our study, the mean graft bending angle was 113.9°, which is less acute than the mean angle (108.4°) reported by Yoon et al. [26]. Although we used an accessory AM portal, we first performed 4.5 mm reaming for a suspensory fixation system to generate a less acute graft bending angle and then tried reaming in the lateral femoral condyle in a less perpendicular trajectory while pushing back a thick reamer suitable for the graft size as far as possible. A sharp graft bending angle at the edge of the femoral tunnel entrance would load much stress on the graft, which could cause graft immaturation or failure, so it should be carefully applied in a flexible reamer system [19,34].

The mean femoral tunnel length (35.2 ± 3.1 mm) of the present study was longer than that of the rigid reamer system and similar to that of previous studies that used the flexible reamer system (Table 4). An advantage of the flexible reamer is that a desirable femoral tunnel length can be secured even without having knee flexion of 120° or greater [11,12]. Hence, if it is possible to generate a 30 mm or longer femoral tunnel, it should be better not to make a tunnel acute graft bending by hyperflexion for elongation of the tunnel. In the current study, a fixed loop suspensory device was used for 35 mm or longer femoral tunnels, whereas an adjustable loop suspensory device was utilized for those shorter than 35 mm to maintain a 20 mm or longer graft within the tunnel. It is known that there should be no clinical difference between them [35]. In comparison with the existing rigid reamer system, the application of the flexible reamer system not only secured a longer femoral tunnel length but also had fewer incidences of posterior wall breakage, which should be considered that it had overcome the weaknesses of the existing transportal technique. Some authors showed that there were only two cases of posterior 334 wall breakage-one in the flexible reamer group ($n = 25$) and one in the rigid reamer group ($n = 25$) [36]. However, their mean femoral tunnel position (deep to shallow) was 32.9% for the flexible reamer group and 32.8% for the rigid reamer group. Our femoral tunnel position was deeper since it was slightly closer to the AM bundle. In order to make a femoral tunnel close to the AM bundle, the risk of breakage is inevitably increased because it is close to the poster wall. Care should be taken to prevent poster wall breakage from occurring, even if the possibility of poster wall breakage is lower than that of the rigid reamer.

By analyzing 3D CT and MRI performed in previous studies, the present study investigated not only femoral tunnel geometry but also graft inclination. To date, there have been no reports of the long-term clinical effects of flexible reamers. Since this study generated tunnels using anatomic femoral footprints with the application of the flexible reamer system and was able to reproduce graft inclination close to native ACL, it should be considered significant, allowing the expectation of desirable long-term clinical outcomes.

This study is a comprehensive evaluation of 3D CT and MRI after ACLR in a relatively homogeneous group of 60 patients at a single institution. Based on the study results, when using a flexible reamer, it is possible to create an anatomically consistent femoral tunnel within a short surgery time, and because the graft bending angle is not acute, we believe that satisfactory radiological examination results, such as CT and MRI, can be obtained once one becomes familiar with this technique.

The current study had some limitations. First, this study was retrospective in design, and there was no control group. Second, since few studies have investigated the femoral tunnel geometry of ACLR, studies comparable to the radiological results of this study and their results have been insufficient. The reason for analyzing previous studies in the results is solely to supplement the data analysis of previous research, which may be insufficient in a case series. Third, this study did not assess the heterogeneity of the patient's characteristics and the risk of bias in the included papers. Fourth, no clinical outcomes were included because this study analyzed 3D CT and MRI data right after surgery. Therefore, even a satisfactory radiological outcome should not be predicated on desirable clinical outcomes. Further research is needed on this. Fifth, while the femoral graft bending angle can be changed depending on the knee motion, this study evaluated the patients only in static states by CT, so it has a limitation in evaluating in vivo clinical significance. Finally, at least 1 year of postoperational MRI follow-up is required to evaluate the effect of the femoral geometry and graft inclination on graft maturation.

5. Conclusions

ACLR using a flexible reamer system allowed for an anatomic femoral tunnel location and a comparable graft inclination to that of the native ACL. In addition, it achieved a tolerable femoral graft bending angle and femoral tunnel length.

Author Contributions: Conceptualization, D.-W.L.; methodology, D.-H.L. and Y.-J.W.; software, J.-H.K. and D.-H.L.; validation, D.-H.L. and Y.-J.W.; formal analysis, D.-W.L. and S.-G.M.; investigation, D.-H.L. and Y.-J.W.; resources, W.-J.K.; data curation, D.-W.L. and S.-G.M.; writing—original draft preparation, D.-H.L.; writing—review and editing, D.-W.L.; visualization, W.-J.K.; supervision, D.-W.L.; project administration, D.-W.L. All authors have read and agreed to the published version of the manuscript.

Funding: This research received no external funding.

Institutional Review Board Statement: The study was conducted in accordance with the Declaration of Helsinki and approved by the Institutional Review Board (or Ethics Committee) of Konkuk University Medical Center (KUMC 2023-01-001; approved date 4 January 2023).

Informed Consent Statement: Informed consent was obtained from all subjects involved in the study.

Data Availability Statement: The data that support the findings of this study are available on request from the corresponding author.

Conflicts of Interest: The authors declare no conflict of interest.

References

1. Vijayan, S.; Kyalakond, H.; Kulkarni, M.S.; Aroor, M.N.; Shetty, S.; Bhat, V.; Rao, S.K. Clinical outcome of anterior cruciate ligament reconstruction with modified transtibial and anteromedial portal. *Musculoskelet. Surg.* **2021**, *107*, 37–45. [CrossRef] [PubMed]
2. Fernandes, T.L.; Moreira, H.H.; Andrade, R.; Sasaki, S.U.; Bernardo, W.M.; Pedrinelli, A.; Espregueira-Mendes, J.; Hernandez, A.J. Clinical Outcome Evaluation of Anatomic Anterior Cruciate Ligament Reconstruction With Tunnel Positioning Using Gold Standard Techniques: A Systematic Review and Meta-analysis. *Orthop. J. Sport. Med.* **2021**, *9*, 23259671211013327. [CrossRef]
3. Wang, H.; Fleischli, J.E.; Zheng, N.N. Transtibial versus anteromedial portal technique in single-bundle anterior cruciate ligament reconstruction: Outcomes of knee joint kinematics during walking. *Am. J. Sport. Med.* **2013**, *41*, 1847–1856. [CrossRef] [PubMed]
4. Bosco, F.; Giustra, F.; Crivellaro, M.; Giai Via, R.; Lavia, A.D.; Capella, M.; Sabatini, L.; Risitano, S.; Rovere, G.; Masse, A.; et al. Is augmentation the best solution in partial anterior cruciate ligament tears? A literature systematic review and meta-analysis. *J. Orthop.* **2023**, *36*, 11–17. [CrossRef]

5. Bosco, F.; Giustra, F.; Giai Via, R.; Lavia, A.D.; Capella, M.; Sabatini, L.; Risitano, S.; Cacciola, G.; Vezza, D.; Masse, A. Could anterior closed-wedge high tibial osteotomy be a viable option in patients with high posterior tibial slope who undergo anterior cruciate ligament reconstruction? A systematic review and meta-analysis. *Eur. J. Orthop. Surg. Traumatol.* **2022**, 1–14. [CrossRef] [PubMed]
6. Loucas, M.; Loucas, R.; D'Ambrosi, R.; Hantes, M.E. Clinical and Radiological Outcomes of Anteromedial Portal Versus Transtibial Technique in ACL Reconstruction: A Systematic Review. *Orthop. J. Sport. Med.* **2021**, *9*, 23259671211024591. [CrossRef]
7. Zhang, C.; Xu, H.; Li, X.; Wang, Y.; Zhang, Q.; Zhu, Q. Oblique femoral tunnel or oblique graft? A modified anteromedial portal technique to obtain vertical femoral tunnel and oblique graft in anatomic anterior cruciate ligament reconstruction. *Eur. J. Orthop. Surg. Traumatol.* **2013**, *23*, 731–735. [CrossRef]
8. Lubowitz, J.H.; Konicek, J. Anterior cruciate ligament femoral tunnel length: Cadaveric analysis comparing anteromedial portal versus outside-in technique. *Arthroscopy* **2010**, *26*, 1357–1362. [CrossRef]
9. Pastrone, A.; Ferro, A.; Bruzzone, M.; Bonasia, D.E.; Pellegrino, P.; D'Elicio, D.; Cottino, U.; Rossi, R. Anterior cruciate ligament reconstruction creating the femoral tunnel through the anteromedial portal. Surgical technique. *Curr. Rev. Musculoskelet. Med.* **2011**, *4*, 52–56. [CrossRef]
10. Fitzgerald, J.; Saluan, P.; Richter, D.L.; Huff, N.; Schenck, R.C. Anterior Cruciate Ligament Reconstruction Using a Flexible Reamer System: Technique and Pitfalls. *Orthop. J. Sport. Med.* **2015**, *3*, 2325967115592875. [CrossRef]
11. Silver, A.G.; Kaar, S.G.; Grisell, M.K.; Reagan, J.M.; Farrow, L.D. Comparison between rigid and flexible systems for drilling the femoral tunnel through an anteromedial portal in anterior cruciate ligament reconstruction. *Arthroscopy* **2010**, *26*, 790–795. [CrossRef]
12. Steiner, M.E.; Smart, L.R. Flexible instruments outperform rigid instruments to place anatomic anterior cruciate ligament femoral tunnels without hyperflexion. *Arthroscopy* **2012**, *28*, 835–843. [CrossRef] [PubMed]
13. Moran, T.E.; Ignozzi, A.J.; Werner, B.C. Comparing the Use of Flexible and Rigid Reaming Systems Through an Anteromedial Portal for Femoral Tunnel Creation During Anterior Cruciate Ligament Reconstruction: A Systematic Review. *Orthop. J. Sport. Med.* **2021**, *9*, 23259671211035741. [CrossRef] [PubMed]
14. Vadlamudi, A.; Kale, A.; Sharma, J.; Patil, V.; Pai, M. Comparison of Inside-Out and Outside-In Methods of Femoral Tunnel Preparation in Anterior Cruciate Ligament (ACL) Reconstruction Using 3D-CT. *Cureus* **2022**, *14*, e23367. [CrossRef]
15. CarlLee, T.; Ries, Z.; Duchman, K.; Gao, Y.; Wolf, B.; Amendola, A.; Hettrich, C.; Bollier, M. Outside-In vs. Anteromedial Portal Drilling During Primary ACL Reconstruction: Comparison at Two Years. *Iowa Orthop. J.* **2017**, *37*, 117–122. [PubMed]
16. Ahn, J.H.; Jeong, H.J.; Lee, Y.S.; Park, J.H.; Lee, J.H.; Ko, T.S. Graft bending angle is correlated with femoral intraosseous graft signal intensity in anterior cruciate ligament reconstruction using the outside-in technique. *Knee* **2016**, *23*, 666–673. [CrossRef]
17. Li, H.; Liu, S.; Sun, Y.; Li, H.; Chen, S.; Chen, J. Influence of Graft Bending Angle on Graft Maturation, the Femoral Tunnel, and Functional Outcomes by 12 Months After Anterior Cruciate Ligament Reconstruction. *Orthop. J. Sport. Med.* **2019**, *7*, 2325967119882663. [CrossRef] [PubMed]
18. Lee, D.K.; Kim, J.H.; Lee, B.H.; Kim, H.; Jang, M.J.; Lee, S.S.; Wang, J.H. Influence of Graft Bending Angle on Femoral Tunnel Widening After Double-Bundle ACL Reconstruction: Comparison of Transportal and Outside-In Techniques. *Orthop. J. Sport. Med.* **2021**, *9*, 23259671211035780. [CrossRef]
19. Lee, D.W.; Kim, J.G.; Lee, J.H.; Park, J.H.; Kim, D.H. Comparison of Modified Transtibial and Outside-In Techniques in Anatomic Single-Bundle Anterior Cruciate Ligament Reconstruction. *Arthroscopy* **2018**, *34*, 2857–2870. [CrossRef]
20. Hagiwara, K.; Terauchi, M.; Hatayama, K.; Yanagisawa, S.; Ohsawa, T.; Kimura, M. Sagittal Inclination Angle of Graft Is Associated With Knee Stability After Anatomic Anterior Cruciate Ligament Reconstruction. *Arthroscopy* **2021**, *37*, 2533–2541. [CrossRef]
21. Snoj, Z.; Zupanc, O.; Strazar, K.; Salapura, V. A descriptive study of potential effect of anterior tibial translation, femoral tunnel and anterior cruciate ligament graft inclination on clinical outcome and degenerative changes. *Int. Orthop.* **2017**, *41*, 789–796. [CrossRef] [PubMed]
22. Kosy, J.D.; Walmsley, K.; Sharma, A.D.; Gordon, E.A.; Heddon, S.V.; Anaspure, R.; Schranz, P.J.; Mandalia, V.I. A comparison of femoral tunnel placement in ACL reconstruction using a 70 degrees arthroscope through the anterolateral portal versus a 30 degrees arthroscope through the anteromedial portal: A pilot 3D-CT study. *Knee Surg. Relat. Res.* **2020**, *32*, 17. [CrossRef] [PubMed]
23. Bernard, M.; Hertel, P.; Hornung, H.; Cierpinski, T. Femoral insertion of the ACL. Radiographic quadrant method. *Am. J. Knee Surg.* **1997**, *10*, 14–21; discussion 21–12.
24. Forsythe, B.; Kopf, S.; Wong, A.K.; Martins, C.A.; Anderst, W.; Tashman, S.; Fu, F.H. The location of femoral and tibial tunnels in anatomic double-bundle anterior cruciate ligament reconstruction analyzed by three-dimensional computed tomography models. *J. Bone Jt. Surg. Am. Vol.* **2010**, *92*, 1418–1426. [CrossRef]
25. Landis, J.R.; Koch, G.G. The measurement of observer agreement for categorical data. *Biometrics* **1977**, *33*, 159–174. [CrossRef]
26. Yoon, K.H.; Kim, J.H.; Kwon, Y.B.; Kim, E.J.; Lee, S.H.; Kim, S.G. A two-portal technique using a flexible reamer system is a safe and effective method for transportal anterior cruciate ligament reconstruction. *Arch. Orthop. Trauma Surg.* **2020**, *140*, 383–390. [CrossRef]
27. Seo, Y.J.; Song, S.Y.; Im, W.Y.; Kim, Y.S.; Jang, S.W. Effects of flexible reamer on the femoral tunnel characteristics in anterior cruciate ligament reconstruction. *Medicine* **2021**, *100*, e27833. [CrossRef] [PubMed]

28. Park, J.S.; Park, J.H.; Wang, J.H.; Oh, C.H.; Hwang, M.H.; Lee, S.H.; Kim, J.G. Comparison of femoral tunnel geometry, using in vivo 3-dimensional computed tomography, during transportal and outside-in single-bundle anterior cruciate ligament reconstruction techniques. *Arthroscopy* **2015**, *31*, 83–91. [CrossRef]
29. Parkar, A.P.; Adriaensen, M.; Vindfeld, S.; Solheim, E. The Anatomic Centers of the Femoral and Tibial Insertions of the Anterior Cruciate Ligament: A Systematic Review of Imaging and Cadaveric Studies Reporting Normal Center Locations. *Am. J. Sport. Med.* **2017**, *45*, 2180–2188. [CrossRef]
30. Piefer, J.W.; Pflugner, T.R.; Hwang, M.D.; Lubowitz, J.H. Anterior cruciate ligament femoral footprint anatomy: Systematic review of the 21st century literature. *Arthroscopy* **2012**, *28*, 872–881. [CrossRef]
31. Jamsher, M.; Ballarati, C.; Vigano, M.; Hofbauer, M.; Togninalli, D.; Lafranchi, S.; de Girolamo, L.; Denti, M. Graft Inclination Angles in Anterior Cruciate Ligament Reconstruction Vary Depending on Femoral Tunnel Reaming Method: Comparison Among Transtibial, Anteromedial Portal, and Outside-In Retrograde Drilling Techniques. *Arthroscopy* **2020**, *36*, 1095–1102. [CrossRef] [PubMed]
32. Araujo, P.H.; Asai, S.; Pinto, M.; Protta, T.; Middleton, K.; Linde-Rosen, M.; Irrgang, J.; Smolinski, P.; Fu, F.H. ACL Graft Position Affects in Situ Graft Force Following ACL Reconstruction. *J. Bone Jt. Surg. Am.* **2015**, *97*, 1767–1773. [CrossRef] [PubMed]
33. Kim, J.G.; Chang, M.H.; Lim, H.C.; Bae, J.H.; Lee, S.Y.; Ahn, J.H.; Wang, J.H. An in Vivo 3D Computed Tomographic Analysis of Femoral Tunnel Geometry and Aperture Morphology Between Rigid and Flexible Systems in Double-Bundle Anterior Cruciate Ligament Reconstruction Using the Transportal Technique. *Arthroscopy* **2015**, *31*, 1318–1329. [CrossRef] [PubMed]
34. Tashiro, Y.; Gale, T.; Sundaram, V.; Nagai, K.; Irrgang, J.J.; Anderst, W.; Nakashima, Y.; Tashman, S.; Fu, F.H. The Graft Bending Angle Can Affect Early Graft Healing After Anterior Cruciate Ligament Reconstruction: In Vivo Analysis with 2 Years' Follow-up. *Am. J. Sport. Med.* **2017**, *45*, 1829–1836. [CrossRef]
35. Asif, N.; Khan, M.J.; Haris, K.P.; Waliullah, S.; Sharma, A.; Firoz, D. A prospective randomized study of arthroscopic ACL reconstruction with adjustable- versus fixed-loop device for femoral side fixation. *Knee Surg. Relat. Res.* **2021**, *33*, 42. [CrossRef]
36. Kosy, J.D.; Walmsley, K.; Anaspure, R.; Schranz, P.J.; Mandalia, V.I. Flexible reamers create comparable anterior cruciate ligament reconstruction femoral tunnels without the hyperflexion required with rigid reamers: 3D-CT analysis of tunnel morphology in a randomised clinical trial. *Knee Surg. Sport. Traumatol. Arthrosc. Off. J. ESSKA* **2020**, *28*, 1971–1978. [CrossRef]

medicina

MDPI

Article

Non-Anatomic Reconstruction in Multiligament Knee Injuries: A Functional Approach

Mihai Hurmuz [1,2], Cătălin-Adrian Miu [1,2,*], Daniel Ceachir [1,2], Romulus-Fabian Tatu [1,2], Mihai Andrei [2], Bogdan Andor [2], Alexandru Catalin Motofelea [3] and Călin Tudor Hozan [4]

1 Department XV, Discipline of Orthopedics, "Victor Babeş" University of Medicine and Pharmacy Timişoara, Eftimie Murgu Square 2, 300041 Timişoara, Romania; hurmuz.mihai@umft.ro (M.H.); daniel.ceachir@umft.ro (D.C.); tatu.fabian@umft.ro (R.-F.T.)

2 Orthopedics Unit, "Dr. Victor Popescu" Emergency Military Clinical Hospital, Gheorghe Lazăr Street 7, 300080 Timişoara, Romania; my.andrei8@gmail.com (M.A.); andor.bogdan@umft.ro (B.A.)

3 Center for Molecular Research in Nephrology and Vascular Disease, Discipline of Nephrology, Department VII/Internal Medicine II, Faculty of Medicine, "Victor Babeş" University of Medicine and Pharmacy, 300041 Timişoara, Romania; alexandru.motofelea@umft.ro

4 Department of Surgical Disciplines, Faculty of Medicine and Pharmacy, University of Oradea, 410087 Oradea, Romania; chozan@didactic.uoradea.ro

* Correspondence: miu.catalin@umft.ro

Abstract: *Background/Objectives*: Multiligament knee injuries, involving damage to multiple stabilizing structures, present a significant challenge in orthopedic surgery, often resulting in knee instability and compromised function. While anatomic ligament reconstruction has been traditionally advocated, non-anatomic techniques may provide effective alternatives, particularly for patients with moderate functional demands who do not require high-level athletic performance. *Material and methods*: In this study, we assessed the outcomes of a non-anatomic, hybrid surgical approach involving combined arthroscopic and open non-anatomic ligament reconstruction in 60 patients with multiligament knee injuries. Using simplified reconstruction methods for the medial collateral ligament (MCL) and lateral collateral ligament (LCL), we tailored the procedures to the needs of active, non-professional patients. Functional outcomes were evaluated using the International Knee Documentation Committee (IKDC) Questionnaire, Lysholm Knee Scoring Scale, and Knee Injury and Osteoarthritis Outcome Score (KOOS). *Results*: Postoperative improvements were significant, with the total IKDC score increasing from a median of 39.1 preoperatively to 75.9 postoperatively, Lysholm from 61.0 to 87.0, and KOOS from 47.6 to 85.7 ($p < 0.01$). The results demonstrated significant improvements across all scoring systems, with enhanced knee stability, reduced pain, and better quality of life. *Conclusions*: These findings support the feasibility of non-anatomic reconstructions as a practical solution for patients seeking a return to daily activities and recreational sports without the complexity of full anatomic reconstruction.

Keywords: knee instability; ligament reconstruction; arthroscopic; open technique; IKDC Questionnaire; Lysholm Knee Scoring Scale; KOOS

1. Introduction

The sensation of knee instability involves the frequent feeling of the knee "giving way" or "dislocating", often making everyday activities such as climbing stairs and walking on uneven surfaces quite difficult. Knee dislocation, which typically results from significant trauma, is commonly accompanied by other injuries. Consequently, knee instability has a substantial impact on the quality of life of affected individuals [1]. Fortunately, there are several treatment options available to manage this issue [2]. Traditional treatments have involved addressing symptoms conservatively, surgically repairing injured ligaments, or reconstructing them using grafts from the patient's body, a donor, or synthetic materials. More recent techniques aim to repair or replace the knee's stabilizing structures as much as possible [3]. Both of these methods have improved outcomes for daily activities [4,5].

Advancements in technology and medical research are constantly expanding the range of treatment options for knee instability [6]. Cutting-edge techniques, including minimally invasive procedures and regenerative medicine, offer promising alternatives to traditional treatments [7–9]. These innovative approaches not only focus on alleviating symptoms but also on promoting tissue regeneration and enhancing long-term joint stability [10], such as combined anterior cruciate ligament (ACL)/posterior cruciate ligament (PCL) and collateral ligament reconstruction, which have shown promising results in improving knee stability and function [11]

The importance of comprehensive rehabilitation programs for individuals with knee instability cannot be overstated. These programs incorporate a combination of physical therapy, strength training, and proprioception exercises to optimize the recovery process and prevent future knee injuries [12–14]. Additionally, advancements in biomechanics research have led to the development of specialized braces and orthotics designed to provide enhanced support and stability [15].

This study evaluates the outcomes of combining arthroscopic anatomic cruciate ligament reconstruction with open non-anatomic collateral ligament reconstruction techniques tailored to patients with moderate functional demands. The approach focuses on simplified reconstruction methods for collateral ligaments, particularly for the medial collateral ligament (MCL) and lateral collateral ligament (LCL), while maintaining anatomic techniques for ACL and PCL reconstructions. With numerous indications and controversies surrounding combined techniques, this study aims to contribute valuable insights into optimizing surgical strategies for knee instability. With numerous indications and controversies still surrounding combined arthroscopic and open non-anatomic ligament reconstruction techniques, this study could contribute valuable insights to the literature regarding the efficacy of combining these surgical techniques.

Moreover, our objective was to observe the outcomes of non-athletes moderate active patients who underwent surgical treatment using combined arthroscopic and non-anatomic reconstructive procedures, assessing significant improvements in knee function and quality of life as measured by the IKDC Questionnaire, Lysholm Knee Scoring Scale, and KOOS.

These outcomes could guide clinicians in optimizing surgical strategies to enhance recovery and long-term knee stability while improving patient-reported quality of life.

2. Materials and Methods

2.1. Selection Criteria

This retrospective cohort study was conducted from 2019 to 2023, focusing on patients with confirmed multiligament knee injuries who received surgical treatment. The study aimed to evaluate the effectiveness of a combined arthroscopic and open non-anatomic ligament reconstruction technique using a non-anatomic approach tailored for patients with moderate activity levels.

The inclusion criteria encompassed adult patients aged 18 to 60 years with multiligament knee injuries confirmed through clinical examinations and imaging, involving at least two of the major knee ligaments (ACL, PCL, MCL, and LCL). Patients were required to present with chronic injuries (more than six weeks from the time of trauma and not more than 6 months after trauma) and to be physically active, defined as engaging in moderate levels of physical activity prior to the injury. Eligible participants needed to have sufficient overall health to undergo surgical intervention and be compliant with postoperative rehabilitation, as determined by a comprehensive preoperative evaluation. Patients with important comorbidities such as osteoporosis, cancer, autoimmune diseases, or metabolic disorders were excluded from the cohort. Individuals with associated meniscal or chondral injuries requiring repair were also included, taking into account these did not diverge from the primary focus on ligament reconstruction. All patients provided informed consent and agreed to participate in the follow-up evaluations. Patients were excluded if they had acute ligament injuries requiring immediate surgery. These criteria ensured that the sample comprised patients who could benefit from the surgical intervention, thereby enhancing the reliability of the outcomes.

The surgical procedure combined arthroscopic and open techniques, performed by a surgeon with over 10 years of experience in knee arthroscopy and sports traumatology. The arthroscopic procedures included anterior cruciate ligament (ACL) reconstruction, posterior cruciate ligament (PCL) reconstruction, combined cruciate reconstructions, and meniscal surgeries as needed, depending on the specific injury patterns observed in each patient. The average duration of the surgery was approximately 1 h and 30 min. The approach was designed to simplify the reconstruction process by using non-anatomic techniques, prioritizing functional outcomes over exact anatomical replication.

For medial collateral ligament (MCL) reconstruction, we employed two simplified methods: a single-bundle graft technique, which provided adequate valgus stability using autograft tissue anchored proximally to the femur and distally to the tibia, and the Danish technique, which utilized a minimally invasive approach with either an autograft or synthetic graft to enhance medial stability while reducing recovery time.

Lateral collateral ligament (LCL) reconstruction involved three techniques adapted based on the specific patient's needs: the Arciero technique, which utilized an autograft passed through femoral and fibular tunnels to restore lateral stability with minimal surgical exposure; the Larson sling technique, which is also fibula-based and employed an allograft passed through a fibula tunnel and anchored at the femur, emphasizing mechanical stability; and a modified version of the LaPrade technique, where the modifications included reducing the number of surgical tunnels to minimize operative time and using a single-bundle graft instead of a double-bundle approach. These adjustments aimed to simplify the procedure while maintaining adequate lateral support and stability. The modifications were tailored to the functional demands of the patient population studied.

There were also a couple of cases on which a single Achilles allograft was used to reconstruct both the ACL and MCL or the ACL and LCL and ALL. In the cases where the ACL and MCL were reconstructed, the ACL was reconstructed in a standard manner, with the Achilles bone block on the femoral condyle, and after fixing the graft in the tibial tunnel, the remaining allograft was used to reconstruct the MCL. When the ACL and LCL were reconstructed with a single Achilles allograft, the femoral tunnel was created in an OUTSIDE-in technique. The ACL part was fixed with screws on the femoral tunnel and the remaining Achilles allograft was split in two, on the reconstructed LCL limb and the ALL on the other (Figures 1 and 2).

Postoperative care followed a standardized rehabilitation protocol. The initial phase (0–2 weeks) focused on immobilization with a knee brace and limited weight-bearing. This was followed by progressive rehabilitation, including range-of-motion exercises and quadriceps strengthening from weeks 2 to 6. The advanced phase (from week 6 onward) incorporated proprioceptive training and sport-specific exercises, aiming for a gradual return to recreational activities.

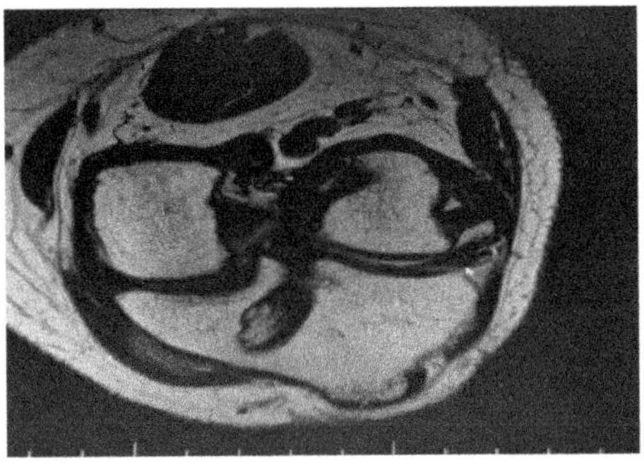

Figure 1. MRI demonstrating a single Achilles allograft used to reconstruct both the ACL and MCL, showing graft positioning and fixation.

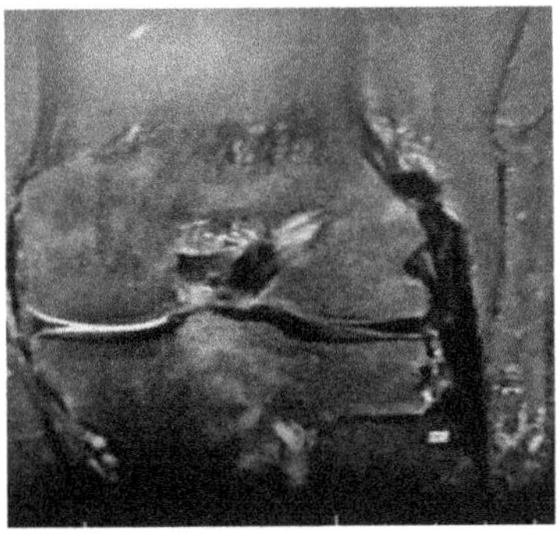

Figure 2. MRI demonstrating a single Achilles allograft used to reconstruct ACL, LCL, and ALL, with clear visualization of the graft distribution.

Clinical assessments such as the Lachman test, Pivot Shift Test (PST), varus stress test (Var), and valgus stress test (Val) were included, ensuring a broader and more objective evaluation of functional outcomes (detailed in the Supplementary Materials).

Clinical outcomes were assessed using three validated scoring systems: the International Knee Documentation Committee (IKDC) Questionnaire, the Lysholm Knee Scoring Scale, and the Knee Injury and Osteoarthritis Outcome Score (KOOS). These scores are extensively utilized and validated instruments for evaluating knee function, symptoms, and patient quality of life. The KOOS is a thorough, self-administered questionnaire that assesses five domains: pain (KOSSP), symptoms (KOSSSy), activities of daily living (KOSSA), sports/recreation (KOSSp), and knee-related quality of life (KOOSQ), rendering it appropriate for monitoring outcomes in patients with knee injuries and osteoarthritis over time [16,17]. These subcategories provide a comprehensive assessment of knee functionality, symptoms, and the impact of knee conditions on daily living and quality of life. The IKDC score, created by the International Knee Documentation Committee, offers a standardized assessment of knee functionality and is commonly utilized in clinical research to evaluate the efficacy of interventions, particularly in cases of ACL and other ligament injuries [18,19]. It encompasses both subjective and objective elements to assess a patient's perceived knee functionality in conjunction with physical examination results. The IKDC (International Knee Documentation Committee) score includes subjective and objective measures of knee function. IKDC3 evaluates the highest level of activity a patient can perform without pain, capturing the functional limitations imposed by knee instability or injury. The Lysholm score, initially developed to assess outcomes after knee ligament surgery, emphasizes eight primary symptoms, such as pain, instability, and functional impairments [20,21]. The Lysholm Knee Scoring Scale consists of eight subsections, each assessing a distinct aspect of knee health. These include the presence and severity of limping, the need for walking aids, instances of knee locking, sensations of instability or "giving way", pain intensity during activities, post-exertion swelling, challenges in stair climbing, and the ability to perform a full squat. Each subsection contributes to the overall score, with higher scores indicating better knee functionality. For example, Lysholm 7 evaluates the patient's ability to ascend stairs, Lysholm 4 measures knee instability, and Lysholm 5 assesses pain intensity. Collectively, these scales offer a comprehensive perspective on knee health and are essential for tracking recovery, evaluating interventions, and measuring patient satisfaction with knee-related therapies.

These tools measured improvements in knee function, pain levels, and overall quality of life. All patients provided written informed consent prior to their participation in the study. The study protocol was reviewed and approved by the institutional ethics committee, with approval reference number 20207/28 August 2024.

2.2. Statistical Analysis

Continuous variables following a normal distribution were presented as means with standard deviation (SD), while non-normally distributed data were presented as medians with interquartile range (IQR). The normality of the distribution was evaluated utilizing the Shapiro–Wilk test. Differences among groups for normally distributed continuous data were assessed utilizing Welch's *t*-test for two groups or ANOVA for more than two groups. Post hoc analyses, when necessary, were conducted utilizing the Bonferroni correction to adjust for multiple comparisons. For non-normally distributed continuous data, the Mann–Whitney U test and the Wilcoxon signed-rank test were employed for two-group comparisons, while the Kruskal–Wallis test was applied for comparisons involving three or more groups. The false discovery rate was applied to adjust for multiple comparisons in the Mann–Whitney U test, Wilcoxon signed-rank test, and Kruskal–Wallis test. Categorical data were analyzed utilizing the χ^2 test or Fisher's exact test, particularly when expected cell counts were below five. Categorical data were reported as frequencies (n) and percentages (%). A priori power analysis was conducted with at least 80% statistical power with a 95% confidence interval. All statistical analyses were performed utilizing R Studio version 3.6.0 using the packages stats, dplyr, coin, multcomp, and pwr. A significant p-value was considered <0.05.

3. Results

The study comprised 60 participants with a median age of 38 years (IQR 32–44), of whom 87% were male (n = 52) and 13% were female (n = 8). Participants predominantly lived in urban regions (60%) as opposed to rural regions (40%). The majority of subjects participated in physical therapy (88%), while a lesser percentage received a combination of physical therapy and hydrotherapy (12%). The median rehabilitation duration was 38 days (IQR 24–40), and the median symptom duration before intervention was 12 months (IQR 8–24), as observed in Table 1.

Table 1. Demographic and clinical characteristics of the study population.

Characteristic	n = 60
Age	38 (32, 44)
Gender	
Female	8 (13%)
Male	52 (87%)

Table 1. *Cont.*

Characteristic	n = 60
BMI (kg/m^2)	29.4 (24.8, 30.0)
Place of residence	
Rural	24 (40%)
Urban	36 (60%)
Type of rehabilitation	
Physical therapy (PT)	53 (88%)
PT + Hydrotherapy	7 (12%)
Duration of rehabilitation (weeks)	38 (24, 40)
Duration of symptoms (months)	12 (8, 24)
Type of work	
Intensive physical work	5 (8.3%)
Moderate physical work	15 (25%)
Sedentary work	40 (67%)
Educational level	
High school	24 (40%)
Post-secondary	7 (12%)
Vocational school	3 (5.0%)
University	26 (43%)
Combinations of reconstructions	
ACL + LCL (single Achilles allograft)	5 (8.3%)
ACL + MCL (single Achilles allograft)	8 (13%)
ACL + LCL (ACL autograft + hamstring allograft)	15 (25%)
ACL + MCL (BTB allograft for ACL and hamstring autograft for MCL)	20 (33%)
ACL + PCL (ACL autograft + PCL Achilles allograft)	4 (6.7%)
ACL + PCL + MCL	6 (10%)
PLC + ACL + MCL (single Achilles allograft for ACL and PLC + hamstring autograft for MCL)	2 (3.3%)

Data are presented as median (interquartile range) for continuous variables and frequency (percentage) for categorical variables. BMI: Body Mass Index; ACL: Anterior Cruciate Ligament; LCL: Lateral Collateral Ligament; MCL: Medial Collateral Ligament; PCL: Posterior Cruciate Ligament; PLC Postero-Lateral Corner; PT: Physical Therapy.

The surgical procedure combined arthroscopic and open techniques. The combinations of procedures included ACL + MCL reconstructions (n = 28), ACL + LCL reconstructions (n = 20), and cases involving all four ligaments (n = 25). Specifically, there were four cases of ACL + PCL reconstructions and eight cases of ACL + PCL + MCL reconstructions These combinations were tailored to the specific injury patterns and functional demands of the patients.

The majority of individuals were employed in sedentary positions (67%), while 25% participated in moderate physical work, and merely 8.3% engaged in strenuous physical labor. Educational qualifications differed, with 43% holding a university degree and 40% having finished high school. The median BMI was documented at 29.4 (IQR 24.8–30.0), signifying a predominantly overweight population. ACL and LCL reconstructions were performed in five patients (8.3%), highlighting the relatively low prevalence of injuries involving these two ligaments. Similarly, ACL and MCL reconstructions were performed in eight patients (13%), indicating a moderate frequency for this combination. The most common reconstructions were ACL with LCL, seen in 15 cases (25%), and ACL with MCL, observed in 20 cases (33%), suggesting that these combinations account for the majority of ligament injuries requiring surgical intervention.

Less frequently, ACL and PCL reconstructions were performed in four patients (6.7%), reflecting a lower occurrence of simultaneous anterior and posterior cruciate ligament injuries. More complex reconstructions, such as ACL, PCL, and MCL, were required in six patients (10%). The rarest combination, involving PCL, ACL, and MCL, was performed in only two patients (3.3%).

These findings suggest that while injuries combining ACL with either LCL or MCL dominate, more complex patterns requiring triple ligament reconstructions are considerably less common. This distribution provides valuable insights into injury prevalence and may help guide clinical decisions and surgical planning.

Functional Outcomes: Preoperative Versus Postoperative

The comparative analysis of preoperative and postoperative conditions utilizing diverse clinical scores revealed significant enhancements post-intervention, as seen in Table 2. All components of the International Knee Documentation Committee (IKDC) scores exhibited significant changes, with *p*-values consistently below 0.013, indicating substantial enhancements in knee functionality. For instance, IKDC1 exhibited an elevation from a preoperative median of 1.0 to a postoperative range of 2.0–4.0, indicating improved knee function and stability. IKDC6 specifically assesses locking or catching symptoms of the knee. In this study, there was no statistically significant change observed in IKDC6 scores, indicating that these symptoms were less responsive to the intervention. The overall IKDC score demonstrated a significant increase, rising from a preoperative median of 32.6–45.2 to a postoperative range of 69.5–95.4 (F-statistic = 67.64, $p < 0.013$). These results highlight a substantial improvement in knee functionality, probably due to the intervention.

Table 2. Preoperative and postoperative IKDC scores.

	n	Preoperatory Status	Postoperatory Status	Test Statistic
		(*n* = 30)	(*n* = 30)	
IKDC1	60	1.0 1.0 1.0	2.0 2.5 4.0	$F_{1,58} = 33.43, p < 0.01$ [1]
IKDC2	60	0.0 4.0 5.0	8.0 9.0 9.1	$F_{1,58} = 44.06, p < 0.01$ [1]
IKDC3	60	1.0 4.0 5.0	8.0 9.0 10.0	$F_{1,58} = 57.70, p < 0.01$ [1]
IKDC4	60	1.0 2.0 2.0	2.0 3.0 3.1	$F_{1,58} = 18.42, p < 0.01$ [1]
IKDC5	60	1.0 1.0 2.0	1.0 2.5 4.0	$F_{1,58} = 18.13, p < 0.01$ [1]
IKDC6	60	0.0 1.0 1.0	1.0 1.0 1.0	$F_{1,58} = 3.13, p = 0.08$ [1]
IKDC7	60	0.0 1.0 2.0	2.0 3.0 3.1	$F_{1,58} = 45.71, p < 0.01$ [1]
IKDC8	60	1.0 1.0 1.0	2.0 2.5 4.0	$F_{1,58} = 26.19, p < 0.01$ [1]
IKDC9	60	12.0 14.5 17.2	25.0 30.0 33.2	$F_{1,58} = 60.03, p < 0.01$ [1]
IKDC10	60	2.0 4.0 5.0	7.9 8.0 10.0	$F_{1,58} = 29.31, p < 0.01$ [1]
Total IKDC	60	31.0 39.1 44.1	69.5 75.9 95.4	$F_{1,58} = 70.66, p < 0.01$ [1]

IKDC: International Knee Documentation Committee score. Data are presented as median (25th percentile, 75th percentile). [1]. Wilcoxon Signed-Rank Test.

The Lysholm Knee Scoring Scale demonstrated statistically significant enhancements in most items postoperatively ($p < 0.01$) (Table 3), signifying diminished pain and enhanced knee function. LYSHOLM7 exhibited an elevation in scores from a preoperative median range of 0.0–6.0 to a postoperative range of 9.7–10.0 ($p < 0.013$), indicating diminished symptoms and improved knee stability. The total Lysholm score exhibited substantial improvement, increasing from a preoperative range of 48.0–73.0 to a postoperative range of 73.6–93.2 ($p < 0.01$). The increase in scores signifies substantial postoperative enhancements, indicating improved knee functionality and alleviation of symptoms.

The KOOS demonstrated significant postoperative enhancements across various sub-domains (Table 4). KOOSP1, which evaluates symptoms and pain, diminished from a preoperative range of 2.0–3.0 to a postoperative range of 0.0–3.0 ($p < 0.01$), indicating a reduction in pain levels. Correspondingly, KOOSA1, indicative of daily living activities, decreased from a preoperative median of 1.0 to 0.0 postoperatively ($p < 0.013$), underscoring improved functionality in executing routine tasks. The total KOOS score significantly increased, from a preoperative median of 42.9–67.3 to a postoperative range of 63.1–89.3

($p < 0.013$), indicating substantial enhancements in knee symptoms, pain alleviation, and quality of life following the intervention.

Table 3. Preoperative and postoperative Lysholm scores.

	n	Preoperatory Status (n = 30)	Postoperatory Status (n = 30)	Test Statistic
LYSHOLM1	60	3.0 3.0 3.0	3.0 5.0 5.0	$F_{1,58} = 19.96, p < 0.01$ [1]
LYSHOLM2	60	0.0 2.0 5.0	5.0 5.0 5.0	$F_{1,58} = 39.21, p < 0.01$ [1]
LYSHOLM3	60	9.7 10.0 15.0	15.0 15.0 15.0	$F_{1,58} = 13.11, p < 0.01$ [1]
LYSHOLM4	60	10.0 15.0 20.0	20.0 20.0 25.0	$F_{1,58} = 29.30, p < 0.01$ [1]
LYSHOLM5	60	10.0 15.0 20.0	19.6 20.0 25.0	$F_{1,58} = 7.50, p = 0.01$ [1]
LYSHOLM6	60	0.0 6.0 10.0	6.0 6.0 10.0	$F_{1,58} = 0.08, p = 0.78$ [1]
LYSHOLM7	60	0.0 2.0 6.0	9.7 10.0 10.0	$F_{1,58} = 41.39, p < 0.01$ [1]
LYSHOLM8	60	0.9 1.0 4.0	4.0 4.5 5.0	$F_{1,58} = 20.44, p < 0.01$ [1]
Total Lysholm	60	48.0 61.0 73.0	73.6 87.0 93.2	$F_{1,58} = 33.53, p < 0.01$ [1]

Lysholm: Lysholm Knee Scoring Scale. Data are presented as median (25th percentile, 75th percentile). [1.] Wilcoxon Signed-Rank Test.

Table 4. Preoperative and postoperative KOSS scores.

	n	Preoperatory Status (n = 30)	Postoperatory Status (n = 30)	Test Statistic
KOOSP1	60	2.0 3.0 3.0	0.0 1.0 3.0	$F_{1,58} = 12.80, p < 0.01$ [1]
KOOSP2	60	2.0 3.0 3.0	0.0 0.0 1.1	$F_{1,58} = 27.93, p < 0.01$ [1]
KOOSP3	60	1.9 3.0 3.0	0.0 0.0 1.0	$F_{1,58} = 36.77, p < 0.01$ [1]
KOOSP4	60	1.0 2.0 3.0	0.0 0.0 1.0	$F_{1,58} = 17.27, p < 0.01$ [1]
KOOSP5	60	0.0 2.0 3.0	0.0 0.0 0.0	$F_{1,58} = 38.50, p < 0.01$ [1]
KOOSP6	60	1.9 3.0 3.0	0.0 0.0 2.0	$F_{1,58} = 41.11, p < 0.01$ [1]
KOOSP7	60	0.0 1.0 3.0	0.0 0.0 1.0	$F_{1,58} = 5.28, p = 0.03$ [1]
KOOSP8	60	0.0 0.0 2.0	0.0 0.0 1.0	$F_{1,58} = 3.18, p = 0.08$ [1]
KOOSP9	60	0.0 2.0 2.0	0.0 0.0 1.0	$F_{1,58} = 10.40, p < 0.01$ [1]
KOOSSy1	60	0.0 2.0 3.0	0.9 1.0 1.0	$F_{1,58} = 8.52, p < 0.01$ [1]
KOOSSy2	60	1.0 1.0 3.0	0.0 0.0 1.0	$F_{1,58} = 13.53, p < 0.01$ [1]
KOOSSy3	60	1.0 2.0 3.0	0.0 1.5 2.0	$F_{1,58} = 4.24, p = 0.04$ [1]
KOOSSy4	60	0.9 1.0 3.0	0.0 0.0 1.0	$F_{1,58} = 17.24, p < 0.01$ [1]
KOOSSy5	60	0.9 1.0 1.2	0.0 3.5 4.0	$F_{1,58} = 2.74, p = 0.10$ [1]
KOOSSy6	60	0.0 1.0 2.0	1.0 3.0 4.0	$F_{1,58} = 13.59, p < 0.01$ [1]
KOOSA1	60	1.0 2.0 2.0	0.0 0.0 1.0	$F_{1,58} = 60.41, p < 0.01$ [1]
KOOSA2	60	1.0 1.5 3.0	0.0 0.0 1.0	$F_{1,58} = 38.56, p < 0.01$ [1]
KOOSA3	60	0.0 1.0 2.0	0.0 0.0 1.0	$F_{1,58} = 3.95, p = 0.05$ [1]
KOOSA4	60	1.0 1.0 3.0	0.0 0.0 1.0	$F_{1,58} = 23.17, p < 0.01$ [1]
KOOSA5	60	0.0 2.0 2.0	0.0 0.0 2.0	$F_{1,58} = 14.86, p < 0.01$ [1]
KOOSA6	60	1.0 1.0 1.1	0.0 0.0 0.0	$F_{1,58} = 24.65, p < 0.01$ [1]
KOOSA7	60	1.0 2.0 2.0	0.0 0.0 0.0	$F_{1,58} = 135.79, p < 0.01$ [1]
KOOSA8	60	1.0 1.0 2.0	0.0 0.0 0.0	$F_{1,58} = 30.10, p < 0.01$ [1]
KOOSA9	60	0.9 1.0 2.0	0.0 0.0 0.0	$F_{1,58} = 21.88, p < 0.01$ [1]
KOOSA10	60	1.0 2.0 2.0	0.0 0.0 0.0	$F_{1,58} = 50.83, p < 0.01$ [1]
KOOSA11	60	1.0 1.0 2.0	0.0 0.0 0.1	$F_{1,58} = 41.07, p < 0.01$ [1]
KOOSA12	60	1.0 1.0 2.0	0.0 0.0 0.1	$F_{1,58} = 41.97, p < 0.01$ [1]
KOOSA13	60	1.0 1.0 2.0	0.0 0.0 0.1	$F_{1,58} = 54.22, p < 0.01$ [1]
KOOSA14	60	0.9 1.0 2.0	0.0 0.0 1.0	$F_{1,58} = 7.94, p = 0.01$ [1]
KOOSA15	60	0.9 1.0 2.0	0.0 0.0 1.0	$F_{1,58} = 25.85, p < 0.01$ [1]
KOOSA16	60	1.0 2.0 4.0	0.0 1.0 2.0	$F_{1,58} = 18.62, p < 0.01$ [1]

Table 4. *Cont.*

	n	Preoperatory Status	Postoperatory Status	Test Statistic
		(n = 30)	(n = 30)	
KOOSA17	60	1.0 1.0 2.1	0.0 0.0 1.0	$F_{1,58} = 21.55$, $p < 0.01$ [1]
KOOSSp1	59	2.0 3.0 3.0	0.0 0.5 1.0	$F_{1,57} = 76.20$, $p < 0.01$ [1]
KOOSSp2	60	2.0 3.0 3.0	0.0 1.0 1.2	$F_{1,58} = 25.21$, $p < 0.01$ [1]
KOOSSp3	60	2.9 3.0 4.0	1.0 1.0 1.1	$F_{1,58} = 50.60$, $p < 0.01$ [1]
KOOSSp4	60	3.0 4.0 4.0	0.0 1.0 2.0	$F_{1,58} = 72.36$, $p < 0.01$ [1]
KOOSSp5	60	2.0 3.0 4.0	0.0 1.0 2.0	$F_{1,58} = 25.41$, $p < 0.01$ [1]
KOOSQ1	60	3.0 4.0 4.0	1.0 3.0 4.0	$F_{1,58} = 11.63$, $p < 0.01$ [1]
KOOSQ2	60	2.9 4.0 4.0	1.0 2.0 3.0	$F_{1,58} = 23.79$, $p < 0.01$ [1]
KOOSQ3	60	3.0 4.0 4.0	0.9 1.0 2.0	$F_{1,58} = 45.72$, $p < 0.01$ [1]
KOOSQ4	60	2.0 3.0 4.0	1.0 1.0 2.0	$F_{1,58} = 25.53$, $p < 0.01$ [1]
KooS total	60	42.9 47.6 65.5	63.1 85.7 89.3	$F_{1,58} = 55.92$, $p < 0.01$ [1]

Data are presented as median (25th percentile, 75th percentile), [1.] Wilcoxon Signed-Rank Test.

Although the majority of items in the IKDC, Lysholm, and KOOS scales demonstrated substantial enhancements, a few anomalies were identified. For example, LYSHOLM6 (swelling) and KOOSP8 exhibited no notable alterations, with p-values exceeding the significance threshold. Notwithstanding these exceptions, the majority of measures in this study achieved statistical significance, underscoring the intervention's efficacy.

The analysis of preoperative and postoperative results indicates significant enhancements across various metrics post-intervention. The findings from Table 3 indicate substantial postoperative enhancements in knee function, pain alleviation, and daily functionality across all three assessment instruments.

All subdomains of the IKDC scores, with the exception of IKDC6 ($p = 0.08$), demonstrated statistically significant improvements ($p < 0.01$). IKDC1 exhibited an enhancement from a preoperative median of 1.0 to a postoperative range of 2.0–4.0 ($p < 0.01$). This trend persisted across additional subdomains, notably IKDC3, which rose from a median of 1.0 (4.0, 5.0) preoperatively to 8.0 (9.0, 10.0) postoperatively ($p < 0.01$), signifying substantial improvements in knee function and stability. The cumulative IKDC score highlights these advancements, increasing from a preoperative median of 31.0 (39.1, 44.1) to 69.5 (75.9, 95.4) postoperatively, with a $p < 0.01$, thereby affirming a comprehensive improvement in knee health following the intervention.

The study findings demonstrate significant enhancements in knee function, pain alleviation, and overall quality of life post-intervention, evaluated through the IKDC, Lysholm, and KOOS scoring systems. Postoperative scores significantly improved across all three tools when compared to preoperative scores, with the majority of p-values falling below 0.01, underscoring the intervention's effectiveness.

4. Discussion

This study's findings indicate that patients who undergo surgical treatment using a combined arthroscopic and open non-anatomic ligament reconstruction technique have markedly enhanced knee function, alleviated pain, and improved participants' quality of life, as evidenced by elevated scores on the IKDC, Lysholm, and KOOS scales.

When comparing ACL + ALL reconstruction to ACL + MCL or ACL + LCL reconstructions, prior research suggests that different ligament combinations address distinct instability patterns. For instance, Sonnery-Cottet et al. (2015) documented significant improvements in knee stability and function following simultaneous ACL and anterolateral ligament (ALL) reconstruction [22], as evidenced by enhancements in the Lysholm, IKDC, and pivot shift scores [11]. Similarly, studies by Noyes et al. [23] reported that ACL + MCL reconstructions are particularly effective in managing valgus instability, while ACL + LCL reconstructions are necessary for addressing varus instability and postero-lateral corner deficiencies. Furthermore, a systematic review and meta-analysis by Lima et al. (2021) found that combined ACL and ALL reconstruction resulted in better postoperative clinical outcomes compared to isolated ACL reconstruction, particularly in reducing residual pivot shift and rerupture rates [24].

However, this study's emphasis on non-anatomic reconstruction highlights a critical distinction from anatomic techniques. While anatomic reconstructions aim to replicate native ligament biomechanics, non-anatomic methods prioritize functional stability and operative simplicity. This approach is particularly advantageous for patients who do not require high-level athletic performance, as it minimizes surgical time and postoperative rehabilitation challenges while delivering comparable functional outcomes.

In comparison to anatomic collateral ligament reconstructions, non-anatomic approaches, as employed in this study, simplify surgical techniques and reduce operative time while still yielding comparable functional outcomes [23]. For example, Ardern et al. found that anatomic ACL + MCL reconstructions resulted in slightly better stability metrics but required longer rehabilitation durations and were associated with higher surgical complexity. Our findings align with these studies, as the combination of ACL + non-anatomic collateral ligament reconstructions demonstrated significant improvements in IKDC, Lysholm, and KOOS scores [25]. The choice of ligament combinations should be tailored to the patient's specific instability patterns, activity level, and functional demands and allograft availability.

In orthopedic settings, quality-of-life assessments are often underemphasized compared to other medical fields.

The significance of the IKDC score as a measure of knee functionality and quality of life is thoroughly documented in the literature. Williams et al. (2020) emphasized that elevated IKDC scores following ACL reconstruction were associated with enhanced quality of life, reinforcing the notion that IKDC is a reliable metric for assessing the impact of surgical procedures on knee health and patient-reported outcomes [10]. Our study similarly demonstrated an elevation in the total IKDC score from a median of 31.0 to 69.5, indicating enhancements in both knee stability and overall quality of life for patients following surgery.

A systematic review by Filbay et al. (2022) affirmed that untreated or inadequately treated ACL and meniscal injuries can adversely affect long-term quality of life, physical activity, and economic productivity [1]. Our findings substantiate the effectiveness of prompt and thorough surgical intervention, as postoperative KOOS scores in our study demonstrated improved quality of life and diminished symptoms and pain. This underscores the essential function of comprehensive surgical methods, such as combined ligament reconstruction, in alleviating the detrimental impacts of knee instability on daily activities and quality of life.

Furthermore, Yanardag et al. (2021) discovered that pain, balance, and gait function substantially influence the quality of life in individuals suffering from knee and hip pain [4]. This finding corresponds with our study's results in the Lysholm and KOOS scores, where we noted significant enhancements in symptoms and pain levels postoperatively, indicating that diminished pain and enhanced stability can markedly influence patient-reported quality of life. The Lysholm score notably improved from a median of 48.0 preoperatively to 73.6 postoperatively, demonstrating that surgical intervention not only restores physical knee function but also mitigates pain, thereby enhancing patients' quality of life.

Innovative therapies for knee instability are progressing, as demonstrated by Körner et al. (2020), who highlighted the advantages of integrating advanced rehabilitation protocols with surgical intervention [5]. In our study, patients underwent a combination of physical therapy and, for some, hydrotherapy postoperatively, which likely facilitated the notable enhancements in functionality and pain levels. This corresponds with Körner's findings, highlighting the significance of a multidisciplinary approach in improving post-operative recovery and ensuring long-term joint stability. Our findings emphasize the importance of optimizing postoperative management strategies, such as physical therapy and hydrotherapy, in facilitating recovery and improving functional outcomes. While pharmacological interventions, such as NSAIDs, may play a role in other clinical settings, this study focused exclusively on physical rehabilitation as the primary modality for postoperative care.

By combining these treatment modalities with proper nutrition and lifestyle modifications, individuals with knee instability can experience a significant improvement in their overall quality of life. It is crucial to note that a multidisciplinary approach is of great importance in effectively managing knee instability [26,27].

This study illustrates notable enhancements in knee functionality and quality of life after combined ligament reconstruction.

5. Limitations

This study has certain limitations that should be acknowledged. The predominance of male participants (87%) restricts the ability to evaluate gender differences in outcomes, and future research should address this imbalance to ensure broader generalizability. Additionally, the relatively small sample size and short-term follow-up period limit the scope of our findings. Expanding the cohort to include more diverse populations and conducting studies with longer follow-up durations will be critical for validating these results. Moreover, while we focused on non-anatomic reconstruction within a single cohort, the absence of a control group prevents direct comparisons with anatomic reconstruction techniques. Future studies should incorporate comparative analyses to provide more comprehensive insights. Future studies with extended follow-ups (5–10 years or longer) will be critical to assessing the durability of joint stability, functional outcomes, and the potential onset of osteoarthritis. Notwithstanding these constraints, the findings align with the current literature supporting comprehensive surgical and rehabilitation strategies for knee injuries [4,6,12]. Furthermore, reliance on subjective outcome measures, such as IKDC, Lysholm, and KOOS scores, highlights the need for additional objective assessments, such as biomechanical evaluations and imaging studies, to enhance the robustness of the findings [18,19].

6. Conclusions

This study indicates that the combination of arthroscopic and open non-anatomic ligament reconstruction markedly enhances knee function, alleviates pain, and improves the quality of life for individuals with knee instability.

Supplementary Materials: The following supporting information can be downloaded at: https://www.mdpi.com/article/10.3390/medicina61010053/s1, Details of the clinical assessments (Lachman, PST, Var, and Val tests) alongside objective MRI findings to provide additional clarity and transparency.

Author Contributions: Conceptualization, M.H. and C.-A.M.; methodology, M.H., C.-A.M. and R.-F.T.; software, D.C.; validation, M.H., C.-A.M., R.-F.T. and M.A.; formal analysis, D.C. and M.H.; investigation, M.A. and B.A.; resources, A.C.M. and C.T.H.; data curation, M.H., C.-A.M. and D.C.; writing—original draft preparation, C.-A.M. and M.H.; writing—review and editing, M.H., R.-F.T. and B.A.; visualization, D.C., A.C.M. and C.-A.M.; supervision, C.-A.M., C.T.H. and R.-F.T.; project administration, M.H. and C.-A.M.; funding acquisition, C.T.H. and C.-A.M. All authors have read and agreed to the published version of the manuscript.

Funding: We would like to acknowledge "Victor Babeș" University of Medicine and Pharmacy Timișoara for their support in covering the costs of publication for this research paper.

Institutional Review Board Statement: The study protocol was reviewed and approved by the institutional ethics committee, with approval reference number 20207/28 August 2024.

Informed Consent Statement: Informed consent was obtained from all subjects involved in the study.

Data Availability Statement: The data supporting the results of this study are available from the corresponding author upon reasonable request.

Conflicts of Interest: The authors declare no conflicts of interest.

References

1. Filbay, S.R.; Skou, S.T.; Bullock, G.S.; Le, C.Y.; Räisänen, A.M.; Toomey, C.; Ezzat, A.M.; Hayden, A.; Culvenor, A.G.; Whittaker, J.L.; et al. Long-Term Quality of Life, Work Limitation, Physical Activity, Economic Cost and Disease Burden Following ACL and Meniscal Injury: A Systematic Review and Meta-Analysis for the OPTIKNEE Consensus. *Br. J. Sports Med.* **2022**, *56*, 1465–1474. [CrossRef] [PubMed]
2. Grassi, A.; Olivieri Huerta, R.A.; Lucidi, G.A.; Agostinone, P.; Dal Fabbro, G.; Pagano, A.; Tischer, T.; Zaffagnini, S. A Lateral Extra-Articular Procedure Reduces the Failure Rate of Revision Anterior Cruciate Ligament Reconstruction Surgery Without Increasing Complications: A Systematic Review and Meta-Analysis. *Am. J. Sports Med.* **2024**, *52*, 1098–1108. [CrossRef]
3. Yang, H.Y.; Cheon, J.H.; Choi, J.H.; Song, E.K.; Seon, J.K. Combined Anterior Cruciate Ligament and Anterolateral Ligament Reconstruction Decreases Passive Anterior Tibial Subluxation Compared With Isolated Anterior Cruciate Ligament Reconstruction Despite Similar Rotational Stability and Clinical Outcomes. *Arthrosc. J. Arthrosc. Relat. Surg.* **2023**, *39*, 2513–2524. [CrossRef]
4. Yanardag, M.; Şimşek, T.T.; Yanardag, F. Exploring the Relationship of Pain, Balance, Gait Function, and Quality of Life in Older Adults with Hip and Knee Pain. *Pain Manag. Nurs.* **2021**, *22*, 503–508. [CrossRef] [PubMed]
5. Körner, D.; Ateschrang, A.; Schröter, S.; Aurich, M.; Becher, C.; Walther, M.; Gottschalk, O.; Bangert, Y.; Ettinger, S.; Plaass, C.; et al. Concomitant Ankle Instability Has a Negative Impact on the Quality of Life in Patients with Osteochondral Lesions of the Talus: Data from the German Cartilage Registry (KnorpelRegister DGOU). *Knee Surg. Sports Traumatol. Arthrosc.* **2020**, *28*, 3339–3346. [CrossRef] [PubMed]
6. Nazzal, E.M.; Keeling, L.E.; Ryan, P.M.; Herman, Z.J.; Hughes, J.D. The Role of Lateral Extra-Articular Tenodesis in Anterior Cruciate Ligament Reconstruction and Treatment of Rotatory Knee Instability: A Scoping Review. *Curr. Rev. Musculoskelet. Med.* **2023**, *16*, 235–245. [CrossRef] [PubMed]
7. Marx, R.G.; Jones, E.C.; Allen, A.A.; Altchek, D.W.; O'Brien, S.J.; Rodeo, S.A.; Williams, R.J.; Warren, R.F.; Wickiewicz, T.L. Reliability, Validity, and Responsiveness of Four Knee Outcome Scales for Athletic Patients. *J. Bone Joint Surg. Am.* **2001**, *83*, 1459–1469. [CrossRef]
8. Calanna, F.; Duthon, V.; Menetrey, J. Rehabilitation and Return to Sports after Isolated Meniscal Repairs: A New Evidence-Based Protocol. *J. Exp. Orthop.* **2022**, *9*, 80. [CrossRef] [PubMed]
9. Guarino, A.; Farinelli, L.; Iacono, V.; Screpis, D.; Piovan, G.; Rizzo, M.; Mariconda, M.; Zorzi, C. Lateral Extra-Articular Tenodesis and Anterior Cruciate Ligament Reconstruction in Young Patients: Clinical Results and Return to Sport. *Orthop. Rev.* **2022**, *14*, 33696. [CrossRef] [PubMed]
10. Williams, T.; Burley, D.; Evans, L.; Robertson, A.; Hardy, L.; Roy, S.; Lewis, D. The Structural Validity of the IKDC and Its Relationship with Quality of Life Following ACL Reconstruction. *Scand. J. Med. Sci. Sports* **2020**, *30*, 1748–1757. [CrossRef]
11. Sonnery-Cottet, B.; Thaunat, M.; Freychet, B.; Pupim, B.H.B.; Murphy, C.G.; Claes, S. Outcome of a Combined Anterior Cruciate Ligament and Anterolateral Ligament Reconstruction Technique With a Minimum 2-Year Follow-Up. *Am. J. Sports Med.* **2015**, *43*, 1598–1605. [CrossRef] [PubMed]
12. van Grinsven, S.; van Cingel, R.E.H.; Holla, C.J.M.; van Loon, C.J.M. Evidence-Based Rehabilitation Following Anterior Cruciate Ligament Reconstruction. *Knee Surg. Sports Traumatol. Arthrosc.* **2010**, *18*, 1128–1144. [CrossRef]
13. Kruse, L.M.; Gray, B.; Wright, R.W. Rehabilitation after Anterior Cruciate Ligament Reconstruction: A Systematic Review. *J. Bone Joint Surg. Am.* **2012**, *94*, 1737–1748. [CrossRef] [PubMed]
14. Adams, D.; Logerstedt, D.; Hunter-Giordano, A.; Axe, M.J.; Snyder-Mackler, L. Current Concepts for Anterior Cruciate Ligament Reconstruction: A Criterion-Based Rehabilitation Progression. *J. Orthop. Sports Phys. Ther.* **2012**, *42*, 601–614. [CrossRef] [PubMed]
15. Xiao, Z.; Li, G. The Effect of Wuqinxi Exercises on the Balance Function and Subjective Quality of Life in Elderly, Female Knee Osteoarthritis Patients. *Am. J. Transl. Res.* **2021**, *13*, 6710–6716.
16. Roos, E.M.; Lohmander, L.S. The Knee Injury and Osteoarthritis Outcome Score (KOOS): From Joint Injury to Osteoarthritis. *Health Qual. Life Outcomes* **2003**, *1*, 64. [CrossRef] [PubMed]

17. Paradowski, P.T.; Bergman, S.; Sundén-Lundius, A.; Lohmander, L.S.; Roos, E.M. Knee Complaints Vary with Age and Gender in the Adult Population. Population-Based Reference Data for the Knee Injury and Osteoarthritis Outcome Score (KOOS). *BMC Musculoskelet. Disord.* **2006**, *7*, 38. [CrossRef]
18. Anderson, A.F.; Irrgang, J.J.; Kocher, M.S.; Mann, B.J.; Harrast, J.J.; International Knee Documentation Committee. The International Knee Documentation Committee Subjective Knee Evaluation Form: Normative Data. *Am. J. Sports Med.* **2006**, *34*, 128–135. [CrossRef] [PubMed]
19. Irrgang, J.J.; Anderson, A.F.; Boland, A.L.; Harner, C.D.; Kurosaka, M.; Neyret, P.; Richmond, J.C.; Shelborne, K.D. Development and Validation of the International Knee Documentation Committee Subjective Knee Form. *Am. J. Sports Med.* **2001**, *29*, 601–613. [CrossRef] [PubMed]
20. Briggs, K.K.; Steadman, J.R.; Hay, C.J.; Hines, S.L. Lysholm Score and Tegner Activity Level in Individuals with Normal Knees. *Am. J. Sports Med.* **2009**, *37*, 898–901. [CrossRef] [PubMed]
21. Kocher, M.S.; Steadman, J.R.; Briggs, K.K.; Sterett, W.I.; Hawkins, R.J. Reliability, Validity, and Responsiveness of the Lysholm Knee Scale for Various Chondral Disorders of the Knee. *J. Bone Joint Surg. Am.* **2004**, *86*, 1139–1145. [CrossRef] [PubMed]
22. Sonnery-Cottet, B.; Daggett, M.; Helito, C.P.; Fayard, J.-M.; Thaunat, M. Combined Anterior Cruciate Ligament and Anterolateral Ligament Reconstruction. *Arthrosc. Tech.* **2016**, *5*, e1253–e1259. [CrossRef] [PubMed]
23. Noyes, F.R. *Noyes' Knee Disorders: Surgery, Rehabilitation, Clinical Outcomes E-Book*; Elsevier Health Sciences: Amsterdam, The Netherlands, 2009; ISBN 978-1-4377-2118-8.
24. Ariel de Lima, D.; de Lima, L.L.; de Souza, N.G.R.; de Moraes Perez, R.A.; Sobrado, M.F.; Guimarães, T.M.; Helito, C.P. Clinical Outcomes of Combined Anterior Cruciate Ligament and Anterolateral Ligament Reconstruction: A Systematic Review and Meta-Analysis. *Knee Surg. Relat. Res.* **2021**, *33*, 33. [CrossRef] [PubMed]
25. Ardern, C.L.; Webster, K.E.; Taylor, N.F.; Feller, J.A. Return to the Preinjury Level of Competitive Sport after Anterior Cruciate Ligament Reconstruction Surgery: Two-Thirds of Patients Have Not Returned by 12 Months after Surgery. *Am. J. Sports Med.* **2011**, *39*, 538–543. [CrossRef] [PubMed]
26. Inderhaug, E.; Stephen, J.M.; Williams, A.; Amis, A.A. Biomechanical Comparison of Anterolateral Procedures Combined With Anterior Cruciate Ligament Reconstruction. *Am. J. Sports Med.* **2017**, *45*, 347–354. [CrossRef] [PubMed]
27. Borque, K.A.; Jones, M.; Laughlin, M.S.; Balendra, G.; Willinger, L.; Pinheiro, V.H.; Williams, A. Effect of Lateral Extra-Articular Tenodesis on the Rate of Revision Anterior Cruciate Ligament Reconstruction in Elite Athletes. *Am. J. Sports Med.* **2022**, *50*, 3487–3492. [CrossRef] [PubMed]

medicina MDPI

Article

Comparison of Proximal Tibiofibular Joint Detachment with Tibial-Sided Osteotomy for Fibular Untethering in Lateral Closing-Wedge High Tibial Osteotomy: A Cadaveric Study

Ryu Kyoung Cho [1], Keun Young Choi [1], Dai-Soon Kwak [2], Man Soo Kim [1] and Yong In [1,*]

[1] Department of Orthopaedic Surgery, Seoul St. Mary's Hospital, College of Medicine, The Catholic University of Korea, Seoul 06591, Republic of Korea; dreamer1222@naver.com (R.K.C.); heaxagon@hanmail.net (K.Y.C.); kms3779@naver.com (M.S.K.)

[2] Catholic Institute for Applied Anatomy, Department of Anatomy, College of Medicine, The Catholic University of Korea, Seoul 06591, Republic of Korea; daisoon@catolic.ac.kr

* Correspondence: iy1000@catholic.ac.kr

Abstract: *Background and Objectives:* Proximal tibiofibular joint detachment (PTFJD) is a fibular untethering procedure during lateral closing-wedge high tibial osteotomy (LCWHTO) for varus knee osteoarthritis. However, the PTFJD procedure is technically demanding, and confirmation of clear joint separation is not straightforward. The aim of this study was to compare the degree of completion and safety of PTFJD versus tibial-sided osteotomy (TSO); this latter procedure is our novel technique for fibular untethering during LCWHTO. *Materials and Methods:* Sixteen fresh frozen cadaver knees from eight cadavers were included in the study. Among the eight pairs of knees, one knee was randomly assigned to undergo PTFJD and the other knee to undergo TSO, which separates the fibula by osteotomizing the lateral cortex of the proximal tibia at the medial side of the proximal tibiofibular joint for fibular untethering during LCWHTO. After each procedure with LCWHTO, the posterior compartment of each knee was dissected to compare the degree of procedural completion and the distance from the posterior detachment or osteotomy site to posterior neurovascular structures between PTFJD and TSO groups. The pass-through test crossing the separation site from anterior to posterior using an osteotome was also performed to evaluate the protective effect of the muscular structures of the posterior compartment. *Results:* In the PTFJD group, four of eight cases (50%) showed fibular head fractures rather than division of the proximal tibiofibular joint. In contrast, in all TSO cases, the lateral cortex of the proximal tibia was clearly osteotomized from the medial side of the posterior proximal tibiofibular joint. Distances from the posterior detachment or osteotomy site to the common peroneal nerve, popliteal artery, and anterior tibial artery in the PTFJD and TSO groups were 20.8 $\pm$ 3.3 mm and 22.9 $\pm$ 3.6 mm (p = 0.382), 11.0 $\pm$ 2.4 mm and 9.8 $\pm$ 2.8 mm (p = 0.382), and 14.8 $\pm$ 1.9 mm and 14.9 $\pm$ 2.5 mm (p = 0.721), respectively. In the pass-through test, an osteotome was able to pass anteriorly to posteriorly in all eight PTFJD group cases. However, the osteotome was blocked posteriorly by the popliteus muscle in the TSO group cases, indicating protection of posterior neurovascular structures during the TSO procedure. *Conclusions:* TSO, a novel fibular untethering procedure for LCWHTO, resulted in clear separation of the fibula from the lateral tibial cortex, and protection of posterior neurovascular structures by the popliteus muscle during the procedure. We anticipate that our novel surgical technique will provide more clear-cut and safer fibular untethering for LCWHTO.

Keywords: lateral closing-wedge high tibial osteotomy; proximal tibiofibular joint; fibular shaft osteotomy; proximal tibiofibular joint detachment; tibial-sided osteotomy

1. Introduction

High tibial osteotomy (HTO) is a joint-preserving procedure that is widely accepted as an effective surgical option for young patients with isolated medial compartment osteoarthritis (OA) in the varus knee [1]. Although medial opening-wedge high tibial osteotomy (MOWHTO) using a modern locking plate system has become popular [2,3], lateral closing-wedge high tibial osteotomy (LCWHTO) has obvious benefits when a large correction is needed [4]. It has the strengths of quicker rehabilitation, better initial stability, no need for a bone graft, and maintenance of patellar position and tibial slope [5–8]. Moreover, better clinical outcomes have also been reported in patients following LCWHTO compared to MOWHTO [9].

However, LCWHTO has the disadvantage that it requires a fibular untethering procedure for osteotomy gap closing such as fibular shaft osteotomy (FSO) or proximal tibiofibular joint detachment (PTFJD) [10–13]. In FSO, an additional incision is required to perform osteotomy of the fibular shaft, which can lead to non-union at the osteotomy site [14], and there is the risk of fatality due to peroneal nerve injury [15,16]. In contrast, peroneal nerve injury is uncommon during PTFJD [11,17]. However, confirmation of clear proximal tibiofibular joint (PTFJ) separation is not straightforward, especially because the posterior part is a blind spot. In normal PTFJD procedures, repeated osteotomy is performed until PTFJ separation is confirmed.

The anatomy of the PTFJ is complex. The anterior capsule of the PTFJ is stabilized by the anterior tibiofibular ligament, which consists of three broad bands, while the posterior joint capsule is supported by the posterior proximal tibiofibular ligament, which consists of two thick bands [18,19]. This complicated anatomy can cause incomplete separation of the PTFJ during LCWHTO. In addition, although the incidence is low, popliteal neurovascular bundle injuries have been reported after LCWHTO [20–22].

Given this uncertainty and these complications of PTFJD, our group devised an alternative fibular untethering procedure, tibial-sided osteotomy (TSO), which separates the fibula and tibial bone fragment from the lateral cortex of the proximal tibia nearby the medial side of PTFJ. The purpose of this study was to compare the degree of completion and safety of PTFJD and TSO during LCWHTO.

2. Materials and Methods

In our study, 16 knees from eight fresh cadavers (three males and five females) were used. Mean age was 80.4 ± 9.1 years (range, 62–93 years). All knees were grossly intact with no history of injury or surgery to the knee joint or PTFJ. Specimens were maintained in a frozen state at −20 °C and allowed to thaw at room temperature for 24 h before dissection. One knee of each cadaver was randomly assigned to the PTFJD group and the other knee to the TSO group by simple randomization. After the designated fibular untethering procedure, LCWHTO was performed in all knees. All surgeries were carried out by two orthopaedic surgeons (Drs. RKC and KYC) together to reduce technical error. This study was approved by the Institutional Cadaver Research Committee of our Institution (research number: MC23EADI0064, IRB review date: 21 July 2023). All donors or their authorized representatives provided written informed consent for use of the cadaver and agreed to the utilization of related materials in the research.

All surgical techniques were performed on the cadaver identically to how they would have been performed in a living patient. An oblique longitudinal incision was made 1 cm below the fibular head on the anterior aspect of the knee toward the tibial tuberosity, and an additional incision was made in the lower-leg fascia. Using a knife and a periosteal elevator, the periosteum was dissected from below Gerdy's tubercle to below the outer border of the tibial tuberosity. The tibialis anterior muscle and periosteum were retracted laterally to prevent neurovascular injury. Both PTFJD and TSO were performed at a knee flexion angle of 90° to reduce the risk of peroneal nerve injury. PTFJD was carried out using the traditional method. After retracing the tibialis anterior muscle, the anterior proximal tibiofibular ligament (PTFL) was identified. The anterior PTFL was divided and the PTFJ was detached using an osteotome repeatedly toward the posterior PTFL until the tibia and fibula were separated under the image intensifier (Figure 1A). For TSO, a Kirschner wire was inserted at a position 5 mm medially from the lateral cortex of the proximal tibia near the PTFJ. After creating a chevron-shaped saw pattern in the anterior tibial cortex along the inserted Kirschner wire, osteotomy to the posterior tibial cortex was commenced using an osteotome (Figure 1B). The TSO procedure was completed after confirming that the thin lateral tibial bone fragment that attached to the PTFJ was separated from the tibia under the image intensifier.

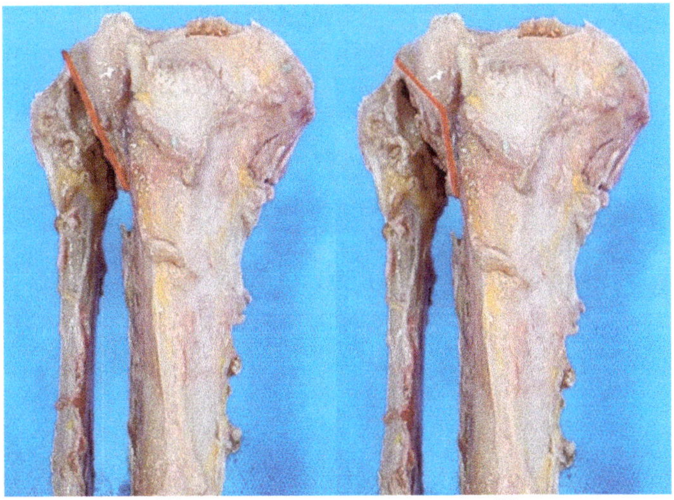

(A) (B)

Figure 1. (**A**) Proximal tibiofibular joint detachment and (**B**) tibial-sided osteotomy. The red lines indicate the sites of fibular untethering following each of the two procedures.

Regardless of the PTFJ separation method, LCWHTO was performed in the same manner with the knee in extension. All LCWHTOs were fixed using a TOMOFIX^{TM} Lateral High Tibia Plate (DePuy Synthes, Zuchwil, Switzerland). The correction angle goal was set to 10° regardless of the varus deformity of the cadaver. After checking the position of the plate where four screws each could be fixed proximally and distally, two anterior and posterior Kirschner wires were inserted toward the medial target point (20 mm distally to the proximal medial tibial joint surface) parallel to the tibial plateau. Subsequently, two additional anterior and posterior Kirschner wires were inserted 10 mm below the previously inserted Kirschner wires. A biplanar osteotomy, which consisted of a tibial tubercle osteotomy and upper and lower tibial osteotomies, was performed using a saw and chisels. After removing the bone fragment, valgus force was applied to close the gap between the upper and lower tibial cut surfaces. While applying valgus force to maintain the contact, eight screws were fixed.

To compare the degree of completion of each procedure, anatomic dissection of the posterior compartment of the knee was performed. Skin and subcutaneous tissue were dissected through an inverted L-shaped incision, exposing the underlying popliteal fossa. Lateral posterior structures were dissected to find the PTFJ and common peroneal nerve in its location beneath the biceps femoris. After laterally retracting the common peroneal nerve, the origin of the lateral head of the gastrocnemius was identified and sacrificed to provide broad exposure of the deep structures on the lateral aspect of the posterior joint, including the arcuate ligament and popliteus muscle. After retracting the popliteus muscle, the degree of procedure completion could be assessed. The objective was clear detachment of the posterior PTFJ in the PTFJD group or clear separation of the bone fragment from the posterolateral cortex of the tibia in the TSO group.

The safety of each procedure was evaluated by measuring the positional relationship between the detachment or osteotomy site and posterior neurovascular structures of the knee in millimeters using a surgical ruler. In the PTFJD and TSO groups, the actual posterior detachment or osteotomy site served as the reference point for measuring distances to posterior neurovascular structures. Distances from each reference point to the common peroneal nerve, popliteal artery, and anterior tibia artery were measured.

The pass-through test was performed to identify the protective effect of the popliteus muscle in each procedure. An osteotome was passed through the detachment or osteotomy site anteriorly to posteriorly to evaluate whether the osteotome was stopped by the popliteus muscle or not.

Statistical Analyses

All calculated data are shown as means with standard deviations using the SPSS statistical software (SPSS 28; SPSS Inc., Chicago, IL, USA). Chi-square and Fisher's exact test were used to determine the significance of differences in categorical or dichotomized data between groups, while t-tests and Mann–Whitney U tests were used to determine the significance of differences in continuous variables between groups. Statistical significance was accepted at $p < 0.05$ for all analyses.

3. Results

PTFJD and TSO with LCWHTO were completed without incomplete closing in all knees. The degree of completion of each procedure was investigated by anatomic dissection of the posterior compartment of the knee. In the PTFJD group, the posterior PTFJ was clearly separated in 50% of cases (Figure 2A). However, in the remaining four cases, a fibular head fracture was observed after PTFJD rather than the intended PTFJ separation (Figure 2B). In contrast, posterior osteotomy was consistently observed at the posterolateral cortex of the tibia in all eight cases (100%) (Figure 3). In other words, the degree of procedural completion was more reliable in the TSO group (100%) than in the PTFJD group (50%) ($p = 0.21$). Including four fibular head fracture cases, a total of five cases showed articular surface injury of the fibular head in the PTFJD group (62.5%). However, the PTFJ was intact in all TSO cases (100%) ($p = 0.007$).

Table 1 shows the average distances from the posterior detachment or osteotomy site to the common peroneal nerve, popliteal artery, and anterior tibial artery. Distances in the PTFJD group from the posterior detachment site to the common peroneal nerve and anterior tibial artery tended to be smaller, but without statistical significance ($p = 0.382$ and $p = 0.721$, respectively). Conversely, the popliteus artery was closer to the osteotomy site in the TSO group, again without statistical significance ($p = 0.382$).

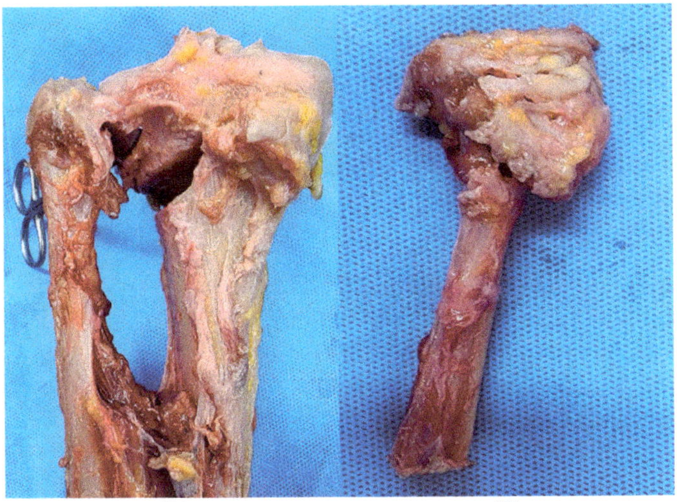

(**A**) (**B**)

Figure 2. (**A**) Posterior aspect of a knee after PTFJD showing clear separation of the PTFJ. (**B**) A fibular head fracture case involving articular cartilage after PTFJD.

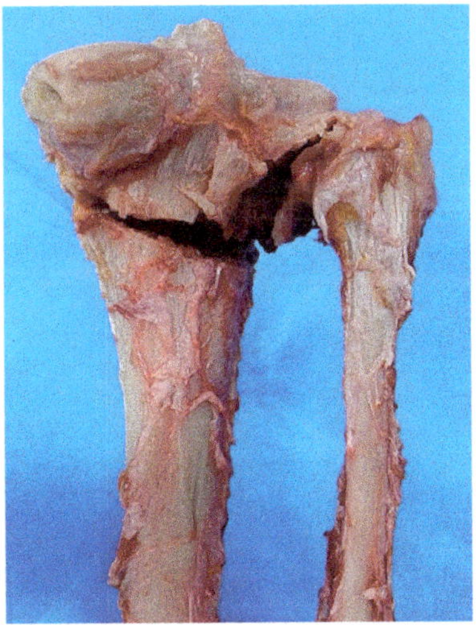

Figure 3. Posterior aspect of a knee showing separation of fibula with tibial bone fragment after TSO.

Table 1. Distances to posterolateral neurovascular structures from the posterior detachment or osteotomy site after PTFJD and TSO.

	PTFJ Detachment (n = 8)	Tibia-Sided Osteotomy (n = 8)	*p*-Value
Distance to common peroneal nerve (mm)	20.8 ± 3.3	22.9 ± 3.6	0.382
Distance to popliteus artery (mm)	11.0 ± 2.4	9.8 ± 2.8	0.382
Distance to anterior tibial artery (mm)	14.8 ± 1.9	14.9 ± 2.5	0.721

PTFJD: proximal tibiofibular joint detachment. PTFJ: proximal tibiofibular joint. PTFL: proximal tibiofibular ligament. TSO: tibial-side osteotomy.

The popliteus muscle covers the posterior aspect of the tibia but does not extend to cover the posterior PTFJ. Substantial differences between the two surgical techniques were uncovered. In the case of PTFJD, because of the absence of popliteus muscle coverage of the posterior PTFJ, an osteotome passed through the PTFJ without popliteus muscle protection in all eight cases. In contrast, the osteotome was blocked by the popliteus muscle while passing the osteotomy site in all eight cases, indicating that the popliteus muscle plays a crucial role protecting posterior neurovascular structures during TSO, a fibular untethering procedure (Figure 4).

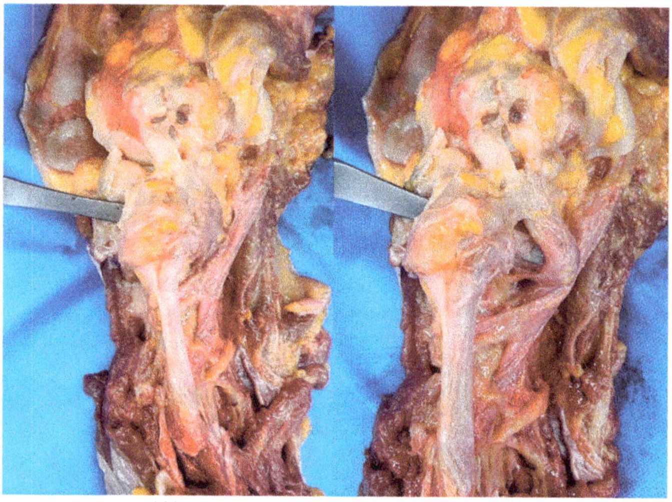

(A) (B)

Figure 4. The protective effect of the popliteus muscle. (**A**) Before entry of the osteotome; (**B**) protected appearance after penetration of the osteotome.

4. Discussion

As mentioned in the introduction, HTO has been considered an effective surgical option for patients with medial knee osteoarthritis (OA) with varus deformity [1]. Moreover, numerous studies report high levels of patient satisfaction and excellent clinical outcomes following HTO [23], with significant advancements continuously being made in the technique. Recently, HTO has increasingly been performed in combination with various cartilage procedures, such as microfracture [24], bone marrow aspirate concentrate (BMAC) [25], human umbilical cord blood-derived mesenchymal stem cells (hUCB-MSC) [26], and collagen augmentation [27]. When HTO is combined with cartilage procedures, second-look arthroscopy often reveals cartilage regeneration, accompanied by excellent clinical outcomes [28]. Takeuchi et al. [29] introduced a new hybrid closing HTO to complement the shortcomings of traditional LCWHTO, and fibular untethering is also required in this technique. The TSO procedure introduced in this study is expected to perform fibular untethering more precisely and safely.

The most important finding of this study is that our novel surgical technique, namely TSO, allowed for the procedural completion of fibular untethering by preserving the PTFJ. In our conventional PTFJD procedure, there was articular surface damage of the fibular head in 62.5% of cases. In addition, the TSO procedure was safer than PTFJD because of the protective effect of the popliteus muscle, as the separation point is more medial than in the PTFJD procedure.

Peroneal nerve dysfunction is a serious complication that can occur after LCWHTO [30,31], with reported rates of symptomatic peroneal nerve injury ranging between 3.3 and 20% [16,30]. While unlikely, there exists the possibility of peroneal nerve damage if the osteotomy is conducted with bias toward the fibula. The average distance from the division site of the common peroneal nerve into the superficial peroneal nerve and deep peroneal nerve to the posterolateral tip of the fibular head has been reported to be 20.7 mm [32]. Although the reference points were different in the study discussed above compared to our study, we observed that the distance from the posterior osteotomized site to the common peroneal nerve was similar in both the PTFJD and TSO groups. The distances mentioned above suggest a potential risk if PTFJD is performed biased toward the fibula. However, TSO has the advantage of reducing the possibility of peroneal nerve damage compared to PTFJD, as the osteotomy is directed toward the tibia. Although we did not find a statistically significant difference between the two groups due to our limited sample size given that this was a cadaveric study, the distance from the common peroneal nerve was numerically greater in the TSO group than in the PTFJD group. Therefore, additional research with a larger sample size is needed to determine if this difference is meaningful.

As mentioned above, LCWHTO is a useful surgical treatment to correct isolated medial OA with varus knee requiring large correction [4]. However, this procedure can result in injury of the popliteal neurovascular bundle, with reported rates of injury around the popliteal artery of between 0.4% and 9.8% [30,33]. Ricardo et al. reported a case of popliteal artery injury after LCWHTO leading to secondary neurological injury [20]. Although popliteal neurovascular injury is rare, this complication can be catastrophic. In our study, the TSO group was closer to the popliteal artery than the PTFJD group; this is likely because the posterior osteotomy site of the tibia was positioned more medially. As shown in the pass-through test results of this study, the popliteus muscle had a protective effect in the TSO procedure. Therefore, we believe that there are no safety concerns when performing TSO if the posterior osteotomy site of the tibia is located medially.

The anterior tibial artery, one of the terminal branches of the popliteal artery, is vulnerable during LCWHTO. Injury of the anterior tibial artery may occur when performing PTFJD using an osteotome. In fact, one study [22] reported a pseudoaneurysm due to anterior tibial arterial injury after LCWHTO. As mentioned in the previous paragraph, PTFJD can cause damage to the fibular head rather than achieving precise division of the PTFJ. Furthermore, even if a surgeon precisely separates the PTFJ, the risk of anterior tibial arterial injury may be increased. In our study, we found no significant difference in distance to the anterior tibial artery between the TSO and PTFJD groups. However, using our new technique, the probability of anterior tibial arterial injury was significantly reduced due to the protective effect of the popliteus muscle. To the best of our knowledge, although many surgeons have performed FSO or PTFJD in LCWHTO, no previous study has systematically evaluated the role of the popliteus muscle. Elucidation of the protective effect of the popliteus muscle would hopefully allow for safer PTFJ manipulation when performing LCWHTO.

PTFJ has been called the fourth compartment of the knee joint [17,20,34]. Although it is a small joint, if there is a pathologic lesion, it can cause lateral knee pain. In fact, Murat et al. reported that PTFJ pathologies result in lateral knee pain [35,36]. The case report of Enrique et al. stated that injury of the PTFJ caused unexplained lateral knee pain after LCWHTO [37]. On bone SPECT CT to detect arthritic changes, "hot" uptake by the PTFJ was noted along with iatrogenic perforation of the screw; osteoarthritis subsequently developed. This suggests that injury of the PTFJ, including PTFJ articular cartilage, can progress to osteoarthritis. There were no cases of PTFJ injury, including the cartilage, after TSO. Conversely, PTFJ cartilage injury was identified in five of eight knees (62.5%)

after PTFJD ($p = 0.007$). In other words, by performing osteotomy biased toward the tibia without causing injury to the PTFJ, TSO is likely to be associated with a lower likelihood of experiencing lateral knee pain due to PTFJ injury after LCWHTO than PTFJD.

The two representative methods of proximal tibial osteotomy are MOWHTO and LCWHTO. Many studies have reported that there is no significant difference between the two techniques in terms of clinical outcomes or radiographic alignment [38]. As mentioned in the introduction, with the development of the locking plate system, many surgeons are preferring MOWHTO because it is relatively easier to perform than LCWHTO [2,3], and it has several advantages [5]. However, although MOWHTO has many merits and LCWHTO is technically challenging, it is crucial to carefully select the appropriate osteotomy based on the specific condition of the patient. For example, if the correction angle is large, MOWHTO may result in a leg length longer than that of the contralateral limb [4], making LCWHTO a more suitable option. In the case of MOWHTO, patella baja may occur [39], and rotational changes can lead to anterior knee pain. Therefore, LCWHTO may be more advantageous for patients with patellofemoral arthritis [40]. Additionally, the choice between the two techniques should be guided by the presence or absence of ACL or PCL deficiency [41], ensuring appropriate selection for each patient. To achieve optimal clinical outcomes, the selection between the two surgical methods should be tailored to the patient's specific condition. Therefore, our new surgical technique can be appropriately utilized when LCWHTO is required in the situations mentioned above.

This study had several limitations, mainly due to our utilization of a cadaveric model. First, the preparation of each specimen may not have precisely replicated natural knee conditions. Second, only cadavers of Korean origin were utilized. Hence, there is the potential for ethnic selection bias in the data. Third, the majority of specimens did not represent knees with isolated medial compartment osteoarthritis requiring more than 10 degrees of correction. Fourth, the number of cadaver samples was relatively small. Fifth, as the correction angle of 10 degrees was uniformly applied to all cadavers, the correction was not individualized to the unique characteristics of each cadaver's knee joint; thus, diversity was not adequately taken into account.

5. Conclusions

We demonstrated that our innovative surgical technique, TSO, which involves tibia-biased osteotomy during PTFJ manipulation in LCWHTO, is a more precise and safer procedure than conventional PTFJD. We attribute this not only to the tibia-biased osteotomy, which enhances the efficacy of procedural completion and diminishes the likelihood of common peroneal nerve damage, but also to the protective effect of the popliteus muscle, which safeguards the posterior neurovascular structures. TSO offers a more precise and safer approach to manipulating the PTFJ during fibular untethering in LCWHTO than PTFJD.

Author Contributions: Conceptualization, Y.I.; data curation, R.K.C., D.-S.K., K.Y.C. and M.S.K.; investigation, R.K.C., D.-S.K. and Y.I.; software, R.K.C., D.-S.K., K.Y.C. and M.S.K.; supervision, Y.I.; visualization, R.K.C.; writing—original draft, R.K.C.; writing—review and editing, R.K.C. and Y.I. All authors have read and agreed to the published version of the manuscript.

Funding: This research received no external funding.

Institutional Review Board Statement: The study was conducted in accordance with the Declaration of Helsinki, and approved by the Institutional Review Board of Seoul St. Mary's Hospital (approval code: MC23EADI0064m, approval date: 21 July 2023).

Informed Consent Statement: Informed consent was obtained from all subjects involved in the study.

Data Availability Statement: The data presented in this study are available on request from the corresponding author.

Conflicts of Interest: The authors declare no conflicts of interest.

References

1. Gomoll, A.H. High tibial osteotomy for the treatment of unicompartmental knee osteoarthritis: A review of the literature, indications, and technique. *Phys. Sportsmed.* **2011**, *39*, 45–54. [CrossRef]
2. Hui, C.; Salmon, L.J.; Kok, A.; Williams, H.A.; Hockers, N.; van der Tempel, W.M.; Chana, R.; Pinczewski, L.A. Long-term survival of high tibial osteotomy for medial compartment osteoarthritis of the knee. *Am. J. Sports Med.* **2011**, *39*, 64–70. [CrossRef] [PubMed]
3. Miller, B.S.; Joseph, T.A.; Barry, E.M.; Rich, V.J.; Sterett, W.I. Patient satisfaction after medial opening high tibial osteotomy and microfracture. *J. Knee Surg.* **2007**, *20*, 129–133. [CrossRef] [PubMed]
4. Kim, J.I.; Kim, B.H.; Lee, K.W.; Lee, O.; Han, H.S.; Lee, S.; Lee, M.C. Lower Limb Length Discrepancy After High Tibial Osteotomy: Prospective Randomized Controlled Trial of Lateral Closing Versus Medial Opening Wedge Osteotomy. *Am. J. Sports Med.* **2016**, *44*, 3095–3102. [CrossRef] [PubMed]
5. Murray, R.; Winkler, P.W.; Shaikh, H.S.; Musahl, V. High Tibial Osteotomy for Varus Deformity of the Knee. *J. Am. Acad. Orthop. Surg. Glob. Res. Rev.* **2021**, *5*, e21.00141. [CrossRef] [PubMed]
6. Amendola, A.; Bonasia, D.E. Results of high tibial osteotomy: Review of the literature. *Int. Orthop.* **2010**, *34*, 155–160. [CrossRef]
7. Brouwer, R.W.; Bierma-Zeinstra, S.M.; van Raaij, T.M.; Verhaar, J.A. Osteotomy for medial compartment arthritis of the knee using a closing wedge or an opening wedge controlled by a Puddu plate. A one-year randomised, controlled study. *J. Bone Jt. Surg. Br.* **2006**, *88*, 1454–1459. [CrossRef]
8. Gooi, S.G.; Chan, C.X.Y.; Tan, M.K.L.; Lim, A.K.S.; Satkunanantham, K.; Hui, J.H.P. Patella Height Changes Post High Tibial Osteotomy. *Indian J. Orthop.* **2017**, *51*, 545–551. [CrossRef]
9. van Egmond, N.; van Grinsven, S.; van Loon, C.J.; Gaasbeek, R.D.; van Kampen, A. Better clinical results after closed- compared to open-wedge high tibial osteotomy in patients with medial knee osteoarthritis and varus leg alignment. *Knee Surg. Sports Traumatol. Arthrosc.* **2016**, *24*, 34–41. [CrossRef]
10. Kurosaka, M.; Tsumura, N.; Yoshiya, S.; Matsui, N.; Mizuno, K. A new fibular osteotomy in association with high tibial osteotomy (a comparative study with conventional mid-third fibular osteotomy). *Int. Orthop.* **2000**, *24*, 227–230. [CrossRef]
11. Aydoğdu, S.; Yercan, H.; Saylam, C.; Sur, H. Peroneal nerve dysfunction after high tibial osteotomy. An anatomical cadaver study. *Acta Orthop. Belg.* **1996**, *62*, 156–160. [PubMed]
12. Coventry, M.B. Osteotomy about the knee for degenerative and rheumatoid arthritis. *J. Bone Jt. Surg. Am.* **1973**, *55*, 23–48. [CrossRef]
13. Soejima, O.; Ogata, K.; Ishinishi, T.; Fukahori, Y.; Miyauchi, R. Anatomic considerations of the peroneal nerve for division of the fibula during high tibial osteotomy. *Orthop. Rev.* **1994**, *23*, 244–247. [PubMed]
14. Ramanoudjame, M.; Vandenbussche, E.; Baring, T.; Solignac, N.; Augereau, B.; Gregory, T. Fibular nonunion after closed-wedge high tibial osteotomy. *Orthop. Traumatol. Surg. Res.* **2012**, *98*, 863–867. [CrossRef] [PubMed]
15. Preston, C.F.; Fulkerson, E.W.; Meislin, R.; Di Cesare, P.E. Osteotomy about the knee: Applications, techniques, and results. *J. Knee Surg.* **2005**, *18*, 258–272. [CrossRef] [PubMed]
16. Wootton, J.R.; Ashworth, M.J.; MacLaren, C.A. Neurological complications of high tibial osteotomy--the fibular osteotomy as a causative factor: A clinical and anatomical study. *Ann. R. Coll. Surg. Engl.* **1995**, *77*, 31–34.
17. Özcan, Ö.; Eroglu, M.; Boya, H.; Kaya, Y. Proximal tibiofibular joint pain versus peroneal nerve dysfunction: Clinical results of closed-wedge high tibial osteotomy performed with proximal tibiofibular joint disruption. *Knee Surg. Sports Traumatol. Arthrosc.* **2017**, *25*, 2936–2941. [CrossRef]
18. Marchetti, D.C.; Moatshe, G.; Phelps, B.M.; Dahl, K.D.; Ferrari, M.B.; Chahla, J.; Turnbull, T.L.; LaPrade, R.F. The Proximal Tibiofibular Joint: A Biomechanical Analysis of the Anterior and Posterior Ligamentous Complexes. *Am. J. Sports Med.* **2017**, *45*, 1888–1892. [CrossRef]
19. Scarciolla, L.; Herteleer, M.; Turquet, E.; Badr, S.; Demondion, X.; Jacques, T.; Cotten, A. Anatomical study of the proximal tibiofibular ligaments using ultrasound. *Insights Imaging* **2021**, *12*, 27. [CrossRef]
20. Santos-Pereira, R.; Aleixo, C.; Bernardes, M.; Costa, A.; Fontes-Lebre, J.; Carvalho, P.J. Popliteal Artery Pseudoaneurysm after Closing Wedge High Tibial Osteotomy. *J. Orthop. Case Rep.* **2019**, *9*, 38–41.
21. Vena, G.; D'Adamio, S.; Amendola, A. Complications of osteotomies about the knee. *Sports Med. Arthrosc. Rev.* **2013**, *21*, 113–120. [CrossRef] [PubMed]
22. Sawant, M.R.; Ireland, J. Pseudo-aneurysm of the anterior tibial artery complicating high tibial osteotomy—A case report. *Knee* **2001**, *8*, 247–248. [CrossRef] [PubMed]

23. Cho, R.K.; Kim, M.S.; Choi, K.Y.; In, Y. Is severe medial knee osteoarthritis a risk factor for dissatisfaction following medial open-wedge high tibial osteotomy in patients 55 years of age or younger? *Orthop. Traumatol. Surg. Res.* **2024**, 104121. [CrossRef] [PubMed]
24. Lee, O.S.; Lee, S.H.; Mok, S.J.; Lee, Y.S. Comparison of the regeneration of cartilage and the clinical outcomes after the open wedge high tibial osteotomy with or without microfracture: A retrospective case control study. *BMC Musculoskelet. Disord.* **2019**, *20*, 267. [CrossRef]
25. Keeling, L.E.; Belk, J.W.; Kraeutler, M.J.; Kallner, A.C.; Lindsay, A.; McCarty, E.C.; Postma, W.F. Bone Marrow Aspirate Concentrate for the Treatment of Knee Osteoarthritis: A Systematic Review. *Am. J. Sports Med.* **2022**, *50*, 2315–2323. [CrossRef]
26. Park, Y.B.; Ha, C.W.; Lee, C.H.; Yoon, Y.C.; Park, Y.G. Cartilage Regeneration in Osteoarthritic Patients by a Composite of Allogeneic Umbilical Cord Blood-Derived Mesenchymal Stem Cells and Hyaluronate Hydrogel: Results from a Clinical Trial for Safety and Proof-of-Concept with 7 Years of Extended Follow-Up. *Stem Cells Transl. Med.* **2017**, *6*, 613–621. [CrossRef]
27. Kim, M.S.; Koh, I.J.; Choi, Y.J.; Pak, K.H.; In, Y. Collagen Augmentation Improves the Quality of Cartilage Repair After Microfracture in Patients Undergoing High Tibial Osteotomy: A Randomized Controlled Trial. *Am. J. Sports Med.* **2017**, *45*, 1845–1855. [CrossRef]
28. Han, J.H.; Jung, M.; Chung, K.; Jung, S.H.; Choi, C.H.; Kim, S.H. Effects of concurrent cartilage procedures on cartilage regeneration in high tibial osteotomy: A systematic review. *Knee Surg. Relat. Res.* **2024**, *36*, 13. [CrossRef]
29. Takeuchi, R.; Ishikawa, H.; Miyasaka, Y.; Sasaki, Y.; Kuniya, T.; Tsukahara, S. A novel closed-wedge high tibial osteotomy procedure to treat osteoarthritis of the knee: Hybrid technique and rehabilitation measures. *Arthrosc. Tech.* **2014**, *3*, e431–e437. [CrossRef]
30. Atrey, A.; Morison, Z.; Tosounidis, T.; Tunggal, J.; Waddell, J.P. Complications of closing wedge high tibial osteotomies for unicompartmental osteoarthritis of the knee. *Bone Jt. Res.* **2012**, *1*, 205–209. [CrossRef]
31. Aydogdu, S.; Cullu, E.; Araç, N.; Varolgüneş, N.; Sur, H. Prolonged peroneal nerve dysfunction after high tibial osteotomy: Pre- and postoperative electrophysiological study. *Knee Surg. Sports Traumatol. Arthrosc.* **2000**, *8*, 305–308. [CrossRef] [PubMed]
32. Grechenig, P.; Hohenberger, G.; Maier, M.; Grechenig, C.; Holweg, P.; Vielgut, I.; Weiglein, A.; Gänsslen, A. The articular branch of the peroneal nerve to the proximal tibiofibular joint descends at a mean height of approximately 18 mm distal to the postero-lateral tip of the fibular head. *Knee Surg. Sports Traumatol. Arthrosc.* **2021**, *29*, 1232–1237. [CrossRef] [PubMed]
33. Efe, T.; Ahmed, G.; Heyse, T.J.; Boudriot, U.; Timmesfeld, N.; Fuchs-Winkelmann, S.; Ishaque, B.; Lakemeier, S.; Schofer, M.D. Closing-wedge high tibial osteotomy: Survival and risk factor analysis at long-term follow up. *BMC Musculoskelet. Disord.* **2011**, *12*, 46. [CrossRef] [PubMed]
34. Gil-Melgosa, L.; Valentí, A.; Suárez, Á.; Montiel, V. Proximal tibiofibular joint changes after closed-wedge high tibial osteotomy. Are they relevant? *Knee* **2020**, *27*, 1585–1592. [CrossRef]
35. Bozkurt, M.; Yilmaz, E.; Akseki, D.; Havitcioğlu, H.; Günal, I. The evaluation of the proximal tibiofibular joint for patients with lateral knee pain. *Knee* **2004**, *11*, 307–312. [CrossRef] [PubMed]
36. Semonian, R.H.; Denlinger, P.M.; Duggan, R.J. Proximal tibiofibular subluxation relationship to lateral knee pain: A review of proximal tibiofibular joint pathologies. *J. Orthop. Sports Phys. Ther.* **1995**, *21*, 248–257. [CrossRef] [PubMed]
37. Testa, E.A.; Haeni, D.L.; Behrens, G.; Hirschmann, M.T. Unexplained proximal tibiofibular joint pain after high tibial osteotomy. *Indian J. Orthop.* **2014**, *48*, 335–338. [CrossRef]
38. Duivenvoorden, T.; Brouwer, R.W.; Baan, A.; Bos, P.K.; Reijman, M.; Bierma-Zeinstra, S.M.; Verhaar, J.A. Comparison of closing-wedge and opening-wedge high tibial osteotomy for medial compartment osteoarthritis of the knee: A randomized controlled trial with a six-year follow-up. *J. Bone Jt. Surg. Am.* **2014**, *96*, 1425–1432. [CrossRef]
39. Bin, S.I.; Kim, H.J.; Ahn, H.S.; Rim, D.S.; Lee, D.H. Changes in Patellar Height After Opening Wedge and Closing Wedge High Tibial Osteotomy: A Meta-analysis. *Arthroscopy* **2016**, *32*, 2393–2400. [CrossRef]
40. Kim, J.I.; Kim, B.H.; Han, H.S.; Lee, M.C. Rotational Changes in the Tibia After High Tibial Valgus Osteotomy: A Comparative Study of Lateral Closing Versus Medial Opening Wedge Osteotomy. *Am. J. Sports Med.* **2020**, *48*, 3549–3556. [CrossRef]
41. Agostinone, P.; Lucidi, G.A.; Dal Fabbro, G.; Di Paolo, S.; Pagano, A.; Viotto, M.; Neri, M.P.; Grassi, A.; Zaffagnini, S. Satisfactory long-term outcomes for combined anterior cruciate ligament reconstruction and lateral closing wedge high tibial osteotomy. *Knee Surg. Sports Traumatol. Arthrosc.* **2023**, *31*, 4399–4406. [CrossRef]

medicina

MDPI

Article

The Effectiveness and Safety of Tibial-Sided Osteotomy for Fibula Untethering in Lateral Close-Wedge High Tibial Osteotomy: A Novel Technique with Video Illustration

Keun Young Choi, Man Soo Kim and Yong In *

Seoul St. Mary's Hospital, The Catholic University of Korea, Seoul 06591, Republic of Korea; heaxagon@hanmail.net (K.Y.C.); kms3779@naver.com (M.S.K.)
* Correspondence: iy1000@catholic.ac.kr

Abstract: *Background and Objectives*: Despite its advantages, lateral close-wedge high tibial osteotomy (LCWHTO) requires proximal tibiofibular joint detachment (PTFJD) or fibular shaft osteotomy for gap closing. These fibula untethering procedures are technically demanding and not free from the risk of neurovascular injuries. Our novel fibula untethering technique, tibial-sided osteotomy (TSO) near the proximal tibiofibular joint (PTFJ), aims to reduce technical demands and the risk of injury to the peroneal nerve and popliteal neurovascular structures. The purposes of this study were to introduce the TSO technique and compare the complexity and safety of TSO with those of radiographic virtual PTFJD, which is defined based on radiographic landmarks representing the traditional PTFJD technique. *Materials and Methods*: Between March and December 2023, 13 patients who underwent LCWHTO with TSO for fibula untethering were enrolled. All patients underwent MRI preoperatively and CT scanning postoperatively. The location of the TSO site on the postoperative CT scans was matched to preoperative MRI to measure the shortest distance to the peroneal nerve and popliteal artery. These values were compared with estimates of the distance between the PTFJ and neurovascular structures in the radiographic virtual PTFJD group. The protective effect of the popliteus muscle was evaluated by extending the osteotomy direction toward the posterior compartment of the knee. *Results*: The TSO procedure was straightforward and reproducible without producing incomplete gap closure during LCWHTO. On axial images, the distances between the surgical plane and the peroneal nerve or popliteal artery were significantly longer in the TSO group than in the radiographic virtual PTFJD group (both $p = 0.001$). On coronal and axial MRI, the popliteus muscle covered the posterior osteotomy plane in all patients undergoing TSO but did not cover the PTFJD plane in the radiographic virtual PTFJD group. *Conclusions*: Our novel TSO technique for fibula untethering during LCWHTO is reproducible and reduces the risk of neurovascular injury by placing the separation site more medially than in the PTFJD procedure.

Keywords: lateral close-wedge high tibial osteotomy; protective effect; popliteus muscle; popliteal neurovascular structure; peroneal nerve; recurrent branch of anterior tibial artery

1. Introduction

Valgus-producing high tibial osteotomy (HTO) is a well-accepted treatment modality in active patients with varus malalignment and symptomatic medial unicompartmental osteoarthritis (OA) of the knee [1]. Traditionally, lateral close-wedge HTO (LCWHTO), introduced by Coventry et al. [2], has been considered the gold standard osteotomy procedure for patients with varus knee alignment. However, medial open-wedge HTO (MOWHTO) has recently surpassed LCWHTO in terms of the number of procedures performed [3]: MOWHTO is easier to perform and tends to more reproducibly acquire an adjustable alignment change [4]. While LCWHTO has certain advantages when compared to MOWHTO, including greater initial postoperative stability, a faster return to weight bearing, favorable bone union, greater ability to address large correction with a lower risk of nonunion, less leg-length discrepancy (LLD), and lower risk of patellofemoral OA and increased tibial slope [5], the LCWHTO procedure can be technically demanding and may not allow precise adjustment [6]. Furthermore, LCWHTO requires an additional fibula untethering procedure that poses a risk of injury to the common peroneal nerve and/or popliteal neurovascular structures that must be considered when selecting a treatment option for varus malaligned medial OA, especially for novice surgeons [7].

Three surgical options to manage the fibula in LCWHTO have been described: proximal tibiofibular joint detachment (PTFJD), fibular head resection, and fibular shaft osteotomy [2,3,8,9]. Although the surgeon generally selects the preferred option, PTFJD has been reported to have the debatable risk of lateral laxity [8,10,11], iatrogenic fibular head fracture resulting in early postoperative proximal tibiofibular joint (PTFJ) arthritis [3]. In addition, fibular head resection requires an additional procedure to reattach the biceps femoris tendon and lateral collateral ligament to the fibular neck and may pose an increased risk of injury to the common peroneal nerve [3,9]. Furthermore, fibular shaft osteotomy was also reportedly associated with a greater risk of nonunion of the fibula shaft, peroneal nerve palsy, and pain at the osteotomy site [5,8,9,12].

We devised a novel tibial-sided osteotomy (TSO) technique for fibula untethering during LCWHTO, (Video S1) that is technically straightforward and reduces the risk of injury to the peroneal nerve and/or popliteal neurovascular structures. Thus, the purposes of this study were to introduce our novel TSO technique and compare the safety of the TSO and radiographic virtual PTFJD techniques by measuring the distances from the surgical site to the neurovascular structures using preoperative MRI and postoperative CT scans.

2. Materials and Methods

2.1. Patients

Between March and December 2023, we prospectively enrolled 13 consecutive patients 70 years of age or younger with isolated medial compartment OA of the knee who were scheduled to undergo an LCWHTO procedure performed by a single surgeon. All radiographic evaluations were conducted retrospectively. The HTO procedure was contraindicated if a patient had symptomatic OA in the lateral compartment or the patellofemoral joint of the knee, inflammatory arthritis, a flexion contracture of 15° or more, knee range of motion less than 120°, joint instability, or a history of knee joint infection [13]. At our institution, the decision to perform MOWHTO or LCWHTO was mainly based on the amount of correction required, which was calculated from preoperative standing radiographs of the lower extremities. Usually, an LCWHTO was performed in patients with a correction angle of 13° or more, an excessive tibial slope, or LLD, or for patients in which there was a risk of aggravation of patellofemoral OA. During the study period, 18 MOWHTOs were performed. The average preoperative hip–knee–ankle (HKA) axis was 11.0. The mean medial proximal tibia angle (MPTA) and mechanical lateral distal femur angle (mLDFA) were 80.7 and 87.6, respectively. The mean correction angle of the patients who underwent MOWHTO was 9.4° (range 6−12°), and that of the patients who underwent LCWHTO was 14.8° (9−18.5°). A patient with a correction angle of 9° underwent LCWHTO because of an acute skin wound on the medial side of the proximal tibia. The mean age of the study cohort was 57.8 years (54−63 years), and there were 2 males and 11 females. These

13 patients underwent MRI evaluation preoperatively to identify intraarticular pathologies, including meniscal tears and cartilage defects. The study design was approved by the institutional review board of our hospital (MC23EADI0064). All patients were informed about the requirements of the study and provided informed consent. This study was supported by the Research Fund of Seoul St. Mary's Hospital, the Catholic University of Korea.

2.2. Surgical Technique

The patient was placed in the supine position on the operating table with an appropriate tourniquet applied over the cast padding. The surgical procedure was performed under general anesthesia with the tourniquet inflated to 300 mmHg. In our institution, LCWHTO was routinely performed under general anesthesia. And a torniquet was also routinely used with 300 mmHg pressure to prevent unintended bleeding. Routine arthroscopic examination was carried out using the anteromedial, anterolateral, and superomedial portals. An arthroscopic examination of all three compartments was performed, and the status of the menisci was determined using a probe.

For biplanar LCWHTO, a curvilinear incision was made between Gerdy's tubercle and the fibular head and extended distally following the anterior crest of the tibia, and the tibialis anterior muscle was dissected subperiosteally. First, the PTFJ and anterior proximal tibiofibular ligament (PTFL) were exposed. Our novel technique for fibula untethering was performed utilizing an additional mini-osteotomy on the tibial side of the PTFJ. For this procedure, a Kirschner wire (K-wire) was inserted under fluoroscopic guidance starting at the tibial cortex at a point 5 mm medial to the PTFJ to secure the PTFJ articular cartilage and anterior PTFL. The K-wire was guided parallel to the joint line on the sagittal plane and about 30° oblique medially on the coronal plane towards the popliteus muscle. By leaving the osteotomy plane covered by the popliteus muscle, this placement was found to preserve the PTFJ and not injure the popliteal vessels. Using a sagittal saw, a guiding fissure was made from the near cortex of the proximal tibia to the cancellous bone (Figure 1). After sawing to the near cortex, TSO of the far cortex was performed using a curved osteotome. By levering the osteotome in a medial-to-lateral direction under the fluoroscope, separation of the tibia and the small tibial-side bone fragment with the fibula head could be confirmed, which indicated complete untethering of the fibula (Video S1 and Figure 2). Patients included in this study were confined to a normal degree LDFA and small MTPA with varus malalignment. So, the Paley's center of rotation of angulation (CORA) was on the proximal metaphyseal area of the tibia. The LCWHTO is an established surgical procedure accepted as one of the gold standard procedures for correcting medial compartment OA with tibia vara. The starting point was located between proximal and distal holes of a TOMOFIX^{TM} Lateral High Tibia Plate (DePuy Synthes, Zuchwil, Switzerland) to ensure the proper location of the plate. And the ending point was 1 cm below the medial plateau of the proximal tibia to avoid MCL injury. The TOMOFIX^{TM} Lateral High Tibia Plate was placed temporarily, and the level of proximal tibial osteotomy was marked with a surgical marking pen. Two K-wires were placed at the level of the tibial plateau. The location of the distal tibial osteotomy was marked according to preoperative calculations of the size of the bone wedge to remove. Two additional K-wires were inserted heading to the hinge point. Posterior to the tibial tubercle, an oblique coronal osteotomy procedure was performed following the line extending from the patella tendon. The proximal and distal tibial osteotomies were performed using a sagittal saw along each of the two K-wires to preserve the far medial cortex and periosteum. The wedge of bone was removed using a pituitary rongeur, and the far medial cortex was carefully drilled with a K-wire and decorticated using an osteotome. A valgus force was gently applied to the level of the osteotomy until the upper and lower osteotomy surfaces contacted each other. A cable was used for an intraoperative assessment of the alignment. The proximal and distal parts were rigidly fixed with a TOMOFIX^{TM} Lateral High Tibia Plate and screws. Figure 3 shows preoperative and postoperative radiographs.

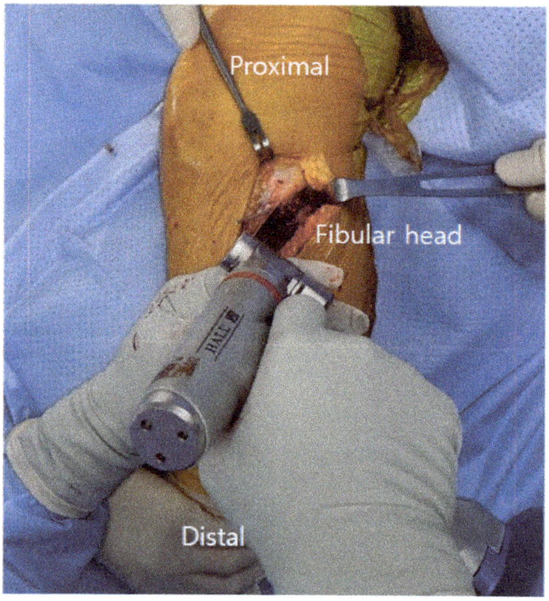

Figure 1. The left knee is shown. A guiding Kirschner wire was inserted 5 mm medial to the PTFJ to secure the articular cartilage and anterior PTFL. Using a sagittal saw, a guiding fissure was made from the near cortex of the proximal tibia to the cancellous bone. PTFJ: proximal tibiofibular joint; PTFL: proximal tibiofibular ligament.

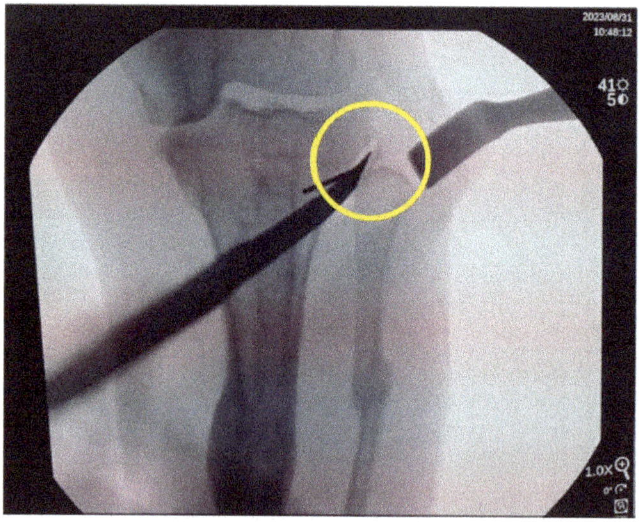

Figure 2. Under fluoroscopic imaging, a small freely movable detached bone fragment was identified at the tibial side (yellow circle).

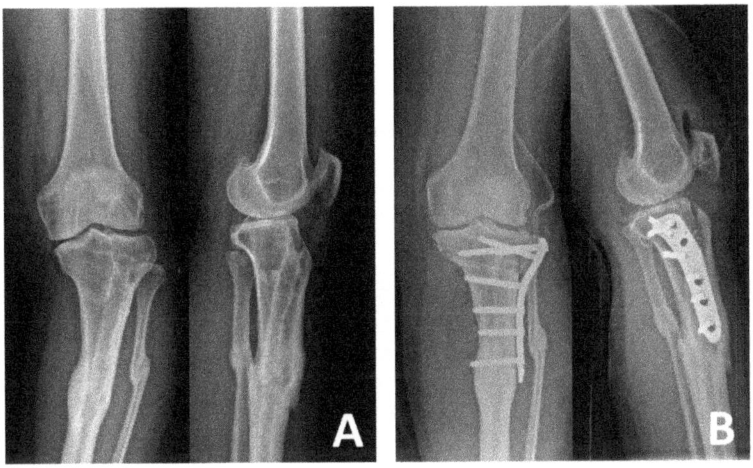

Figure 3. Preoperative (**A**) and postoperative (**B**) radiographs of a 42-year-old female patient who underwent LCWHTO using the TSO technique. LCWHTO: lateral close-wedge high tibial osteotomy; TSO: tibial-sided osteotomy.

A quadriceps-setting exercise and continuous passive motion began on the first postoperative day. Partial weight bearing with crutches was allowed 4 weeks after surgery, and full weight bearing was started 6 weeks after surgery. The same protocol was applied to all patients, including those who underwent meniscal or cartilage procedures.

2.3. Evaluation

To evaluate the safety and ease of performing our novel TSO for fibula untethering, a radiographic virtual conventional PTFJD group was set as the control group.

The radiographic virtual PTFJD group was defined based on radiographic landmarks. If an ideal genuine PTFJD procedure was performed, the dissociation plane should be located between the anterior PTFJ to the posterior end of the PTFJ. According to this hypothesis, evaluations of the radiographic virtual PTFJD group were conducted while assuming the dissociation plane was located on the extended line from the anterior to posterior PTFJ.

With their consent, postoperative CT scans were performed on all 13 patients to identify the position and status of the osteotomy. The TSO plane was determined on the postoperative CT scan, and the corresponding radiographic virtual plane was identified on the preoperative MRI of the same patient to measure the distance from the surgical plane to the peroneal nerve and popliteal artery that were not definitively seen on the postoperative CT scan (Figure 4A,B). The position of neurovascular structures can be evaluated more accurately using MRI. However, during the MRI scan, even though the metal reduction protocol is adapted, the artifact can disturb authors locating the positions of the neurovascular structures. So, the plane of TSO was evaluated on the postoperative CT scan, and it was embedded to the preoperative MRI. The shortest distance from the extended line of the TSO plane (TSO group) or PTFJ (PTFJD group) to the peroneal nerve and popliteal artery wall were measured on axial images. Although PTFJD was not actually performed in the control group, PTFJD could be assured because the PTFJ could be identified on both the CT scan and MRI (Figure 4B).

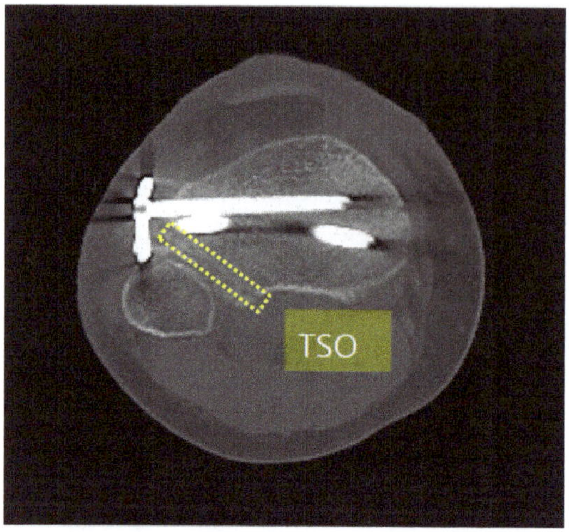

(**A**)

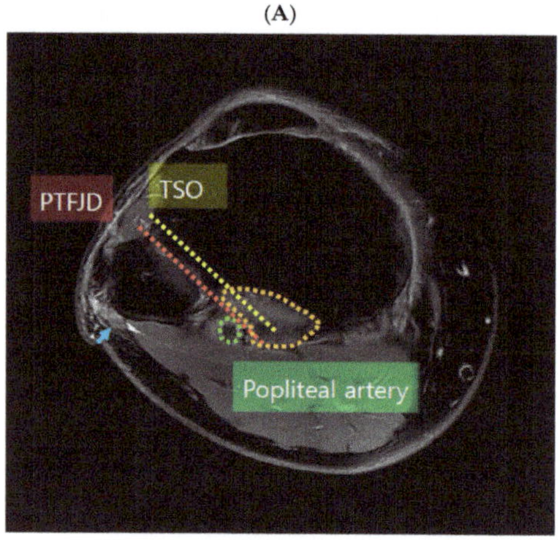

(**B**)

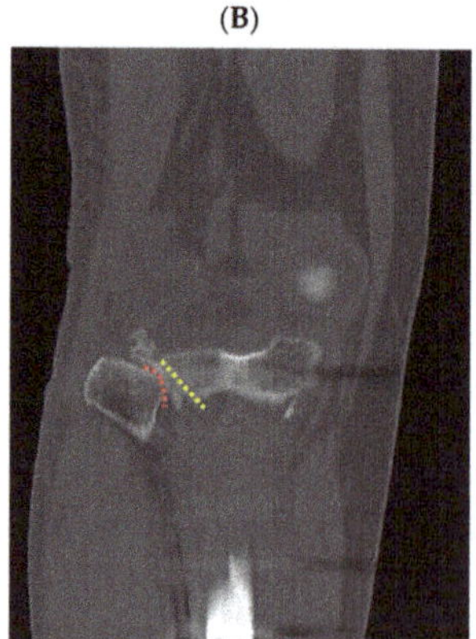

(**C**)

Figure 4. *Cont.*

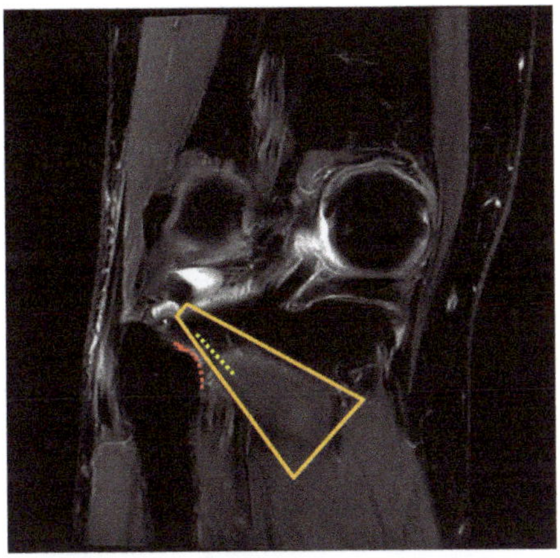

(**D**)

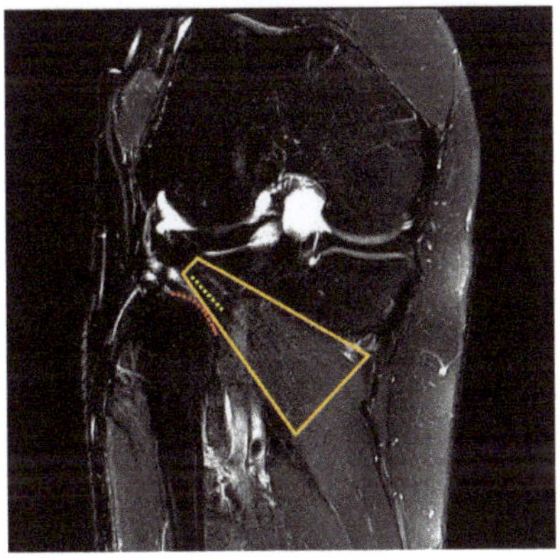

(**E**)

Figure 4. (**A**) An axial image from the postoperative CT scan. On CT scans with the knee in full extension, the osteotomy plane (yellow dotted box) adjacent to the proximal tibiofibular joint is located on the more medial side parallel to the proximal tibiofibular joint. TSO: tibial-sided osteotomy. (**B**) On the axial MRI of the knee in full extension, the TSO plane (yellow dotted line), defined on the corresponding postoperative CT scan, is located more medially than the PTFJD plane (red dotted line) and located farther from the peroneal nerve (blue arrow). A line extending from the TSO plane is covered by the popliteus muscle (orange dotted line), whereas the PTFJD is not, indicating that the popliteus muscle does not protect the popliteal neurovascular structures during PTFJD with the knee positioned in full extension. TSO: tibial-sided osteotomy; PTFJD: proximal tibiofibular joint detachment. (**C**) On the coronal image of the postoperative CT with the knee in full extension, the TSO plane (yellow dotted line) aside the PTFJ (red dotted line) is confirmed. TSO: tibial-side osteotomy; PTFJ: proximal tibiofibular joint. (**D**) On the coronal MRI of the knee in full extension, the TSO plane (yellow dotted line) defined on the corresponding postoperative CT scan is located more medially compared to the PTFJD plane (red dotted line). The TSO plane is covered by the popliteus muscle (orange line), whereas the PTFJD is not, indicating that the popliteus muscle does not protect the popliteal neurovascular structures during PTFJD with the knee positioned in full extension. TSO: tibial-side osteotomy; PTFJD: proximal tibiofibular joint detachment. (**E**) Flex 90 MRI. On the coronal MRI of the knee in 90-degree flexion, the TSO plane (yellow dotted line) defined on the corresponding postoperative CT scan is located more medially than the PTFJD plane (red dotted line). The TSO plane is covered by the popliteus muscle (orange line), whereas the PTFJD is not, indicating that the popliteus muscle does not protect the popliteal neurovascular structures during PTFJD with the knee positioned in 90-degree flexion. TSO: tibial-side osteotomy; PTFJD: proximal tibiofibular joint detachment.

The popliteus muscle is known to have a debatable potential to protect the popliteal neurovascular structures during a corrective osteotomy procedure [14]. This protective effect by the popliteus muscle against the osteotome toward the posterior neurovascular structure during the TSO or PTFJD was evaluated on coronal and axial MRI and matched with the postoperative CT scan images (Figure 4A–D).

2.4. Image Analyses

Two orthopedic surgeons performed all measurements retrospectively in a step-by-step manner. The final values were the averages of the two evaluations. Each researcher assessed every radiographic variable on two occasions at least two weeks apart. Intra- and inter-observer reliability for each measurement was expressed as an intraclass correlation coefficient (ICC).

First, the two orthopedic surgeons assessed the postoperative CT images of the knee, which were used as reference standards for the TSO or radiographic virtual PTFJD plane. The reviewers evaluated the three-dimensional direction and depth of the TSO plane or radiographic virtual PTFJD plane. The starting and end points of the TSO or PFTJ were estimated on axial images. Second, the two orthopedic surgeons evaluated the preoperative MRI images obtained using axial and coronal fat-saturated proton density (PD)-weighted turbo spin-echo sequences and sagittal T2-weighted turbo spin-echo sequences. Third, the corresponding CT and MRI data sets were reviewed by the two orthopedic surgeons. To evaluate the risk of injury to neurovascular structures, the osteotomy or detachment plane identified on the CT scans was embedded in the MRI images on axial and coronal views. For an exact side-by-side comparison, distances from the joint line were matched in both images.

2.5. Statistical Analyses

All variables are presented as the mean ± standard deviation. The Mann–Whitney U-test was used to compare the distances from the TSO site or PTFJ to the peroneal nerve and popliteal artery. The protective effect of the popliteus muscle was expressed as a percentage, and the significance of differences between the groups was evaluated using the chi-square test. All statistical analyses were performed using SPSS® (IBM® Corp, Armonk, NY, USA, version 24), and significance was set at $p < 0.05$.

3. Results

The TSO procedure was technically straightforward and did not result in incomplete separation. Separation of the osteotomy site could be confirmed fluoroscopically by levering the tibial bone fragment and fibula head laterally using an osteotome. Complete closure of the tibial osteotomy gap was achieved in all 13 cases, avoiding incomplete closure that may occur when the fibula is untethered incompletely. The mean HKA axis and MPTA were changed from 11.0 to 2.0 and from 80.7 to 89.5 after operation.

The distance from the TSO or PTFJD plane to the peroneal nerve on the axial images was significantly longer in the TSO group than the PTFJD group ($p = 0.001$; Table 1). The distance from the TSO or PTFJD plane to the popliteal artery was also significantly longer in the TSO group than the PTFJD group ($p < 0.001$). The intra- and inter-observer reliability for all radiographic measurements was considered acceptable, ranging from 0.81 to 0.99 and from 0.81 to 0.96, respectively.

In all patients in the TSO group, the osteotomy plane was covered by the popliteus muscle in the coronal and axial images. However, in the PTFJD group, the detachment plane was not covered by the popliteus muscle in the coronal or axial plane in all cases (Figure 4D).

Table 1. Distances from popliteal artery or peroneal nerve to osteotomy plane.

	TSO Group	PTFJD Group	p Value
Distance from popliteal artery	8.5 ± 3.4	0.7 ± 1.5	<0.001
Distance from peroneal nerve	26.1 ± 2.8	21.7 ± 2.6	0.001

TSO: tibial-side osteotomy; PTFJD: proximal tibiofibular joint detachment.

4. Discussion

The most important finding of this study is that our novel TSO technique is technically straightforward while enabling effective fibular untethering, and it can be performed safely, reducing the risk of peroneal nerve and popliteal neurovascular injury.

Despite evident advantages, the decision to perform LCWHTO as an option to correct medial unicompartmental OA with varus alignment should not be made lightly, especially for novice surgeons, given that the procedure requires additional manipulation of the PTFJ or fibula shaft [7]. Due to the inevitably greater risk of injury to the peroneal nerve and popliteal neurovascular structures when performing an LCWHTO procedure to treat medial unicompartmental OA with varus alignment compared with an MOWHTO, many surgeons are hesitant to choose LCWHTO as their surgical option. While many patients can be treated with an MOWHTO, LCWHTO should be considered among the surgical options, especially for patients with a large correction gap, patients at risk of patellofemoral OA, those with an excessive tibial slope, or for patients for which there are concerns about LLD due to unilateral surgery [5].

Various surgical approaches for fibular untethering have been used to perform LCWHTO safely, including fibular shaft osteotomy, PTFJD, and fibular head resection [2,3,8,9]. However, to the best of our knowledge, to date, no technique has been reported to secure the PTFJ articular cartilage and maintain a safe distance to posterolateral neurovascular structures. Previously reported methods for PTFJ in LCWHTO have several technical and clinical limitations. Fibular shaft osteotomy is technically demanding because it requires an additional incision to perform osteotomy of the fibular shaft, and there is a risk of nonunion of the osteotomy site [6]; in addition, the risk of peroneal nerve injury, a fatal complication, is not negligible [9,12]. The PTFJD technique limits the correction angle of LCWHTO [6], which reduces the reproducible gap correction and is also associated with a greater risk of TKA conversion than the fibular head resection technique [15].

In terms of surgical straightforwardness, our novel TSO technique has several advantages over PTFJD. In the process of PTFJD, the anterior and posterior PTFLs should be dissociated to prevent incomplete LCWHTO. If dissociation is incomplete, elevation of the fibula head is limited, and closure of the osteotomy gap is also limited by the remnant tethering effect of the PTFL. It is not possible to definitively prove that the PTFJL has been dissociated during the PTFJD procedure: in such circumstances, the surgeon may repetitively apply a dissociating force to the PTFJ with a blunt osteotome, increasing the risk of iatrogenic popliteal neurovascular injury beyond the popliteus muscle or fibula head fracture. In contrast, during the TSO procedure, surgeons can confirm whether the tibial-side osteo-fragment is freely movable or not by using an image intensifier in real time within the operation room, thus simplifying fibula untethering during LCWHTO and improving the reproducibility of the procedure.

Additionally, unlike PTFJD, during the TSO procedure, surgeons can estimate the depth of the osteotomy using haptic sensing and can therefore feel the osteotome advance through the far cortex, allowing them to stop advancing the osteotome. The surgeon is also able to feel the K-wire penetrate the near cortex and cancellous bone and make contact with the far cortex. In contrast, during the PTFJD procedure, surgeons are not able to employ tactile exploration as the osteotome penetrates into deeper layers. These differences in the utility of the tactile sense could provide the beneficial effect of lessening excessive advancement of the surgical device to a deep layer (Table 2).

Table 2. Benefits and limitations.

Benefits	Limitations
Reduced risk of iatrogenic peroneal nerve injury because of relative anatomical location	Risk of iatrogenic injury of PTFJ articular cartilage due to incomplete TSO and/or incorrect direction of TSO
Possible protection of underlying popliteus vessel by popliteal muscle	Possible risk of iatrogenic PTFJ injury due to iatrogenic fracture, especially in patients with osteoporosis
Reduced risk of anterior tibial artery recurrent branch injury because osteotomy plane is located farther away	
Fewer morbidities than for PTFJD, including PTFJ articular cartilage injury or iatrogenic fibula head fracture	
Surgeons can use haptic sense to estimate advancement depth of surgical devices	

TSO: tibial-sided osteotomy, PTFJ: proximal tibiofibular joint, PTFJD: proximal tibiofibular joint detachment.

To simplify the TSO technique, we recommend several technical tips. It is important to identify the border of the PTFJ to prevent unintended injury to the PTFJ articular cartilage and neurovascular bundle. The PTFJ can be identified more easily if blunt dissection of the anterior PTFL is performed; excessive dissection with a sharp scalpel should be avoided because it could cause injury to the PTFL and articular cartilage of the PTFJ. We also recommend inserting the guiding K-wire 5 mm medial to the PTFJ to sufficiently secure the bone fragment and avoid anterior PTFL injury. The creation of an excessively large bony fragment should also be avoided in order to prevent iatrogenic proximal tibia articular fracture. The guiding K-wire should not penetrate the far cortex of the proximal tibia in order to avoid penetrating the popliteal neurovascular structures. We also advise that the oscillating saw should not be advanced farther than the far cortex, and the final detachment of the far cortex should be performed with an osteotome. Finally, complete detachment should be confirmed using an image intensifier.

When compared with the PTFJD procedure, the novel TSO procedure improves safety by moving the osteotomy site farther from the neurovascular structure and allowing the popliteus muscle to provide protective cover. The shortest distances from the TSO or PTFJD plane to the peroneal nerve and popliteal artery were significantly farther in the TSO group. Moving the surgical site farther away from the neurovascular structure reduces the risk of neurovascular injury. In addition, the TSO technique may better protect the recurrent branch of the anterior tibial artery (ATA); the ATA arises from the popliteal artery just below the popliteus muscle and pierces or passes above the interosseous membrane in a posterior-to-anterior direction, giving rise to the anterior tibial recurrent artery, which ascends from the aperture and anastomoses with the genicular arteries [16]. In the TSO procedure, the osteotomy line is positioned farther from the PTFJ and interosseous membrane and should therefore also be farther from the recurrent branch of the ATA; however, we were unable to confirm positioning because the tiny ATA could not be identified in postoperative MRI, and further studies utilizing angio-CT or cadaver studies are required.

Our novel technique also has a protective effect due to the mechanical blocking effect of the popliteus muscle. According to the findings reported by Parker et al., the popliteal neurovascular bundle is thought to be protected by the popliteus muscle and the posterior tibialis muscle [14]. However, our MRI findings with the knee in full extension or at 90° flexion (a position that many surgeons prefer when performing LCWHTO) indicate that the popliteus muscle does not properly cover the posterior PFTJ in the coronal and sagittal planes. The inferior margin of the popliteus muscle is more proximal than the posterior PFTJ and does not provide any protective cover beyond the PTFJ. However, with our novel technique, the osteotomy line lies more medially and parallel to the PTFJ and is fully covered by the popliteus muscle (Figure 4B,D). Moreover, in the axial plane, the popliteal vessel located on the extended line of the PTFJ is positioned more laterally than the TSO line (Figure 4B), which may elevate the risk of injury to the neurovascular bundle during the dissociation of the PTFJ with the osteotome. However, in the TSO technique, the blunt osteotome is blocked by the popliteus muscle, reducing the risk of popliteal neurovascular injury. As such, by opting for the TSO procedure, inexperienced surgeons may avoid many of the risks presented by the LCWHTO procedure while ensuring effective correction of varus malalignment. Further evaluations, including cadaveric studies or randomized controlled trials with larger cohorts, are required to confirm our findings.

This protective effect could transform LCWHTO. Although some previous studies that included cadaveric angiography reported that during knee flexion, the popliteal neurovascular bundle moves posteriorly at the joint line level [17], other studies employing duplex ultrasound in living patients reported that the popliteal artery is closer to the posterior border of the tibia when the knee is in 90° flexion than in full extension, especially at 1 to 2 cm below the joint line, where coronal osteotomy occurs [18,19]. Notably, MRI studies have reported that knee flexion and the effects of gravity do not guarantee repositioning of the popliteal vessels away from potential harm during surgery [20]. Estimating the exact location of the popliteal artery was not feasible, especially at the level of proximal tibial osteotomy, which is about 2 to 3 cm distal to the joint line [17–20]. In this circumstance, the protective cover provided by the popliteus muscle could be a key pro of our novel technique to improve the safety of the LCWHTO procedure performed by surgeons to treat medial unicompartmental OA.

Our TSO technique does not violate the PTFJ articular cartilage, which is frequently reported in PTFJ detachment, and can reduce the likelihood of iatrogenic fibular head fracture and consequently reduce the risk of peroneal nerve injury. Instead, we separated the PTFJ directly from the tibial side. Fine TSO may be performed using a guiding K-wire and oscillating saw under an image intensifier. By means of this simple TSO technique, surgeons can overcome the risk of PTFJ cartilage injury that may result in lateral knee pain after LCWHTO. Moreover, there is no need for the additional skin incision and soft tissue dissection that are necessary when performing fibular shaft osteotomy procedures, and the TSO technique may reduce the operation time compared to the fibular shaft osteotomy method. These advantages indicate that the TSO procedure is a viable alternative to lateral closure when performing HTO, especially for novice surgeons.

This study had several limitations. First, this study was confined to an Asian population. Thus, these results might not be generalizable to other ethnicities. Second, a radiographic virtual control group was used to compare the anatomical variables of PTFJD with those of our novel technique; however, additional studies using values obtained from real-world PTFJD procedures are required. In addition, the genuine PTFJD plane could not be confirmed on the postoperative CT because it does not leave a confirmable trace in the radiologic test. Together, these limitations may limit the generalizability of our results.

Despite these limitations, our oblique mini-osteotomy of the proximal tibia technique for the PTFJ in LCWHTO can provide a reproducible and safer surgical method, protecting popliteal neurovascular structures and the recurrent branch of ATA. Further validation through additional studies, including cadaveric investigations, is warranted.

Supplementary Materials: The following supporting information can be downloaded at: https://www.mdpi.com/article/10.3390/medicina61010091/s1, Video S1: Lateral closing wedge high tibial osteotomy.

Author Contributions: Conceptualization, Y.I. and K.Y.C.; Data Curation, K.Y.C. and M.S.K.; Investigation, K.Y.C. and Y.I.; Software, K.Y.C. and M.S.K.; Supervision, Y.I.; Visualization, K.Y.C.; Writing—Original Draft, K.Y.C.; Writing—Review and Editing, K.Y.C. and Y.I. All authors have read and agreed to the published version of the manuscript.

Funding: This study was supported by the Research Fund of Seoul St. Mary's Hospital, the Catholic University of Korea (ZC23EISI0862).

Institutional Review Board Statement: The study was conducted in accordance with the Declaration of Helsinki, and approved by the Institutional Review Board of Seoul St. Mary's Hospital. (MC23EADI0064, date of approval: 21 July 2023).

Informed Consent Statement: Informed consent was obtained from all subjects involved in the study. Written informed consent has been obtained from the patient(s) to publish this paper.

Data Availability Statement: The data presented in this study are available upon request from the corresponding author.

Conflicts of Interest: The authors declare no conflicts of interest.

References

1. van Raaij, T.M.; Brouwer, R.W. Proximal Tibial Valgus Osteotomy: Lateral Closing Wedge. *JBJS Essent. Surg. Tech.* **2015**, *5*, e26. [CrossRef]
2. Coventry, M.B. Upper tibial osteotomy for osteoarthritis. *J. Bone Jt. Surg. Am.* **1985**, *67*, 1136–1140. [CrossRef]
3. Torres-Claramunt, R.; Sánchez-Soler, J.F.; Hinarejos, P.; Sala-Pujals, A.; Leal-Blanquet, J.; Monllau, J.C. Proximal Tibiofibular Dislocation in a Closing-Wedge High Tibial Osteotomy Causes Lateral Radiological Gapping of the Knee: A Prospective Randomized Study. *J. Clin. Med.* **2020**, *9*, 1622. [CrossRef] [PubMed]
4. Han, S.B.; Choi, J.H.; Mahajan, A.; Shin, Y.S. Incidence and Predictors of Lateral Hinge Fractures Following Medial Opening-Wedge High Tibial Osteotomy Using Locking Plate System: Better Performance of Computed Tomography Scans. *J. Arthroplast.* **2019**, *34*, 846–851. [CrossRef] [PubMed]
5. Kim, J.I.; Kim, B.H.; Lee, K.W.; Lee, O.; Han, H.S.; Lee, S.; Lee, M.C. Lower Limb Length Discrepancy After High Tibial Osteotomy: Prospective Randomized Controlled Trial of Lateral Closing Versus Medial Opening Wedge Osteotomy. *Am. J. Sports Med.* **2016**, *44*, 3095–3102. [CrossRef] [PubMed]
6. Ramanoudjame, M.; Vandenbussche, E.; Baring, T.; Solignac, N.; Augereau, B.; Gregory, T. Fibular nonunion after closed-wedge high tibial osteotomy. *Orthop. Traumatol. Surg. Res.* **2012**, *98*, 863–867. [CrossRef]
7. Parker, D.A.; Viskontas, D.G.J.S.M.; Review, A. Osteotomy for the early varus arthritic knee. *Sports Med. Arthrosc. Rev.* **2007**, *15*, 3–14. [CrossRef] [PubMed]
8. Park, J.Y.; Kim, J.K.; Han, H.S.; Lee, M.C. Proximal tibiofibular division in lateral closing wedge high tibial osteotomy does not increase varus instability of the knee. *Knee* **2019**, *26*, 1299–1305. [CrossRef] [PubMed]
9. Preston, C.F.; Fulkerson, E.W.; Meislin, R.; Di Cesare, P.E. Osteotomy about the knee: Applications, techniques, and results. *J. Knee Surg.* **2005**, *18*, 258–272. [CrossRef] [PubMed]
10. MacMahon, E. Failure of high tibial osteotomy for varus gonarthrosis. *Proc. Semin. Arthroplast.* **1996**, *7*, 212–218.
11. Shaw, J.A.; Dungy, D.S.; Arsht, S.S. Recurrent varus angulation after high tibial osteotomy: An anatomic analysis. *Clin. Orthop. Relat. Res.* **2004**, *420*, 205–212. [CrossRef] [PubMed]
12. Wootton, J.R.; Ashworth, M.J.; MacLaren, C.A. Neurological complications of high tibial osteotomy--the fibular osteotomy as a causative factor: A clinical and anatomical study. *Ann. R. Coll. Surg. Engl.* **1995**, *77*, 31–34. [PubMed]
13. Kim, M.S.; Koh, I.J.; Sung, Y.G.; Park, D.C.; Han, S.B.; In, Y. Alignment adjustment using the Valgus stress technique can increase the surgical accuracy of novice surgeons during medial opening-wedge high Tibial osteotomy. *BMC Musculoskelet. Disord.* **2021**, *22*, 585. [CrossRef] [PubMed]
14. Georgoulis, A.D.; Makris, C.A.; Papageorgiou, C.D.; Moebius, U.G.; Xenakis, T.; Soucacos, P.N. Nerve and vessel injuries during high tibial osteotomy combined with distal fibular osteotomy: A clinically relevant anatomic study. *Knee Surg. Sports Traumatol. Arthrosc.* **1999**, *7*, 15–19. [CrossRef] [PubMed]

15. Sánchez-Soler, J.; Coelho, A.; Torres-Claramunt, R.; Gasol, B.; Fontanellas, A.; Perelli, S.; Hinarejos, P.; Monllau, J.C. Proximal Tibiofibular Dislocation in Closing-Wedge High Tibial Osteotomy Increases the Risk of Medium and Long-Term Total Knee Replacement. *J. Clin. Med.* **2021**, *10*, 2743. [CrossRef]
16. Sawant, M.R.; Ireland, J. Pseudo-aneurysm of the anterior tibial artery complicating high tibial osteotomy—A case report. *Knee* **2001**, *8*, 247–248. [CrossRef] [PubMed]
17. Kim, J.; Allaire, R.; Harner, C.D. Vascular safety during high tibial osteotomy: A cadaveric angiographic study. *Am. J. Sports Med.* **2010**, *38*, 810–815. [CrossRef]
18. Zaidi, S.H.; Cobb, A.G.; Bentley, G. Danger to the popliteal artery in high tibial osteotomy. *J. Bone Jt. Surg. Br.* **1995**, *77*, 384–386. [CrossRef]
19. Shetty, A.A.; Tindall, A.J.; Qureshi, F.; Divekar, M.; Fernando, K.W. The effect of knee flexion on the popliteal artery and its surgical significance. *J. Bone Jt. Surg. Br.* **2003**, *85*, 218–222. [CrossRef] [PubMed]
20. Smith, P.N.; Gelinas, J.; Kennedy, K.; Thain, L.; Rorabeck, C.H.; Bourne, R.B. Popliteal vessels in knee surgery. A magnetic resonance imaging study. *Clin. Orthop. Relat. Res.* **1999**, *367*, 158–164. [CrossRef]

medicina

MDPI

Article

Assessing the Tibial Tubercle–Posterior Intercondylar Eminence Distance as a Superior Indicator for Patellar Instability and Surgical Planning in Tibial Tubercle Osteotomy

Georgian-Longin Iacobescu [1,2], Antonio-Daniel Corlatescu [1], Octavian Munteanu [2,3,*], Bogdan Serban [1,2], Razvan Spiridonica [2] and Catalin Cirstoiu [1,2]

[1] Department of Orthopedics and Traumatology, University of Medicine and Pharmacy "Carol Davila", 050474 Bucharest, Romania; georgianyak@yahoo.com (G.-L.I.); antonio.corlatescu0920@stud.umfcd.ro (A.-D.C.); bogdan.serban@umfcd.ro (B.S.); catalin.cirstoiu@umfcd.ro (C.C.)

[2] University Emergency Hospital Bucharest, 050098 Bucharest, Romania; rspiridonica@yahoo.com

[3] Department of Anatomy, University of Medicine and Pharmacy "Carol Davila", 050474 Bucharest, Romania

* Correspondence: octavian.munteanu@umfcd.ro

Abstract: *Background and Objectives*: This study aimed to evaluate the tibial tubercle–posterior intercondylar eminence (TT-IC) distance as a diagnostic tool and surgical guide for correcting extensor apparatus misalignment through tibial tubercle osteotomy. *Materials and Methods*: A retrospective analysis was conducted on patients with extensor apparatus misalignment. The TT-IC distance was measured using MRI. Patients underwent tibial tubercle osteotomy, guided by the TT-IC distance for correction. Post-operative outcomes, including alignment, pain scores, and functional recovery, were assessed. *Results*: A significant correlation was found between the TT-IC distance and the degree of extensor apparatus misalignment. Utilizing the TT-IC distance as a surgical guide led to improved alignment in majority of patients. Post-operative outcomes showed reduced pain and enhanced functional recovery. *Conclusions*: The study established the TT-IC measurement as a valuable tool for determining the need for tibial tuberosity osteotomy in patients with patellar instability, particularly those with trochlear dysplasia, by providing a more precise criterion than the traditional TT-TG distance.

Keywords: tibial tubercle–posterior intercondylar eminence (TT-IC); diagnostic imaging; surgical guide; extensor mechanism misalignment; osteotomy

1. Introduction

The surgical indication for tibial tubercle osteotomy (TTO) is based on a tibial tubercle–trochlear groove (TT-TG) distance of 20 mm or more. This standard was proposed by Dejour et al. in 1994 [1]. In patients with trochlear dysplasia, the TT-TG distance is less consistent, especially in those with high-grade dysplasia. The TT-TG values obtained from computed tomography (CT) imaging do not always match those measured by magnetic resonance imaging (MRI), with an average difference ranging between 2.2 and 4.16 mm, according to the literature [2]. As is known, the tibial tubercle osteotomy is used in patients with patellar maltracking caused by the presence of a lateral force vector acting on the extensor apparatus. Dejour et al. highlighted in their studies that patients with a distance greater than 20 mm between the most anterior part of the tibial tubercle and the deepest part of the trochlear groove primarily require medialization of the tibial tubercle to correct the excessive lateralization of the tibial tubercle [1,3,4]. Identifying the deepest point of the trochlear groove is challenging in patients with trochlear dysplasia, especially for those with type C or D trochlear dysplasia. As highlighted by Dejour in his study, the interobserver reproducibility is only 60% [3]. Furthermore, the surgical management of patients with TT-TG values between 16 and 20 mm, who also show other signs of extensor apparatus misalignment, is challenging [1,5]. The reference value for the TT-TG distance determined by MRI is currently unknown and can be influenced by the patient's age or body weight [6].

Patellar maltracking is closely linked to a range of histopathological alterations within the knee joint, with significant impact on the synovial tissues and fat pads. Synovitis and joint effusion are prevalent in these cases, typically presenting in the suprapatellar and infrapatellar recesses. These pathological changes are indicative of inflammatory processes and fluid accumulation, which are key contributors to pain and impaired knee function. Moreover, impingement and edema of the intra-articular fat pads, including the pre-femoral, suprapatellar, and Hoffa's fat pads, are frequently observed. Hoffa's fat pad, located between the patellar tendon and the tibial plateau, is particularly susceptible to inflammation—termed Hoffitis—arising from repetitive microtrauma and mechanical stress during knee motion, thereby exacerbating the clinical manifestations of patellar maltracking. Beyond the involvement of soft tissues, patellar maltracking frequently precipitates tendinopathies, especially within the quadriceps and patellar tendons. These tendinopathies are typically the result of chronic microtrauma, which leads to tendon degeneration and, in more severe instances, partial tears. This condition, commonly referred to as "Jumper's Knee", is prevalent among individuals who engage in repetitive jumping activities. Additionally, patellar chondropathy represents a significant histopathological consequence of maltracking. The aberrant movement of the patella leads to uneven stress distribution across the patellar cartilage, resulting in cartilage softening, fibrillation, and ultimately, chondromalacia, further intensifying knee pain and functional decline [7].

The aim of this study was to determine the correlations between a new parameter, specifically the tibial tubercle to intercondylar posterior arc distance (TT-IC), and the TT-TG distance, as well as other extensor apparatus misalignment parameters associated with trochlear dysplasia, such as the lateral trochlear slope, the trochlear angle, and trochlear facet asymmetry. The study also sought to establish a potential indication for osteotomy in these patients. This study hypothesized that the tibial tubercle–posterior intercondylar eminence (TT-IC) distance is a more reliable and reproducible parameter than the traditionally used tibial tubercle–trochlear groove (TT-TG) distance in guiding the surgical correction of extensor apparatus misalignment, especially in patients with advanced trochlear dysplasia. It is very important to establish a clearer indication for tibial tubercle osteotomy (TTO) in patients with patellar maltracking, particularly those with advanced trochlear dysplasia. Traditional criteria for TTO, based on a tibial tubercle–trochlear groove (TT-TG) distance of 20 mm or more, have limitations in patients with high-grade trochlear dysplasia, where the TT-TG measurements can be inconsistent and unreliable. Considering the variability in TT-TG values, especially in cases with complex anatomical distortions, this study explores the tibial tubercle to intercondylar posterior arc distance (TT-IC) as a potentially more reliable parameter. By examining the correlation between the TT-IC distance and other key misalignment parameters, such as the lateral trochlear slope, trochlear angle, and trochlear facet asymmetry, this study seeks to provide a more precise criterion for surgical intervention. Establishing the TT-IC distance as a potential indicator for osteotomy could offer a more effective and individualized approach to managing patellar maltracking, ultimately improving surgical outcomes in this patient population.

2. Materials and Methods

2.1. Study Participants

This is a retrospective observational study analyzing data from patients diagnosed with extensor apparatus misalignment who underwent tibial tubercle osteotomy between 2016 and 2022 at the Orthopedics and Traumatology Clinic of the Bucharest Emergency University Hospital. Within the study, data from 60 patients diagnosed with extensor apparatus misalignment, who underwent osteotomy surgery between 2016 and 2022, were analyzed. Prior approvals were obtained from the hospital's Ethics Committee, and informed consent was secured from the patients to be included in the study cohort, ensuring adherence to international standards of research ethics and integrity. In our study, the inclusion criteria were patients diagnosed with patellar instability, recurrent luxation, and trochlear dysplasia. Patients were excluded from the study if they had prior surgeries on the knee, non-standard imaging studies, or incomplete clinical records. MRIs were taken preoperatively to accurately assess the TT-IC distance and other relevant anatomical parameters. The study included patients diagnosed with extensor apparatus misalignment and the presence of trochlear dysplasia, specifically characterized by a trochlear angle greater than 140 degrees and a lateral trochlear inclination angle below 11–12 degrees. Eligible patients had undergone tibial tubercle osteotomy between 2016 and 2022 and had available preoperative MRI and CT scans for precise measurement of the TT-PIE and TT-TG distances. Patients were required to have no prior knee surgeries and to possess complete clinical and imaging records to confirm consistency and reliability in the analysis.

All measurements were performed by the same radiologist from the Department of Radiology and Medical Imaging at the University Hospital to establish consistency and minimize inter-observer variability. The imaging assessments, including the TT-TG and TT-IC distance measurements, were conducted with each patient positioned in the supine (dorsal decubitus) position, with the knee flexed at 30 degrees. This specific positioning was chosen to provide optimal visualization of the relevant anatomical landmarks while maintaining a consistent approach across all patients. Ensuring that all measurements were taken under these standardized conditions helped enhance the accuracy and reproducibility of the radiological evaluations.

2.2. Surgical Procedure

The tibial tubercle osteotomy (TTO) procedure was carried out in a standardized manner to maintain uniformity across all patients. The process began with thorough preoperative planning, involving the review of detailed imaging studies, such as CT and MRI, to evaluate the tibial tubercle–trochlear groove (TT-TG) distance. This step was critical for accurately determining the extent of medialization required for the tibial tubercle.

Following the completion of preoperative planning, the patient was placed in a supine position on the operating table with the knee in slight flexion to allow optimal access to the surgical site. The surgical area was then aseptically prepared, and a longitudinal incision was made along the anterior aspect of the knee to expose the tibial tubercle and trochlear groove (Figure 1).

With the surgical site exposed, the osteotomy procedure commenced. The tibial tubercle was carefully cut and mobilized medially according to the preoperative plan. This repositioning was performed to correct the excessive lateralization of the tibial tubercle. After achieving the desired position, the tibial tubercle was fixed securely in place using screws to ensure stability and promote proper healing.

Following the osteotomy and fixation, the incision was meticulously closed in layers to minimize the risk of infection and promote optimal wound healing. A sterile dressing was then applied to protect the surgical site.

Post-operative care involved adhering to standard protocols, including pain management to secure patient comfort, immobilization to facilitate proper healing, and a structured rehabilitation program to restore function and strength to the operated limb. These steps collectively aimed to ensure a successful surgical outcome and a smooth recovery process for all patients.

Post-surgical rehabilitation is essential for restoring knee stability and function in patients with patellar maltracking. The initial phase focused on isometric and isotonic strengthening exercises for the quadriceps, hamstrings, and hip muscles. Isometric exercises are crucial early on, as they activate muscles without significant joint movement, thereby reducing stress on healing tissues. These exercises stabilize the knee, particularly during valgus and rotatory stresses. As recovery progresses, isotonic exercises gradually rebuild muscle strength and endurance, facilitating a transition to more dynamic activities. In the advanced rehabilitation phases, the program introduced semi-squats to enhance the strength and control of the knee extensor mechanism, with careful attention to proper alignment to avoid excessive patellar tendon stress. Progressive jump training was then incorporated to improve eccentric loading, shock absorption, and movement control, which are vital for preventing recurrent patellar dislocation. This structured approach ensures the extensor mechanism is adequately prepared for the functional demands of daily activities and sports [8].

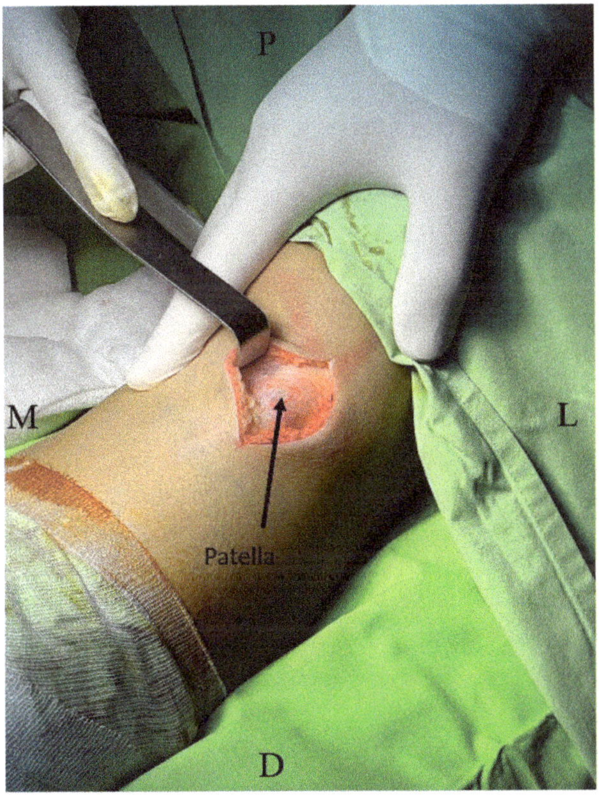

Figure 1. Intraoperative image showing the surgical approach (left knee). M, medial; L, lateral; D, distal; P, proximal.

2.3. Diagnostic Assessments and Measurement Techniques

Patients were assessed using computed tomography (CT) and MRI on the operated limb. Established diagnostic parameters, such as the TT-TG distance, trochlear angle, lateral trochlear slope, and trochlear asymmetry, were determined, along with the TT-IC parameter. The measurement of the distance between the tibial tubercle and the posterior intercondylar arc was conducted as follows: A reference line was drawn tangent to the posterior femoral condyles, with a parallel line considered as the tangent line of the posterior arc, termed the bony landmark of the posterior arc. The bony landmark of the tibial tubercle was identified as the center of the tibial tubercle when the patellar tendon was in close contact with it. Consequently, the TT-IC distance was defined as the distance between two parallel lines passing through the bony edge of the tibial tubercle and the posterior arc, perpendicular to the posterior intercondylar reference line (Figures 2 and 3).

All patients were assessed using high-resolution computed tomography (CT) and magnetic resonance imaging (MRI) of the operated limb. The CT scans were performed using a Siemens CT Definition Edge 128-slice scanner, with a slice thickness set to 1 mm to ensure optimal spatial resolution for detailed identification of bony landmarks. MRI assessments were conducted using a 3 Tesla Siemens Magnetom Vida scanner. For both imaging modalities, standardized patient positioning was maintained: patients were positioned supine with the knee at 30 degrees of flexion to replicate functional alignment and enhance measurement accuracy. The foot was secured in a neutral position using a foot holder to minimize movement. This imaging protocol facilitated precise and reproducible measurements of the TT-TG distance, TT-IC parameter, and other diagnostic parameters, ensuring consistent comparisons across all patients.

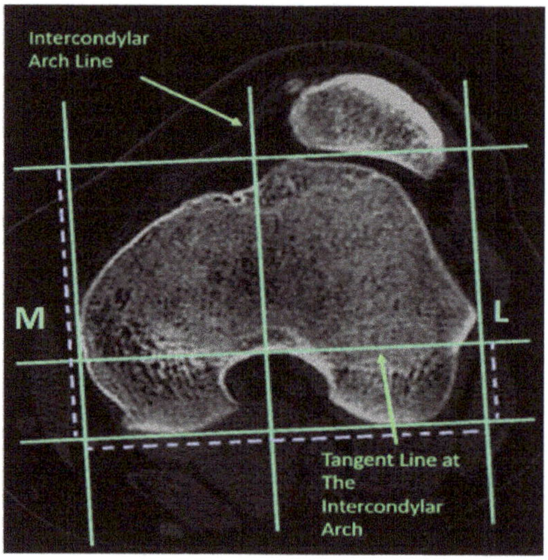

Figure 2. On the CT scan, the tangent line of the posterior arc, the bony landmark at the arc level, and the line of the intercondylar arc were identified (left knee). L, lateral; M, medial.

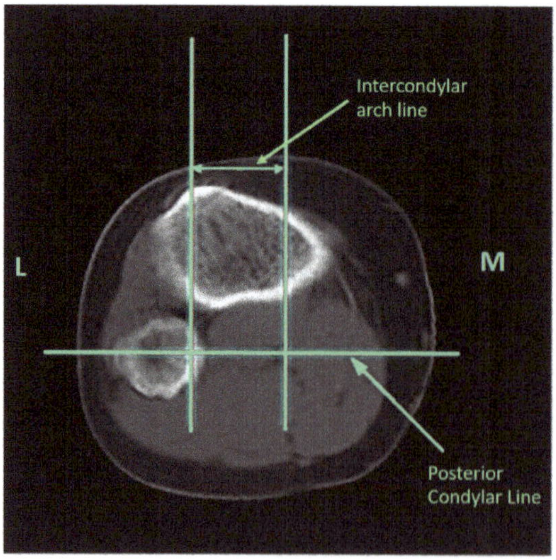

Figure 3. On the CT scan, the tangent line of the posterior arc, the bony landmark at the arc level, and the line of the intercondylar arc were identified (right knee). L, lateral; M, medial.

2.4. Statistical Analysis

The statistical analysis was conducted using IBM SPSS Statistics software, version 21, utilizing a range of statistical tests tailored to the specific data characteristics and research questions. Each test employed had distinct assumptions, which were systematically verified to secure the robustness and validity of the results.

The Mann–Whitney U test was chosen to compare differences between two independent groups when the dependent variable was either ordinal or continuous but did not follow a normal distribution. This non-parametric test's assumptions included that the two groups were independent, the dependent variable was measured on at least an ordinal scale, and the distributions of the groups were similar in shape. Independence was maintained through the study's design, while the shape of the distributions was assessed through visual inspection of histograms to confirm comparability.

For comparing two related samples or repeated measurements within a single sample, the Wilcoxon signed-rank test was employed to evaluate whether the population mean ranks differed. The test's assumptions required that the samples be related (paired) and that the dependent variable be measured at least on an ordinal scale. The relatedness of the samples was inherent to the study's design, and the ordinal nature of the variable was verified during data collection to meet these assumptions.

The chi-squared test was applied to examine the association between two categorical variables. The assumptions for this test required that both variables be categorical, that observations were independent of each other, and that the expected frequency in each cell of the contingency table was at least 5. The independence of observations was ensured by the study's design, while expected frequencies were calculated and confirmed to satisfy the necessary criteria for the test's validity.

To measure the strength and direction of the association between two binary variables, the Phi correlation coefficient was used. This test assumes that both variables are binary and that the sample size is adequate to produce a reliable correlation. These assumptions were met by verifying the binary nature of the variables during data collection and confirming that the sample size was sufficient through a prior sample size calculation to confirm statistical power.

Across all tests, a p-value threshold of less than 0.05 was used to determine statistical significance. Thorough checks were conducted on all assumptions associated with each test, ensuring that the chosen statistical methods were appropriate for the data, thereby enhancing the reliability and interpretability of the study findings.

The sample size for this study was determined through a power analysis. With an effect size of 0.5, a significance level of 0.05, and a power of 0.80, we calculated that 60 patients were necessary to achieve robust statistical validity. This calculation accounted for potential dropouts and aimed to guarantee the study's findings would be statistically significant.

3. Results

The analysis of our patient cohort revealed distinct demographic and clinical patterns. There was a notable predominance of female patients, with approximately 50 females compared to only 10 males, highlighting a skewed gender distribution within the study population. Age-wise, the majority of patients were young adults, predominantly in their mid-20s, with 25 years being the most represented age group (Table 1).

Clinically, variations in the CT tibial tubercle–trochlear groove (TT-TG) distance were observed in relation to the trochlear angle. Patients with a trochlear angle exceeding 140 degrees demonstrated higher median TT-TG distances than those with angles of 140 degrees or less. This indicates that the trochlear angle plays a critical role in influencing the TT-TG distance, a key factor in planning tibial tubercle osteotomy. These findings underscore the importance of accounting for both demographic and anatomical factors when assessing and managing patients with patellar instability and recurrent dislocation (Figures 4 and 5).

Table 1. Demographic characteristics of the study population.

Characteristic	Number (*n*)	Percentage (%)
Total Patients	60	100
Sex Distribution		
Female	50	83.3
Male	10	16.7
Age Distribution		
20–24 years	15	25
25–29 years	30	50
30–34 years	10	16.7
35–40 years	5	8.3
Mean Age (years)	25.57	
Standard Deviation	5.01	

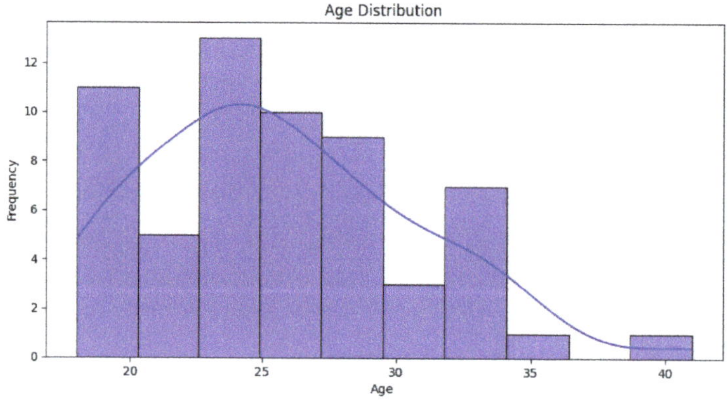

Figure 4. Age distribution. The ages ranged from early 20s to 40 years old. The distribution shows a higher concentration of patients in their mid-20s, with the most frequent age group being 25 years old.

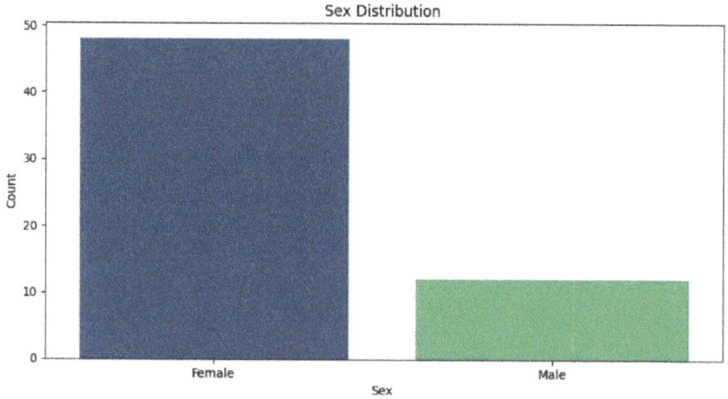

Figure 5. Sex distribution. A significant majority of the patients were female, with approximately 50 female patients compared to around 10 male patients.

The average age of the patients was 25.57 years (standard deviation: 5.013; CI: [24.27; 26.86]). There were no significant differences between genders, but there was a predominantly female distribution, with 80% being women ($n = 48$) and 20% men ($n = 12$). Figure 6 shows the distribution of cases based on the TT-TG and TT-IC distances measured by CT.

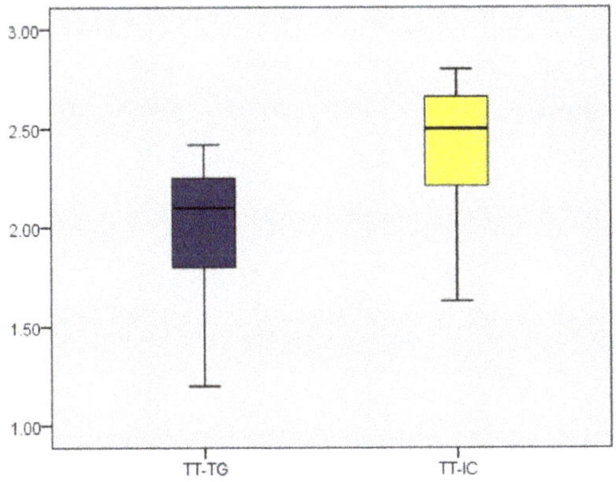

Figure 6. Distribution of cases based on the TT-TG and TT-IC distances measured by CT.

The distribution of cases based on the TT-TG and TT-IC distances measured by CT showed significantly higher values for the TT-IC parameter across the entire patient group compared to the TT-TG values.

3.1. Assessment of the Lateral Trochlear Slope and Its Association with TT-IC by CT

The average value for the TT-IC parameter was 2.42 cm (standard deviation: 0.29; CI: [2.34; 2.49]), with a median value of 2.50 cm. Patients with a lateral trochlear slope of ≤11 degrees (measured by CT) had TT-IC values ranging from 2.10 to 2.80, with an average value of 2.4259 (standard deviation: 0.22; CI: [2.30; 2.54]) and a median value of 2.40. Meanwhile, patients with a lateral trochlear slope of >11 degrees (measured by CT) had TT-IC values between 1.63 and 2.80, with an average of 2.4202 (standard deviation: 0.31; CI: [2.32; 2.51]) and a median value of 2.54. No significant differences were observed between the TT-IC values measured in the patient group with a lateral trochlear slope of ≤11 and the group with a slope of >11 ($p = 0.867$).

Subsequently, we compared the TT-TG and TT-IC values in patients with a lateral trochlear slope of ≤11 ($n = 17$). As previously noted, these patients showed considerably higher TT-IC distances compared to the TT-TG distances (average values: 2.42 vs. 1.95). The application of the Wilcoxon signed-rank test indicated that the differences between TT-IC and TT-TG values were statistically significant ($Z = -3.626$; $p < 0.001$). Significant differences between the TT-TG and TT-IC distances were also found in patients with a lateral trochlear slope of >11 ($n = 42$), with TT-IC values also being notably higher than TT-TG values (average values: 2.42 vs. 2.01; $Z = -5.691$; $p < 0.001$; Figures 7 and 8, Table 2).

Table 2. CT and MRI measurements by trochlear angle.

Measurement	Trochlear Angle ≤ 140° ($n = 27$)	Trochlear Angle > 140° ($n = 23$)	p-Value
TT-TG Distance (CT)	Mean: 2.04 cm (SD: 0.33)	Mean: 1.94 cm (SD: 0.23)	0.056
TT-IC Distance (CT)	Mean: 2.45 cm (SD: 0.32)	Mean: 2.38 cm (SD: 0.23)	0.184
TT-TG Distance (MRI)	Mean: 2.02 cm (SD: 0.36)	Mean: 1.94 cm (SD: 0.23)	0.149
TT-IC Distance (MRI)	Mean: 2.42 cm (SD: 0.35)	Mean: 2.38 cm (SD: 0.24)	0.425

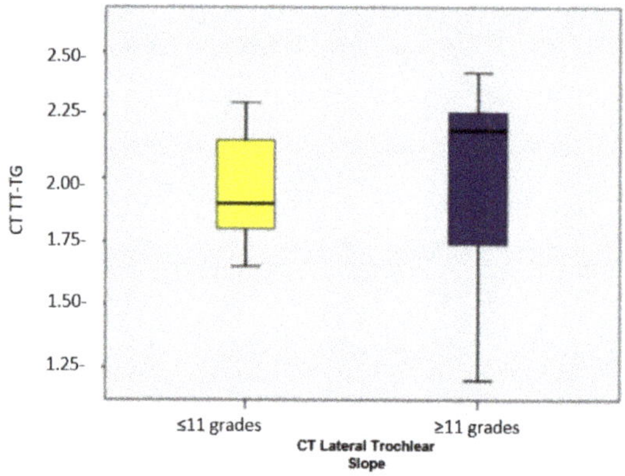

Figure 7. Distribution of cases based on TT-TG in patients with a lateral trochlear slope of <11 degrees and >11 degrees, respectively.

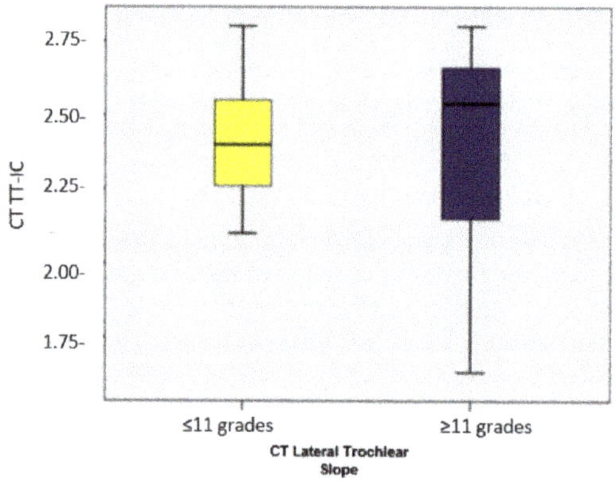

Figure 8. Distribution of cases based on TT-IC in patients with a lateral trochlear slope of <11 degrees and >11 degrees, respectively.

3.2. *Assessing Trochlear Facet Asymmetry and Its Relationship with TT-TG and TT-IC by MRI*

When examining trochlear facet asymmetry, patients displaying this asymmetry (as measured by MRI) had TT-TG values ranging from 1.74 to 2.30, with an average of 1.9867 (standard deviation: 0.20; CI: [1.89; 2.07]) and a median of 1.90 ($n = 21$). In contrast, patients without trochlear facet asymmetry had TT-TG values between 1.20 and 2.42, averaging 1.9886 (standard deviation: 0.37; CI: [1.84; 2.13]) with a median of 2.2 ($n = 29$). There were no statistically significant differences in TT-TG distances between patients with and without trochlear facet asymmetry ($p = 0.510$). For the TT-IC parameter measurements, patients with trochlear facet asymmetry showed values between 2.12 and 2.80, averaging 2.4248 (standard deviation: 0.21; CI: [2.32; 2.52]) with a median of 2.40. Those without this asymmetry had TT-IC values ranging from 1.63 to 2.80, with an average of 2.3972 (standard deviation: 0.36; CI: [2.25; 2.53]) and a median of 2.60. Although patients with trochlear facet asymmetry had slightly higher TT-IC values compared to those without, the differences were not statistically significant ($p = 0.984$). Subsequently, we compared the TT-TG and TT-IC values in patients with trochlear facet asymmetry ($n = 21$). As previously noted, these patients exhibited significantly higher TT-IC distances compared to the TT-TG distances (average values: 2.42 vs. 1.98). The Wilcoxon signed-rank test confirmed that the differences between TT-IC and TT-TG values were statistically significant ($Z = -4.018$; $p < 0.001$; Table 3).

Table 3. Association of TT-IC and TT-TG distances with trochlear facet asymmetry.

Measurement	With Asymmetry (n = 21)	Without Asymmetry (n = 29)	p-Value
TT-TG Distance (MRI)	Mean: 1.99 cm (SD: 0.20)	Mean: 1.99 cm (SD: 0.37)	0.51
TT-IC Distance (MRI)	Mean: 2.42 cm (SD: 0.21)	Mean: 2.40 cm (SD: 0.36)	0.984
TT-TG vs. TT-IC Difference (MRI)	$Z = -4.018; p < 0.001$	$Z = -4.759; p < 0.001$	

Similarly, significant differences between the TT-TG and TT-IC distances were observed in patients without trochlear facet asymmetry (n = 29). The TT-IC values were also notably higher than the TT-TG values (average values: 2.39 vs. 1.98; $Z = -4.759$; $p < 0.001$; Figures 9 and 10).

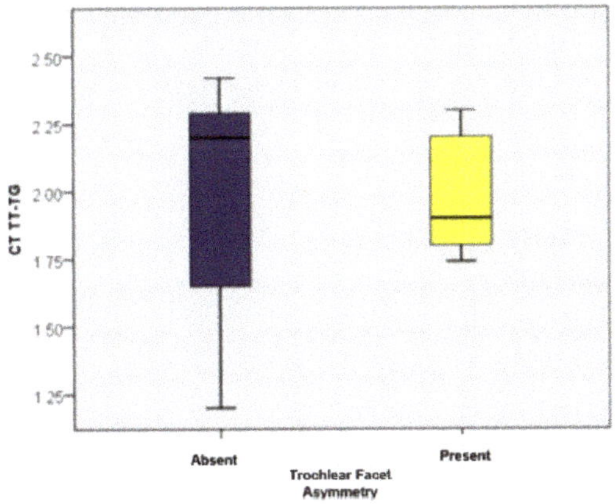

Figure 9. Distribution of cases based on TT-TG values in patients with and without trochlear facet asymmetry.

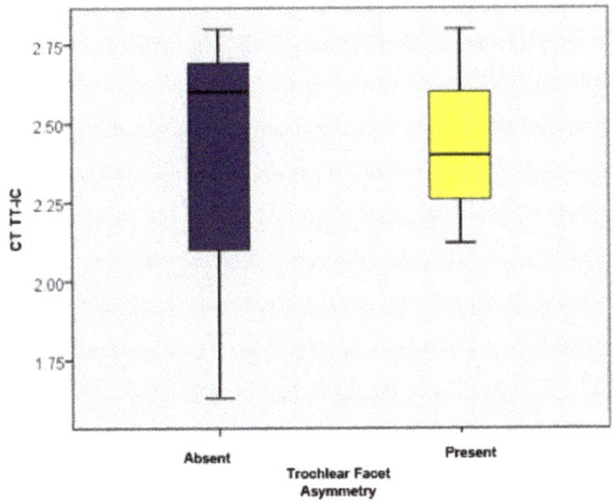

Figure 10. Distribution of cases based on TT-IC values in patients with and without trochlear facet asymmetry.

3.3. Assessment of the Trochlear Angle and Its Correlation with TT-TG and TT-IC by Both CT and MRI

Patients with a trochlear angle of ≤140 degrees (measured by MRI) had TT-TG values ranging from 1.20 to 2.42, with an average of 2.02 (standard deviation: 0.36; CI: [1.87; 2.16]) and a median of 2.24 ($n = 27$). Meanwhile, those with a trochlear angle over 140 degrees had TT-TG values between 1.43 and 2.30, averaging 1.94 (standard deviation: 0.23; CI: [1.84; 2.04]) with a median of 1.90 ($n = 23$). No statistically significant differences in TT-TG distances were observed between the two groups ($p = 0.149$).

Furthermore, patients with a trochlear angle of ≤140 degrees had TT-IC values between 1.63 and 2.80, averaging 2.42 (standard deviation: 0.35; CI: [2.28; 2.56]) with a median of 2.64. In contrast, those with a trochlear angle over 140 degrees had TT-IC values ranging from 1.85 to 2.80, with an average of 2.38 (standard deviation: 0.24; CI: [2.27; 2.49]) and a median of 2.37. No significant differences in TT-IC distances were noted between the two groups ($p = 0.425$).

By comparing the TT-TG and TT-IC values in patients with a trochlear angle of ≤140 degrees ($n = 27$), the Wilcoxon signed-rank test revealed statistically significant differences between TT-IC and TT-TG values ($Z = -4.606$; $p < 0.001$). This emphasized that these patients had notably higher TT-IC distances compared to TT-TG (average values: 2.42 vs. 2.02). Significant differences between TT-TG and TT-IC distances were also found in patients with a trochlear angle over 140 degrees ($n = 23$), with TT-IC values also being significantly higher than TT-TG values (average values: 2.38 vs. 1.94; $Z = -4.200$; $p < 0.001$; Figures 11 and 12).

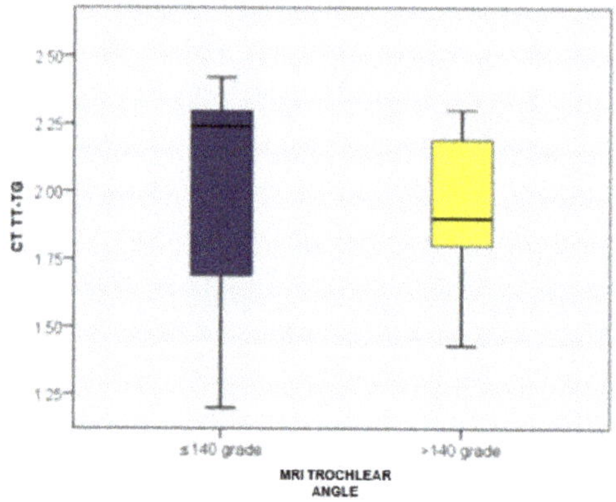

Figure 11. Distribution of cases based on TT-TG values and their association with the trochlear angle, determined by MRI.

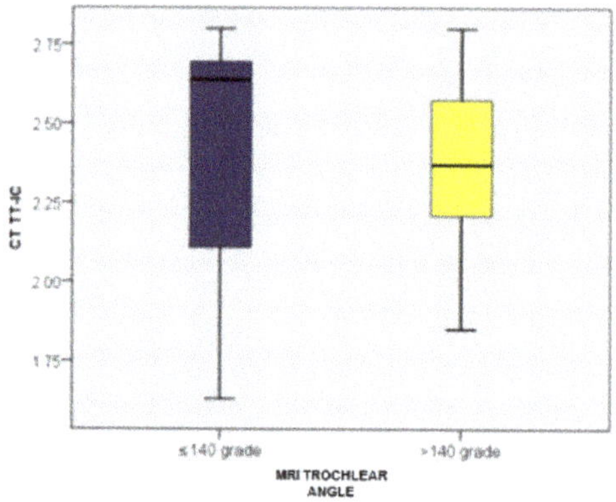

Figure 12. Distribution of cases based on TT-IC values and their association with the trochlear angle, determined by MRI.

Regarding the CT evaluation, in the group with a trochlear angle of ≤140 degrees (measured by CT), TT-TG values ranged from 1.20 to 2.42, with an average of 2.04 (standard deviation: 0.33; CI: [1.92; 2.16]) and a median of 2.20 ($n = 33$). Meanwhile, for those with a trochlear angle over 140 degrees, TT-TG values ranged from 1.43 to 2.30, averaging 1.94 (standard deviation: 0.23; CI: [1.85; 2.03]) with a median of 1.90 ($n = 26$). No statistically significant differences in TT-TG distances were observed between the two groups ($p = 0.056$).

For the TT-IC parameter, patients with a trochlear angle of ≤140 degrees (measured by CT) had values between 1.63 and 2.80, averaging 2.45 (standard deviation: 0.32; CI: [2.33; 2.56]) with a median of 2.60. In contrast, those with a trochlear angle over 140 degrees had TT-IC values ranging from 1.85 to 2.80, averaging 2.38 (standard deviation: 0.23; CI: [2.28; 2.48]) with a median of 2.38. No significant differences in TT-IC distances were noted between the two groups ($p = 0.184$).

Subsequently, we compared the TT-TG and TT-IC values in patients with a trochlear angle of ≤140 degrees ($n = 33$). As previously noted, these patients exhibited significantly higher TT-IC distances compared to the TT-TG distances (average values: 2.45 vs. 2.04). The Wilcoxon signed-rank test confirmed that the differences between TT-IC and TT-TG values were statistically significant ($Z = -5.088$; $p < 0.001$). Similarly, significant differences between the TT-TG and TT-IC distances were observed in patients with a trochlear angle over 140 degrees ($n = 26$), with TT-IC values also being notably higher than TT-TG values (average values: 2.38 vs. 1.94; $Z = -4.461$; $p < 0.001$; Figures 13 and 14).

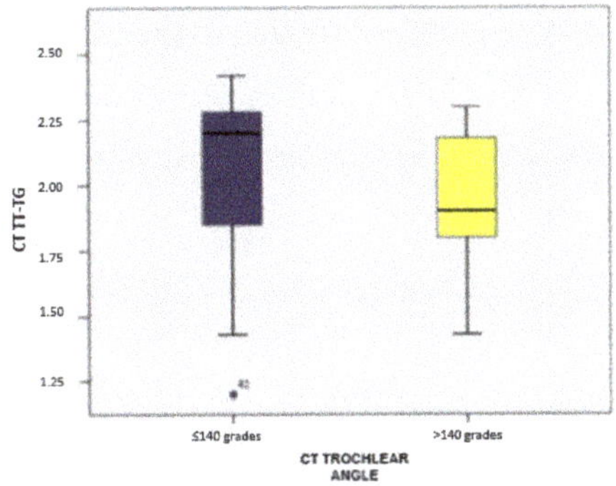

Figure 13. Distribution of cases based on TT-TG values and their correlation with the trochlear angle, determined using CT imaging.

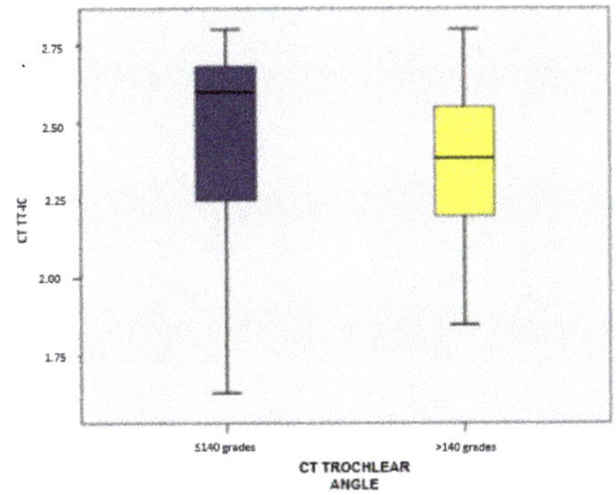

Figure 14. Distribution of cases based on TT-IC values and their correlation with the trochlear angle, determined using CT imaging.

3.4. Evaluation of TT-TG and TT-IC Parameters Using ROC Curves

Both the TT-TG distance and the TT-IC distance showed limited specificity and sensitivity in predicting patients with a lateral trochlear slope of ≤11 degrees. For TT-TG, the AUC was 0.411, with a cut-off value of 1.86 cm, a sensitivity of 56%, and a specificity of

36%. For TT-IC, the AUC was 0.490, with a cut-off value of 2.25 cm, a sensitivity of 75%, and a specificity of 36%. The *p*-values were 0.313 and 0.91, respectively (Figures 15 and 16).

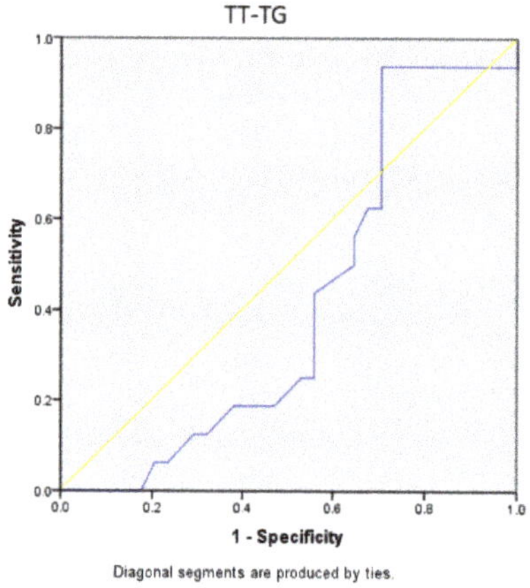

Figure 15. ROC curves for TT-TG distances in patients with a lateral trochlear slope of <11 degrees. The blue line represents the test's performance at different thresholds, with a higher AUC indicating better accuracy, while the yellow diagonal shows random chance, and the goal is for the blue line to be above the yellow one, indicating the test outperforms randomness.

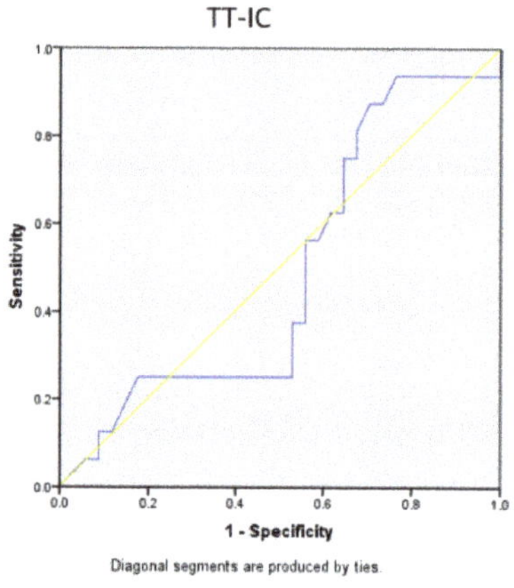

Figure 16. ROC curves for TT-IC distances in patients with a lateral trochlear slope of <11 degrees. The blue line represents the test's performance at different thresholds, with a higher AUC indicating better accuracy, while the yellow diagonal shows random chance, and the goal is for the blue line to be above the yellow one, indicating the test outperforms randomness.

Through the analysis of ROC curves for patients undergoing Elmslie–Trillat medialization osteotomy, both the TT-TG and TT-IC parameters demonstrated high sensitivity and specificity, both statistically significant. The TT-IC distance showed slightly higher values, indicating its predictive power for this type of surgical intervention. For TT-TG, the AUC was 0.778, with a cut-off value of 1.86 cm, a sensitivity of 78%, and a specificity of 62% ($p = 0.001$). For TT-IC, the AUC was 0.787, with a cut-off value of 2.25 cm, a sensitivity of 85%, and a specificity of 62% ($p < 0.0001$; Figures 17 and 18, Table 4).

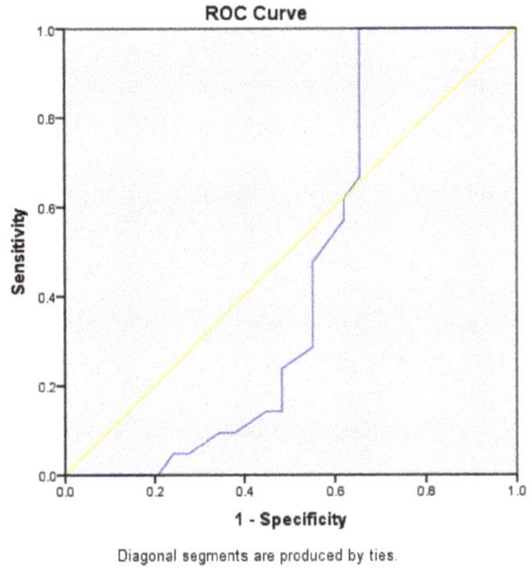

Figure 17. ROC curves for TT-TG distances in patients with Elmslie–Trillat osteotomy. The blue line represents the test's performance at different thresholds, with a higher AUC indicating better accuracy, while the yellow diagonal shows random chance, and the goal is for the blue line to be above the yellow one, indicating the test outperforms randomness.

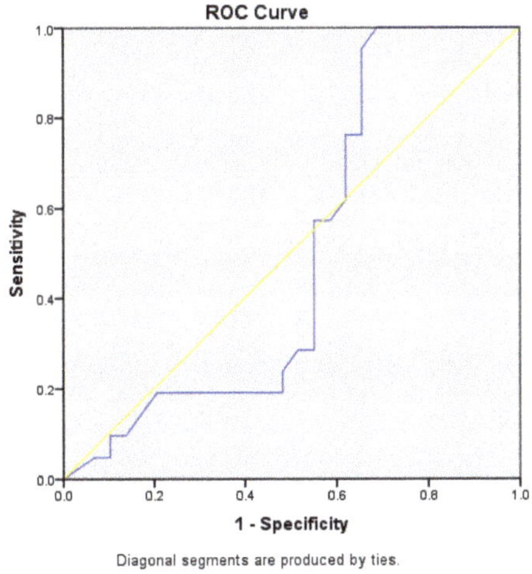

Figure 18. ROC curves for TT-IC distances in patients with Elmslie–Trillat osteotomy. The blue line represents the test's performance at different thresholds, with a higher AUC indicating better accuracy, while the yellow diagonal shows random chance, and the goal is for the blue line to be above the yellow one, indicating the test outperforms randomness.

Table 4. Diagnostic performance of TT-TG and TT-IC distances using ROC analysis.

Parameter	AUC	Cut-Off Value	Sensitivity (%)	Specificity (%)	*p*-Value
TT-TG Distance	0.778	1.86 cm	78	62	0.001
TT-IC Distance	0.787	2.25 cm	85	62	<0.0001

4. Discussion

In our study, the TT-IC benchmark was compared with the traditional TT-TG distance across a cohort of patients, including those with varying degrees of trochlear dysplasia, assessed by metrics such as the lateral trochlear inclination angle, trochlear angle, and trochlear facet asymmetry, as well as those without dysplasia. The findings indicated that TT-IC values were consistently higher than TT-TG values, particularly in patients with dysplasia, suggesting that TT-IC offers greater accuracy in these cases. Both measurements were effective in predicting patellar instability; however, TT-IC demonstrated superior accuracy in the presence of dysplastic trochleae.

The clinical implications of our findings are significant for the management of patellar instability, particularly in patients with trochlear dysplasia. The TT-IC benchmark proved more accurate in assessing tibial tuberosity lateralization in advanced dysplastic cases than the conventional TT-TG distance. This is especially relevant considering the reproducibility challenges associated with TT-TG, which stem from difficulties in identifying the deepest point of the trochlear groove, particularly when the trochlear angle approaches 180 degrees, indicating a flat trochlea. Consequently, the use of TT-IC may provide more reliable data for surgical planning, such as determining the necessity for a medializing tibial tuberosity osteotomy, ultimately contributing to improved patient outcomes.

Subsequent research has determined that an increased TT-TG distance is a predictive marker for patellar instabilities, with a value exceeding 20 mm being the gold standard for formally indicating a medializing tibial tuberosity osteotomy [9]. However, this axial measurement has shown limitations due to its reduced reproducibility, especially in patients with trochlear dysplasia, particularly those with advanced trochlear dysplasia with a trochlear angle nearing 180 degrees—a flat trochlea. This challenge arises from the difficulty in accurately determining the deepest point of the trochlear groove [10–12]. Consequently, there was a need for a new benchmark that could be more effective in determining the lateralization of the tibial tuberosity in patients with advanced trochlear dysplasia.

While our study introduced the TT-IC benchmark as a novel approach, it is essential to recognize that the use of axial measurements for surgical guidance is not a new concept. Previous studies have established that an increased TT-TG (tibial tubercle–trochlear groove) distance serves as a predictive marker for patellar instability and a primary indicator for medializing tibial tuberosity osteotomy. Despite its status as the gold standard, TT-TG has notable limitations, particularly in patients with advanced trochlear dysplasia, prompting the need for alternative benchmarks. Our research addressed these limitations by proposing the TT-IC benchmark, which aims to enhance measurement reliability in specific patient groups.

According to a study by Xu et al., the TT-RA (tibial tubercle–Roman arch) distance was proposed as a more reliable measure for assessing tibial tubercle positioning in patients with patellar dislocation, particularly in cases of trochlear dysplasia. Their findings demonstrated that the TT-RA distance had higher reproducibility than the traditional TT-TG (tibial tubercle–trochlear groove) distance, which is often unreliable due to the difficulty in accurately identifying the deepest point of the trochlear groove in dysplastic trochlea. Xu et al. established a surgical threshold for the TT-RA distance at 26 mm, and they reported excellent intraclass correlation coefficients (ICCs) across all Dejour classifications, indicating its utility for clinical decision-making. Furthermore, the TT-RA distance showed superior diagnostic accuracy over the TT-TG distance, especially in complex trochlear morphologies, supporting its use as a preferred surgical guide [13].

Our findings align with Xu et al.'s conclusion regarding the limitations of the TT-TG distance in patients with advanced trochlear dysplasia and the need for more reliable measurements. However, while Xu et al. recommend the TT-RA distance, our study introduced the TT-IC benchmark, which also demonstrated greater accuracy and reliability, particularly in severe dysplastic cases. Both studies emphasized the necessity of consistent and reproducible metrics across varying trochlear types, but our research further suggested that the TT-IC may offer additional advantages in evaluating tibial tuberosity lateralization in complex presentations [13]. Compared to other axial measurements, the TT-IC distance provides a clearer indication for surgical intervention in patients with complex trochlear dysplasia, as it is less affected by the variability in the trochlear groove's anatomy. This enhances its reproducibility and reliability, particularly in severe dysplastic cases, where the traditional TT-TG distance is less dependable. Our study offered an innovative perspective by introducing a benchmark that considers anatomical variations more comprehensively, potentially improving patient outcomes through better-informed surgical decisions.

The study had its limitations. The first was that the sample size was relatively small, especially when considering patients with high-grade trochlear dysplasia, where the new benchmark showed enhanced accuracy. Second, the study was conducted at a single center, which may limit the applicability of the findings to other populations or clinical settings with different patient demographics or surgical practices.

Future research should address the limitations we found in our study. One key area is to increase the sample size, especially by including more patients with high-grade trochlear dysplasia, to better confirm the accuracy of the TT-IC benchmark. Additionally, it would be beneficial to include anatomical changes at the tibia level in the analysis to provide a more comprehensive understanding of extensor apparatus misalignments. Long-term studies could also help assess the clinical outcomes of using TT-IC for surgical planning and management of patellar instability. By addressing these aspects, future research can improve the diagnostic and treatment methods for patients with patellar instability and trochlear dysplasia.

5. Conclusions

This study laid the groundwork for a new axial measurement that quantifies the degree of tibial tuberosity lateralization in patients with patellar instability. Upon analysis, the new TT-IC benchmark showed higher values compared to TT-TG across all patients, with notably higher values in those with trochlear dysplasia. Therefore, when assessing a patient with patellar instability and trochlear dysplasia, it is essential to consider the TT-IC value alongside the traditional TT-TG distance to accurately determine the need for tibial tuberosity osteotomy. To address the potential indication for osteotomy, our study suggested that the new TT-IC measurement can serve as a critical factor in decision-making for tibial tuberosity osteotomy in patients with patellar instability, particularly in those with concomitant trochlear dysplasia. By demonstrating that the TT-IC values were consistently higher than TT-TG values, especially in patients with trochlear dysplasia, our findings highlighted the importance of incorporating TT-IC into the assessment process. This addition can help identify candidates who may benefit most from osteotomy, providing a clearer, more precise criterion for surgical intervention and improving patient outcomes.

Author Contributions: Conceptualization, A.-D.C., G.-L.I. and C.C.; methodology, G.-L.I., R.S. and A.-D.C.; validation, G.-L.I. and O.M.; formal analysis, A.-D.C. and R.S.; investigation, O.M. and A.-D.C.; resources, O.M., G.-L.I. and B.S.; data curation, G.-L.I., R.S. and A.-D.C.; writing—original draft preparation, A.-D.C. and B.S.; writing—review and editing, A.-D.C. and O.M.; visualization, O.M.; supervision, G.-L.I. and C.C.; project administration, G.-L.I. All authors have read and agreed to the published version of the manuscript.

Funding: Publication of this paper was supported by the University of Medicine and Pharmacy Carol Davila, through the institutional program Publish not Perish.

Institutional Review Board Statement: The study was conducted in accordance with the Declaration of Helsinki and approved by the Ethics Committee of the University Emergency Hospital Bucharest (No. 56457/7 November 2022).

Informed Consent Statement: Written informed consent was obtained from the patients to publish this paper.

Data Availability Statement: All the data processed in this article are part of the research for a doctoral thesis, which is archived in the pathology department at the University Hospital of Bucharest, where the interventions were performed. The original data are available upon reasonable request.

Conflicts of Interest: The authors declare no conflicts of interest.

References

1. Dejour, D.; Le Coultre, B. Osteotomies in Patello-Femoral Instabilities. *Sports Med. Arthrosc. Rev.* **2007**, *15*, 39–46. [CrossRef] [PubMed]
2. Camp, C.L.; Stuart, M.J.; Krych, A.J.; Levy, B.A.; Bond, J.R.; Collins, M.S.; Dahm, D.L. CT and MRI Measurements of Tibial Tubercle–Trochlear Groove Distances Are Not Equivalent in Patients with Patellar Instability. *Am. J. Sports Med.* **2013**, *41*, 1835–1840. [CrossRef] [PubMed]
3. Dejour, D.H.; Mesnard, G.; De Sanctis, E.G. Updated treatment guidelines for patellar instability: "un menu à la carte". *J. Exp. Orthop.* **2021**, *8*, 109. [CrossRef] [PubMed]
4. Catelas, I.; Wimmer, M.A. New Insights into Wear and Biological Effects of Metal-on-Metal Bearings. *J. Bone Jt. Surg.* **2011**, *93* (Suppl. S2), 76–83. [CrossRef]
5. O'Neill, D.B. Open lateral retinacular lengthening compared with arthroscopic release. A prospective, randomized outcome study. *J. Bone Jt. Surg. Am.* **1997**, *79*, 1759–1769. [CrossRef]
6. Vitale, T.E.; Mooney, B.; Vitale, A.; Apergis, D.; Wirth, S.; Grossman, M.G. Physical therapy intervention for medial patellofemoral ligament reconstruction after repeated lateral patellar subluxation/dislocation. *Int. J. Sports Phys. Ther.* **2016**, *11*, 423–435. [PubMed]
7. Pirri, C.; Stecco, C.; Güvener, O.; Mezian, K.; Ricci, V.; Jačisko, J.; Novotný, T.; Kara, M.; Chang, K.-V.; Dughbaj, M.; et al. EURO-MUSCULUS/USPRM Dynamic Ultrasound Protocols for Knee. *Am. J. Phys. Med. Rehabil.* **2023**, *102*, e67–e72. [CrossRef]
8. Cocco, G.; Ricci, V.; Corvino, A.; Abate, M.; Vaccaro, A.; Bernabei, C.; Cantisani, V.; Vallone, G.; Caiazzo, C.; Caulo, M.; et al. Musculoskeletal disorders in padel: From biomechanics to sonography. *J. Ultrasound* **2024**, *27*, 335–354. [CrossRef] [PubMed]
9. Wagner, D.; Pfalzer, F.; Hingelbaum, S.; Huth, J.; Mauch, F.; Bauer, G. The influence of risk factors on clinical outcomes following anatomical medial patellofemoral ligament (MPFL) reconstruction using the gracilis tendon. *Knee Surg. Sports Traumatol. Arthrosc.* **2013**, *21*, 318–324. [CrossRef] [PubMed]
10. Wang, S.; Qin, C.; Jiang, N.; Wang, B.; Wang, L.; Yu, B. Is surgical treatment better than conservative treatment for primary patellar dislocations? A meta-analysis of randomized controlled trials. *Arch. Orthop. Trauma Surg.* **2016**, *136*, 371–379. [CrossRef] [PubMed]
11. Beaufils, P.; Thaunat, M.; Pujol, N.; Scheffler, S.; Rossi, R.; Carmont, M. Trochleoplasty in major trochlear dysplasia: Current concepts. *Sports Med. Arthrosc. Rehabil. Ther. Technol.* **2012**, *4*, 7. [CrossRef] [PubMed]
12. Biedert, R.M. Lengthening Osteotomy with or without Elevation of the Lateral Trochlear Facet. In *Patellofemoral Pain, Instability, and Arthritis*; Dejour, D., Zaffagnini, S., Arendt, E.A., Sillanpää, P., Dirisamer, F., Eds.; Springer: Berlin/Heidelberg, Germany, 2020; pp. 335–341. [CrossRef]
13. Xu, Z.; Zhang, H.; Fu, B.; Mohamed, S.I.; Zhang, J.; Zhou, A. Tibial Tubercle–Roman Arch Distance: A New Measurement of Patellar Dislocation and Indication of Tibial Tubercle Osteotomy. *Orthop. J. Sports Med.* **2020**, *8*, 232596712091487. [CrossRef] [PubMed]

medicina

MDPI

Article

Sex Differences in Sarcopenia in Patients Undergoing Total Knee Arthroplasty for Advanced Knee Osteoarthritis

Oog-Jin Shon [1,2], Gi Beom Kim [1,2,*] and Seong Hyeon Jo [2]

[1] Department of Orthopedic Surgery, College of Medicine, Yeungnam University, 170 Hyonchung-ro, Namgu, Daegu 42415, Republic of Korea; maestro-jin@hanmail.net

[2] Department of Orthopedic Surgery, Yeungnam University Medical Center, 170 Hyonchung-ro, Namgu, Daegu 42415, Republic of Korea; fmsndkfmoo@gmail.com

* Correspondence: donggamgb@hanmail.net; Tel.: +82-53-6203640

Abstract: *Background and Objectives:* The purpose of this study was to compare sex differences in the incidence of sarcopenia, demographic characteristics, and preoperative sarcopenic parameters in patients undergoing TKA for advanced knee osteoarthritis (OA). Moreover, we sought to compare patient-reported outcome measures (PROMs) and the predisposing factors after TKA in patients with sarcopenia by sex through subgroup analysis. *Materials and Methods:* From May 2020 to September 2022, a total of 892 patients who were evaluable for sarcopenia before primary TKA were enrolled. Sarcopenia was defined according to the Asian Working Group for Sarcopenia 2019 criteria. Patients were assessed according to the presence or absence of sarcopenia. After a two-to-one matched-pair analysis for subgroup analysis, 21 knees in men were matched with a corresponding number of knees in women (42), resulting in a total of 63 knees. PROMs were investigated using the Knee Injury and Osteoarthritis Outcome Score, Western Ontario and McMaster Universities Osteoarthritis Index, and the Short Form-12 physical and mental component summary scores. Moreover, the postoperative complications and predisposing factors for male sarcopenia were investigated. *Results:* The prevalence of sarcopenia was 10.9% (97/892), and the prevalence was higher in men (19.6%, 21/107) than in women (9.7%, 76/785). In subgroup analyses, male patients had significantly inferior PROMs up to 12 months after index surgery. Moreover, there was no significant difference in the systemic complications between the two groups. Multivariate binary logistic regression analysis indicated that alcohol consumption, smoking, and higher modified Charlson Comorbidity Index (mCCI) were predisposing factors for male patients with sarcopenia. The prevalence of sarcopenia was higher in male patients undergoing primary TKA. *Conclusions:* When compared with the propensity-matched female group, male patients had inferior PROMs up to 12 months postoperatively. Alcohol consumption, current smoker status, and higher mCCI were predisposing factors for sarcopenia in male patients with advanced knee OA.

Keywords: total knee arthroplasty; sarcopenia; patient-reported outcome measures; sex differences

1. Introduction

Skeletal muscle naturally declines with age, and this loss accelerates after the age of 65, which can increase the risk of poor quality of life, physical disability, and death [1]. Sarcopenia, defined as the loss of muscle mass, strength, and function with aging [2] is known to be an independent risk factor for frailty, falls, and lower extremity fractures [1,3,4]. In 2020, the Asian Working Group for Sarcopenia (AWGS) published updated guidelines based on East Asian and Southeast Asian studies (AWGS 2019) [5]. As sarcopenia has been associated with a variety of total knee arthroplasty (TKA)-related complications including periprosthetic joint infection, its importance should be further emphasized in elderly patients undergoing TKA [6–8].

Elderly women account for about 70–90% of TKA candidates, and their number is gradually increasing due to the aging population. As some studies have reported, especially in Asia, this female predominance is more pronounced [9]. Therefore, to date, most studies related to sarcopenia have focused on elderly women, and their outcomes have mostly addressed these women [10]. However, with the gradual increase in TKA volume [11] and since the number of elderly men who are undergoing TKA is also increasing it has become necessary to pay attention to the results of TKA in the elderly men group. However, few studies have been conducted on the comparison of outcomes after TKA in elderly men and women with sarcopenia and on the risk factors in elderly men with sarcopenia.

The purpose of this study was to compare sex differences in the incidence of sarcopenia, demographic characteristics, and preoperative sarcopenic parameters in patients undergoing TKA for advanced knee OA. Moreover, we also sought to compare PROMs and the predisposing factors after TKA in patients with sarcopenia by sex through subgroup analysis. We hypothesized that (1) the incidence, preoperative parameters, and predisposing factors for sarcopenia in patients undergoing TKA for advanced knee OA would significantly differ between the sexes; (2) when compared with the propensity-matched female control group, inferior improvement would be reported for the male study group.

2. Materials and Methods

2.1. Study Subjects

After obtaining the approval of the institutional review board of our hospital, we conducted a retrospective comparative, single-center study. From May 2020 to September 2022, a consecutive series of 922 patients (1270 knees) who underwent primary TKA were screened. Patients were enrolled who were 60 years of age or older, had symptomatic progressive osteoarthritis (OA) (Kellgren–Lawrence (K–L) grade $\geq$ 3), had a follow-up period of at a minimum of 1 year after index surgery, and were able to be evaluated using preoperative assessments for sarcopenia, including body composition, muscle strength, and physical performance, based on AWGS 2019 criteria (Figure 1) [5].

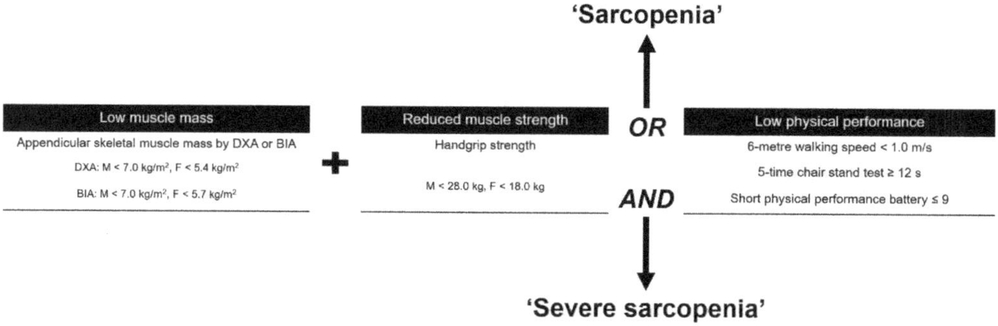

Figure 1. Guideline for the Asian Working Group for Sarcopenia (AWGS) 2020. DXA, dual-energy X-ray absorptiometry; BIA, bioelectrical impedance analysis.

Patients with other diagnoses, such as rheumatoid arthritis or post-traumatic OA, patients who had not been able to walk independently within the previous year because of medical comorbidities (functionally dependent) [12], whose body composition could not be measured because of body metal implants in the appendicular region of the body, and who were severely obese (body mass index (BMI) $\geq$ 35 kg/m^2) were excluded.

2.2. Definition of Sarcopenia

Subjects who had low muscle mass, low muscle strength, and/or low physical performance were classified as having sarcopenia. The skeletal muscle index was measured using whole-body dual-energy X-ray absorptiometry (DXA) (Horizon, Hologic, Bedford, MA, USA) [13]. Appendicular skeletal muscle mass (ASM) was calculated as the sum of arm and leg lean muscle mass [13]. As suggested by Baumgartner et al. [14], ASMI was derived from DXA measurements by dividing ASM by height squared (kg/m^2). Low muscle mass was categorized as ASMI < 5.4 kg/m^2 for women and <7.0 kg/m^2 for men [5]. Isometric handgrip strength was assessed with a grip strength test using a dynamometer (Jamar, Bolingbrook, IL, USA) [15,16]. Low strength was categorized as a handgrip strength < 28 kg for men and <18 kg for women [5]. Physical performance was measured with a walking speed of 6 m; a walking speed of <1.0 m/s for both men and women was defined as low physical performance [5].

2.3. Matched-Pair Analysis

Since attempting to match two untreated subjects to each treated subject would improve precision without a commensurate increase in bias or confounding factors in some settings, we used the two-to-one matched-pair analysis. Based on previous relevant studies [10,17], propensity scores were estimated from multiple logistic regression analyses including all relevant covariates. The matching criteria were age at surgery and BMI. Two-to-one matched-pair analysis was performed using nearest neighbor matching, a propensity score (PS) matching method [18]. All subjects were grouped as either women (F) or men (M), and we conducted matching in the order of the smallest absolute value of the difference in the propensity score (Figure 2).

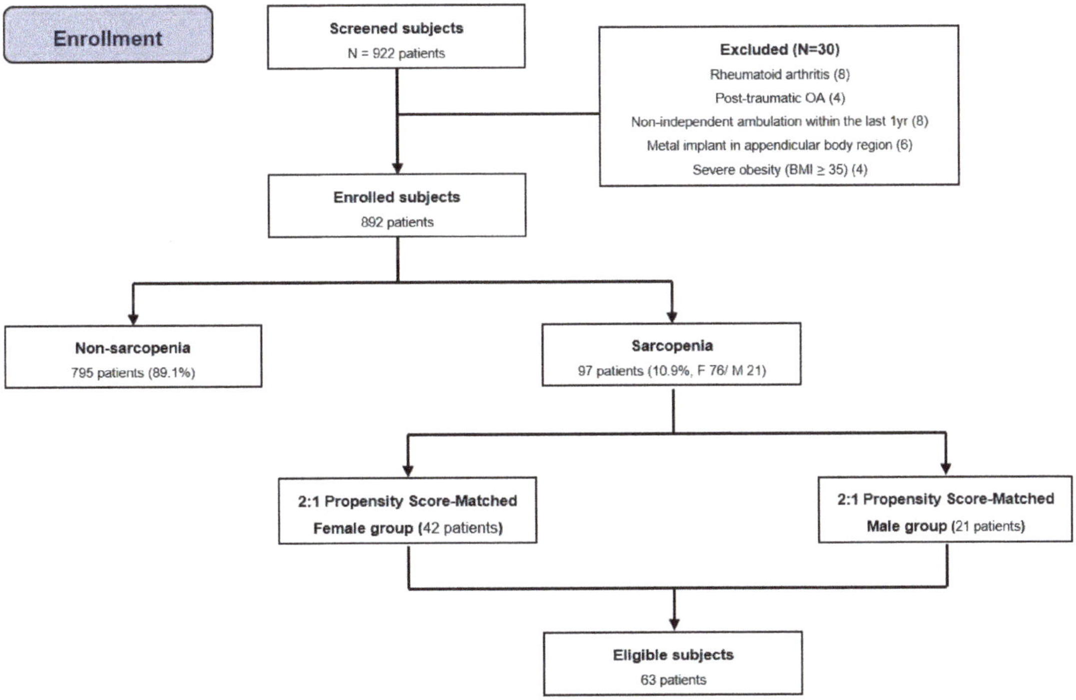

Figure 2. Flow diagram illustrating patient enrollment. Ultimately, 892 patients were enrolled in our study. After 2:1 propensity score matching, 63 patients were analyzed. Note: BMI, body mass index.

When the standardized difference was <0.1 in determining the balance of covariance, it was regarded as balanced matching.

2.4. Operative Details and Postoperative Protocol

All operations were conducted by two experienced orthopedic surgeons in our hospital using the modified gap-balancing technique with the same implant (posterior-stabilized,

Attune® TKA System, Depuy Synthes Inc., Warsaw, IN, USA) [19]. All prostheses were used with cement, and fixed-bearing antioxidant polyethylene inserts were used.

All patients received the same rehabilitation protocol. A closed suction drain was inserted and removed 24 h after the index surgery. The same perioperative pain control protocol was used, including a multimodal drug regimen, intraoperative periarticular injection, and postoperative patient-controlled analgesic device. Postoperative range of motion (ROM) was allowed on the day of surgery. After resolution of acute postoperative pain, partial weight-bearing with a crutch was allowed on the first postoperative day. Full weight-bearing was allowed 2 or 3 weeks after index surgery [20].

2.5. Outcome Assessment

All data were obtained from the institutional electronic medical records. Patient demographic characteristics (including age, sex, BMI, follow-up period, current smoking status, alcohol consumption, and modified Charlson Comorbidity Index (mCCI) [21]); and laboratory data (including hemoglobin (Hb, g/dL) and total protein (TP, g/dL) levels) were compared between the female (F) and male (M) groups. The mCCI was calculated as the sum of the weighted scores for each comorbidity [21] (Table 1).

Table 1. Scoring system for the modified Charlson Comorbidity Index (mCCI) [22].

Variables	Score
Peripheral vascular disease or pain at rest	1
Congestive heart failure	1
Prior myocardial infarction	1
Diabetes mellitus	1
Prior transient ischemic attack or stroke	1
Chronic obstructive pulmonary disease	1
Renal failure	2
Hemiplegia or paraplegia	2
Ascites or esophageal varices	3
Disseminated cancer	6
(Age)	
≤40 years old	0
41–50 years old	1
51–60 years old	2
61–70 years old	3
≥70 years old	4

Note: Different scores were assigned to certain comorbidities and age groups. The final score of the mCCI is the sum of the weighted scores for each comorbidity.

Patients were regularly assessed preoperatively, and at 6 weeks, 6 months, and 12 months postoperatively, and annually thereafter. All clinical outcomes were compared between the groups (group F vs. M).

For assessments of PROMs, the Knee Injury and Osteoarthritis Outcome Score (KOOS) [22], the Western Ontario and McMaster Universities Osteoarthritis Index (WOMAC) [23], and the Short Form (SF)-12 physical and mental component summary scores [24] were investigated. The ROM of the knee joint was assessed using a standardized manual goniometer with a 30 cm long plastic movable arm (from the greater trochanter of the femur to the lateral malleolus) [25]. They were recorded by an independent researcher in the outpatient clinic.

Moreover, the incidence of systemic and specific complications was compared between the groups. Systemic complications were considered such as the worsening of an underlying systemic comorbidity or the development of a new medical problem [26]. Specific complications included the need for postoperative blood transfusion, venous thromboembolism (VTE), periprosthetic joint infection (PJI) [27], and periprosthetic fracture. Patients whose Hb level dropped to less than 7.0 g/dL within 2 weeks of the index surgery received a postoperative blood transfusion [28].

2.6. Statistical Analysis

A statistical evaluation was performed using SPSS version 28 software (IBM Corp, Armonk, NY, USA), and continuous data are expressed as means with range or ± standard deviation. The Kolmogorov–Smirnov test was used to evaluate all dependent variables for normality of distribution and equality of variance. Pearson's two-tailed χ^2 test or Fisher's exact test was used for comparison of proportions between groups. Independent samples *t*-test was performed to detect significant differences between groups. Univariate and multivariate logistic regression analyses were used on categorical and continuous variables to assess for factors impacting the presence of sarcopenia in male patients with end-stage knee OA. For all tests, a p value < 0.05 was considered statistically significant.

3. Results

In total, this study included 892 patients (795 women, 97 men). The average age at surgery was 71.6 years (range, 60–88 years), and the average follow-up period was 24.5 months (range, 12.0–37.0 months) (Table 2).

Table 2. Demographic characteristics according to the presence of sarcopenia.

	Total	Sarcopenia	Non-Sarcopenia	*p* Value
Patients, *n* (%) †	892 (100)	97 (10.9)	795 (89.1)	-
Age (years) *	71.6 (60–88)	75.8 (69–88)	68.7 (60–76)	0.871
Sex, n †				
Female, *n*	785 (88.0)	76 (78.4)	709 (89.2)	0.002
Male, *n*	107 (11.2)	21 (21.6)	86 (10.8)	
BMI (kg/m^2) ‡	26.9 ± 3.7	23.2 ± 3.4	27.5 ± 3.2	<0.001
Mean f/u (mon) *	24.5 (12–37)	24.7 (12–37)	24.4 (12–37)	0.791
Bilaterality, *n* (%) †	381 (42.7)	40 (41.2)	337 (42.4)	0.810
Preop K–L grade, *n* (%) †				
Grade III	226 (25.3)	26 (26.8)	200 (25.2)	0.745
Grade IV	666 (74.7)	71 (73.2)	595 (74.8)	
Current smoker, *n* (%) †	76 (8.5)	12 (12.4)	64 (8.1)	0.165
Alcohol drinker, *n* (%) †	87 (9.8)	15 (15.5)	72 (9.1)	0.060
mCCI †				
2	40 (4.5)	-	40 (5.0)	<0.001
3 and 4	419 (47.0)	7 (7.2)	412 (51.8)	
5–8	316 (35.4)	46 (47.4)	270 (34.0)	
≥9	117 (13.1)	44 (45.4)	73 (9.2)	
Hb level (g/dL) ‡	12.5 ± 2.1	11.1 ± 3.2	12.8 ± 1.0	0.021
Total protein (g/dL) ‡	6.8 ± 1.0	5.9 ± 1.2	7.0 ± 0.9	0.037
ASM index (ASM/height^2), kg/m^2 ‡	6.0 ± 0.6	5.0 ± 0.8	6.3 ± 0.6	0.004
Grip strength, kg ‡	18.0 ± 3.4	16.1 ± 4.5	19.2 ± 3.1	0.030
6 m walking speed, m/s ‡	1.2 ± 0.2	0.8 ± 0.1	1.4 ± 0.2	0.025

Note: BMI, body mass index; f/u, follow-up; Preop, preoperative; K-L, Kellgren–Lawrence; mCCI, modified Charlson Comorbidity Index; Hb, hemoglobin; ASMI, appendicular skeletal muscle mass index. * Values are provided as numbers with ranges. † Values are provided as numbers with percentages. ‡ Values are provided as means ± standard deviations.

The overall prevalence of sarcopenia in this cohort was 10.9% (97/892), and it was more common in male patients (21/107, 19.6%) than in female patients (76/785, 9.7%). After two-to-one matched-pair analysis for subgroup, 21 knees in men were matched with a corresponding number of knees in women (42), resulting in a total of 63 knees (Table 3).

Table 3. Sex differences of demographic characteristics in propensity-matched population.

	2:1 Propensity-Matched Population (n = 63)		
	Female Sarcopenia (n = 42)	**Male Sarcopenia (n = 21)**	**p Value**
Age (years) *	75.6 (70–83)	76.1 (70–82)	0.501
BMI (kg/m^2) ‡	23.0 ± 3.0	23.5 ± 2.9	0.762
Mean f/u (mon) *	24.6 (12–37)	24.6 (12–37)	0.791
Bilaterality, n (%) †	18 (42.9)	9 (42.9)	-
Preop K-L grade, n (%) †			
Grade III	11 (26.2)	5 (23.8)	0.838
Grade IV	31 (73.8)	16 (76.2)	
Current smoker, n (%) †	3 (7.1)	8 (38.1)	0.002
Alcohol drinker, n (%) †	3 (7.1)	10 (47.6)	<0.001
mCCI †			0.022
2	-	-	
3 and 4	6 (9.5)	1 (4.8)	
5–8	28 (54.8)	9 (42.9)	
≥9	8 (35.7)	11(52.4)	
Hb level (g/dL) ‡	9.9 ± 1.3	11.2 ± 1.0	0.021
Total protein (g/dL) ‡	5.2 ± 1.2	5.9 ± 1.2	0.043
ASM index (ASM/height^2), kg/m^2 ‡	4.2 ± 0.5	5.8 ± 0.6	<0.001
Grip strength, kg ‡	15.4 ± 3.3	16.5 ± 3.1	0.021
6 m walking speed, m/s ‡	0.5 ± 0.2	0.9 ± 0.2	0.018

NOTE. BMI, body mass index; f/u, follow-up; Preop, preoperative; K-L, Kellgren–Lawrence; mCCI, modified Charlson Comorbidity Index; Hb, hemoglobin; ASMI, appendicular skeletal muscle mass index. * Values are provided as numbers with ranges. † Values are provided as numbers with percentages. ‡ Values are provided as means ± standard deviations.

In subgroup analyses, male patients with sarcopenia had significantly inferior PROMs up to one year after surgery compared to female patients with sarcopenia (Figure 3A–D).

Meanwhile, there was no significant difference in systemic complications between the two groups (Table 4).

Table 4. Sex differences of systemic and specific complications in propensity-matched cohort.

		Total (n = 63)	**Female (n = 42)**	**Male (n = 21)**	**p-Value**
Systemic	Cardiovascular	2 (3.2)	1 (2.4)	1 (2.4)	0.559
	Pulmonary	4 (6.3)	1 (2.4)	3 (14.3)	0.104
	Gastrointestinal	-	1 (2.3)	-	-
	Hepatic	6 (9.5)	4 (9.5)	2 (9.5)	0.686
	Nephrotic	-	-	-	-
	Endocrinologic	-	-	-	-
	Urologic	13 (20.6)	6 (14.3)	7 (33.3)	<0.001
	Cerebral	2 (3.2)	1 (2.4)	1 (4.8)	0.559
	Delirium	11 (17.5)	9 (21.4)	2 (9.5)	0.085
Specific	Blood transfusion	17 (27.0)	12 (28.6)	5 (23.8)	0.466
	Venous thromboembolism				
	PTE	-	-	-	-
	DVT (proximal)	3 (4.8)	2 (4.8)	1 (4.8)	0.774
	DVT (distal)	6 (9.5)	4 (9.5)	2 (9.5)	0.686
	Infection	2 (3.2)	1 (2.4)	1 (4.8)	0.559
	Periprosthetic fracture	-	-	-	-

Note: PTE, pulmonary thromboembolism; DVT, deep vein thrombosis. Values are provided as number (percentage). DVT was classified as proximal or distal DVT. Thrombi limited to the popliteal vein or above were classified as proximal DVT, and thrombi within the calf vein were classified as distal DVT.

	Preop	6wks	3 mon	6 mon	12 mon	*P* value*
Male group	41.1 ± 2.17	42.0 ± 1.7	49.9 ± 1.7	58.5 ± 1.7	61.9 ± 1.8	0.013
Female group	45.1 ± 2.07	46.4 ± 2.1	55.1± 1.7	60.4 ± 1.7	63.1 ± 1.8	

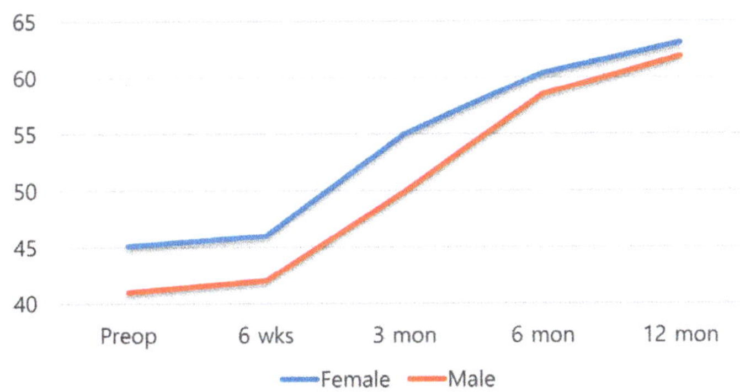

(A)

	Preop	6wks	3 mon	6 mon	12 mon	*P* value*
Male group	53.8 ± 3.4	50.2 ± 3.1	40.9 ± 2.9	29.7 ± 3.0	17.3 ± 2.5	.021
Female group	50.9 ± 2.9	47.8 ± 2.6	33.5 ± 2.5	23.8 ± 2.5	13.3 ± 2.1	

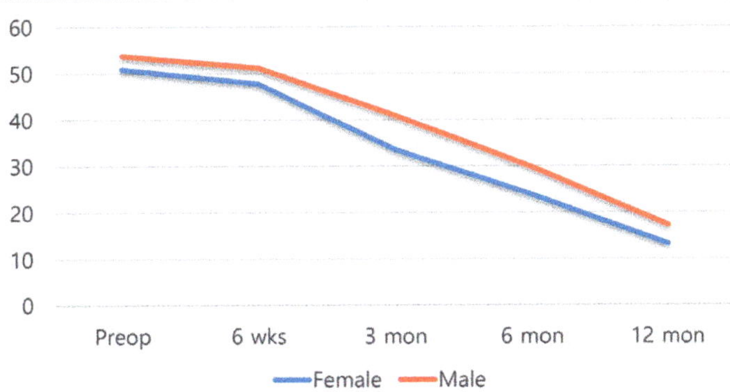

(B)

Figure 3. *Cont.*

	Preop	6wks	3 mon	6 mon	12 mon	*P* value*
Male group	23.2 ± 3.4	34.2 ± 1.9	37.3 ± 2.9	40.3 ± 3.0	41.5 ± 2.5	<0.001
Female group	27.2 ± 2.9	40.5 ± 2.1	44.5 ± 2.5	45.5 ± 2.5	45.6 ± 2.1	

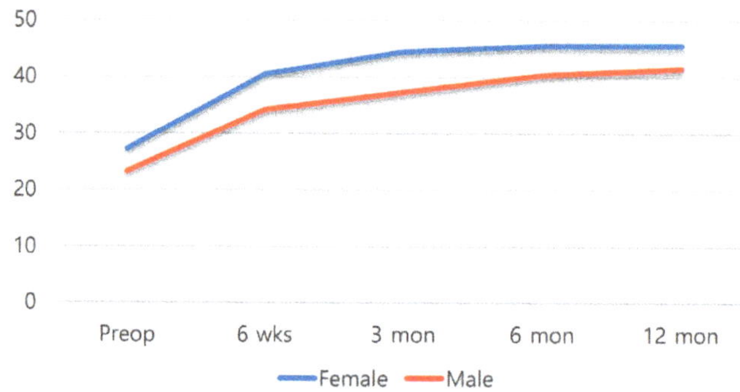

(C)

	Preop	6wks	3 mon	6 mon	12 mon	*P* value*
Male group	55.7 ± 3.4	55.6 ± 1.9	54.3 ± 2.9	55.3 ± 3.0	55.8 ± 2.5	0.435
Female group	56.4 ± 2.9	56.3 ± 2.1	55.8 ± 2.5	55.5 ± 2.5	55.9 ± 2.1	

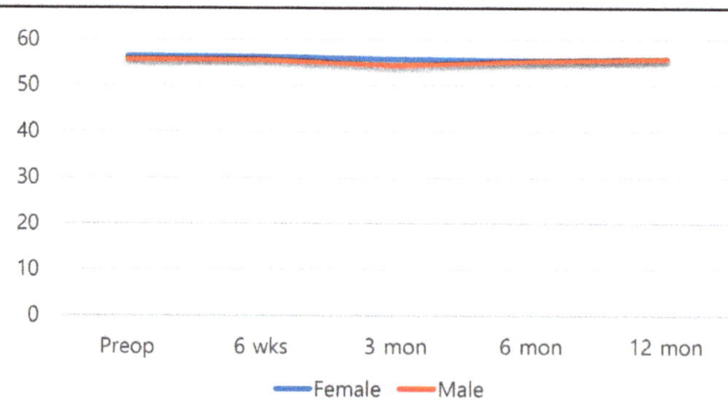

(D)

Figure 3. (**A**) KOOS score. (**B**) WOMAC score. (**C**) SF-12 physical component summary scores. (**D**) SF-12 mental component summary scores. * Independent samples *t*-test was performed to detect significant differences between groups.

The multivariate logistic regression analysis revealed that alcohol consumption and higher mCCI (OR, 1.4; 95% CI, 0.9–1.8; $p = 0.003$), current smoker status (OR, 1.2; 95% CI, 0.9–1.4; $p = 0.019$), and higher mCCI (OR: 1.2; 95% CI: 0.8–1.5; $p = 0.036$) were found to be predisposing risk factors for sarcopenia in male patients (Table 5).

Table 5. Univariate and multivariate logistic regression analyses for the propensity-matched cohort.

Variable	*p* Value		Odds Radio (95% CI)	
	Univariate Analysis	Multivariate Analysis	Univariate Analysis	Multivariate Analysis
Age	0.501		1.8 (0.9–2.7)	
BMI	0.731		1.9 (1.8–2.2)	
Alcohol drinker	<0.001 *	0.003 †	1.5 (0.8–1.7)	1.4 (0.9–1.8)
Current smoker (Preoperative)	<0.001 *	0.019 †	1.3 (1.1–2.5)	1.2 (0.9–1.4)
K–L grade	0.751		1.2 (0.8–1.6)	
mCCI	0.012	0.036 †	1.1 (0.8–1.4)	1.2 (0.8–1.5)
Hb level	0.021 *	0.253	0.8 (0.6–0.9)	0.7 (0.6–0.9)
Total protein	0.037 *	0.302	0.7 (0.5–0.8)	0.6 (0.5–0.8)
ASMI	<0.001 *	0.125	0.7 (0.5–0.8)	0.6 (0.5–0.8)

Note: BMI, body mass index; K-L grade, Kellgren–Lawrence grade; mCCI, modified Charlson Comorbidity Index; Hb, hemoglobin; ASMI, appendicular skeletal muscle index. * Univariate binary logistic regression analysis revealed that alcohol consumption, current smoker status, higher mCCI, preoperative Hb level, total protein, and ASMI were associated with the presence of male sarcopenia. † Multivariate binary logistic regression analysis showed that alcohol consumption, current smoker status, and higher mCCI were found to be predisposing risk factors for the presence of male sarcopenia.

4. Discussion

The most notable finding of the current study was that a propensity score-matched analysis showed inferior PROMs in male patients with sarcopenia undergoing TKA for advanced knee OA up to one year after index surgery. Furthermore, multivariate logistic regression analysis identified alcohol consumption, smoking, and higher mCCI as predisposing risk factors for sarcopenia in male patients in this cohort. To the best of our knowledge, some recent studies have reported the incidence or outcomes of sarcopenia in patients with knee OA [7,17,29]. However, few studies have reported sex differences in patients with sarcopenia undergoing TKA for advanced knee OA. Our study illustrates a higher prevalence of sarcopenia in male patients (19.6%) with end-stage OA of the knee joint compared to female patients (9.7%). This is consistent with the prevalence reported in studies of sarcopenia patients with musculoskeletal disorders. Studies that assessed the effectiveness of TKA in patients with end-stage knee OA with or without sarcopenia showed a high prevalence of sarcopenia in male patients (approximately 41.7%) compared to female patients (30.4%) [7]. Although in different disease entities, studies of sarcopenia in hip and distal radius fracture patients reported from Asia have all reported a higher prevalence in male patients than in female patients [30–32]. Another study analyzing factors associated with sarcopenia reported that male sex and smoking were independently associated with pre-sarcopenia, sarcopenia, and severe sarcopenia [33]. This study reported a higher prevalence of sarcopenia in older males than in females and suggested that the sex differences in prevalence may be due to sex differences in insulin growth factor-1 levels [33,34].

Notably, male patients with sarcopenia showed significantly inferior PROMs up to 1 year after TKA in the present study. Men typically gain an average of 40% more lean body mass and 60% more strength than women over the course of several decades of their lives [35]. As men typically maintain higher levels of physical activity and therefore higher levels of muscle strength than women [36], they may be more susceptible to muscle loss if their activity is reduced by knee OA. Female patients may be less susceptible to the adverse effects of limited physical activity due to knee OA because they are naturally less physically active than male patients. Therefore, for male sarcopenic patients with advanced knee OA, increasing muscle mass through regular exercise, especially resistance or strength training, along with eating a balanced diet that includes adequate proteins are crucial measures to prevent or slow down the progression of sarcopenia.

In the present study, a higher mCCI was found to be one of the predisposing factors for male sarcopenia patients with advanced knee OA. Several studies have reported that the mCCI reflects the overall health status and even the mortality rate based on the multiple comorbidities of a patient [21,37,38]. On average, male sarcopenia patients present poorer overall health status, as measured using the mCCI, which may compromise their ability to recover from muscle loss and physical activity limitations, compared to female patients with similar levels of knee OA. A study comparing mortality rates between the sexes for low-energy proximal femur fractures showed that men had a higher risk of death than women [37]. The study reported that men had a higher mean age-adjusted CCI and that this poorer health status could affect not only the fracture itself but also the ability to recover from the injury. A comparison of our with the multiple comorbidities found to be significantly more common in male sarcopenia with advanced knee OA suggests that a decreased overall health status may predispose these men to poorer functional recovery after TKA.

Lifestyle behaviors such as alcohol consumption and smoking have been identified as risk factors for muscle weakness due to loss of muscle mass and strength [39,40]. Although there is some variation based on nationality and culture, men are much more likely to drink alcohol than women. According to a study based on the 2010–2012 National China Nutrition and Health Survey, the prevalence of alcohol consumption was about four times higher among men than women [41]. Similarly, about 49.8% of adult men and 4.2% of adult women in South Korea were identified as smokers, according to the 2017 World Health Organization report [42]. Our results suggest that alcohol consumption and smoking may have detrimental effects on muscle mass in male patients undergoing TKA for advanced knee OA.

Despite these informative outcomes, there are some limitations associated with our study. First, this study had a relatively small sample size. This may be due to the fact that women more commonly undergo TKA for advanced knee OA in Asia than men [43], so less screening is conducted for sarcopenia in this limited number of male patients. Further studies in larger cohorts or community-dwelling populations are needed to confirm the findings of this study. Second, this study had a short follow-up period, which may have missed significant differences. In addition, the current results are not necessarily indicative of longer-term outcomes. Third, this study was not able to identify underlying causes, such as hormonal changes or reduced physical activity, for the sex differences in sarcopenia. As people age, many factors contribute to the development of sarcopenia, including hormonal changes, reduced physical activity, poor nutrition, and certain health conditions. However, this study showed that alcohol consumption, smoking, and mCCI may be predisposing factors in male sarcopenia patients with advanced knee OA. Further studies are needed to determine the relevance of hormonal or specific physical activity changes in men in relation to the progression of sarcopenia. Fourth, since this study only included patients with limited grades of OA (K-L grade III or IV), the results may not be comparable to those of all male patients with other grades of OA.

5. Conclusions

The prevalence of sarcopenia was higher in male patients undergoing primary TKA. When compared with the propensity-matched female group, male patients had inferior PROMs up to 12 months postoperatively. Alcohol consumption, current smoker status, and higher mCCI were predisposing factors for sarcopenia in male patients with advanced knee OA.

Author Contributions: Conceptualization, G.B.K.; methodology, G.B.K. and O.-J.S.; formal analysis, G.B.K. and S.H.J.; resources, G.B.K.; data curation, G.B.K. and S.H.J.; writing—original draft preparation, G.B.K.; writing—review and editing, G.B.K. and O.-J.S.; visualization, G.B.K.; supervision, O.-J.S.; project administration, G.B.K.; funding acquisition, G.B.K. All authors have read and agreed to the published version of the manuscript.

Funding: This research was supported by Basic Science Research Program through the National Research Foundation of Korea (NRF), funded by the Ministry of Education (2021R1A6A1A03040177).

Institutional Review Board Statement: This study was conducted according to the guidelines of the Declaration of Helsinki and approved by the Institutional Review Board of the Yeungnam University Medical Center (Protocol No. 2022-10-022, date: 14 October 2022).

Informed Consent Statement: Informed consent was obtained from all the subjects involved in this study. Written informed consent has been obtained from the patients to publish this paper.

Data Availability Statement: Data supporting the reported findings are available from the corresponding author upon reasonable request.

Conflicts of Interest: The authors declare no conflicts of interest.

References

1. Evans, W.J. Sarcopenia should reflect the contribution of age-associated changes in skeletal muscle to risk of morbidity and mortality in elderly people. *J. Am. Med. Dir. Assoc.* **2015**, *16*, 546–547. [CrossRef]
2. Cruz-Jentoft, A.J.; Bahat, G.; Bauer, J.; Boirie, Y.; Bruyère, O.; Cederholm, T.; Cooper, C.; Landi, F.; Rolland, Y.; Sayer, A.A. Sarcopenia: Revised european consensus on definition and diagnosis. *Age Ageing* **2019**, *48*, 16–31. [CrossRef] [PubMed]
3. Cruz-Jentoft, A.J.; Baeyens, J.P.; Bauer, J.M.; Boirie, Y.; Cederholm, T.; Landi, F.; Martin, F.C.; Michel, J.-P.; Rolland, Y.; Schneider, S.M. Sarcopenia: European consensus on definition and diagnosisreport of the european working group on sarcopenia in older people. *Age Ageing* **2010**, *39*, 412–423. [CrossRef] [PubMed]
4. Bokshan, S.L.; Han, A.L.; DePasse, J.M.; Eltorai, A.E.; Marcaccio, S.E.; Palumbo, M.A.; Daniels, A.H. Effect of sarcopenia on postoperative morbidity and mortality after thoracolumbar spine surgery. *Orthopedics* **2016**, *39*, e1159–e1164. [CrossRef]
5. Chen, L.-K.; Woo, J.; Assantachai, P.; Auyeung, T.-W.; Chou, M.-Y.; Iijima, K.; Jang, H.C.; Kang, L.; Kim, M.; Kim, S. Asian working group for sarcopenia: 2019 consensus update on sarcopenia diagnosis and treatment. *J. Am. Med. Dir. Assoc.* **2020**, *21*, 300–307.e302. [CrossRef] [PubMed]
6. Goates, S.; Du, K.; Arensberg, M.; Gaillard, T.; Guralnik, J.; Pereira, S. Economic impact of hospitalizations in us adults with sarcopenia. *J. Frailty Aging* **2019**, *8*, 93–99. [CrossRef]
7. Ho, K.K.-W.; Lau, L.C.-M.; Chau, W.-W.; Poon, Q.; Chung, K.-Y.; Wong, R.M.-Y. End-stage knee osteoarthritis with and without sarcopenia and the effect of knee arthroplasty–A prospective cohort study. *BMC Geriatr.* **2021**, *21*, 2. [CrossRef] [PubMed]
8. Babu, J.M.; Kalagara, S.; Durand, W.; Antoci, V.; Deren, M.E.; Cohen, E. Sarcopenia as a risk factor for prosthetic infection after total hip or knee arthroplasty. *J. Arthroplast.* **2019**, *34*, 116–122. [CrossRef]
9. Koh, I.J.; Kim, T.K.; Chang, C.B.; Cho, H.J.; In, Y. Trends in use of total knee arthroplasty in Korea from 2001 to 2010. *Clin. Orthop. Relat. Res.* **2013**, *471*, 1441–1450. [CrossRef]
10. Hwang, D.; Han, H.-S.; Lee, M.C.; Ro, D.H. Low muscle mass is an independent risk factor for postoperative blood transfusion in total knee arthroplasty: A retrospective, propensity score-matched cohort study. *BMC Geriatr.* **2022**, *22*, 218. [CrossRef]
11. Kim, T.W.; Kang, S.-B.; Chang, C.B.; Moon, S.-Y.; Lee, Y.-K.; Koo, K.-H. Current trends and projected burden of primary and revision total knee arthroplasty in Korea between 2010 and 2030. *J. Arthroplast.* **2021**, *36*, 93–101. [CrossRef]
12. Tay, L.; Ding, Y.; Leung, B.; Ismail, N.; Yeo, A.; Yew, S.; Tay, K.; Tan, C.; Chong, M. Sex-specific differences in risk factors for sarcopenia amongst community-dwelling older adults. *Age* **2015**, *37*, 121. [CrossRef]
13. Heymsfield, S.B.; Smith, R.; Aulet, M.; Bensen, B.; Lichtman, S.; Wang, J.; Pierson, R., Jr. Appendicular skeletal muscle mass: Measurement by dual-photon absorptiometry. *Am. J. Clin. Nutr.* **1990**, *52*, 214–218. [CrossRef] [PubMed]
14. Baumgartner, R.N.; Koehler, K.M.; Gallagher, D.; Romero, L.; Heymsfield, S.B.; Ross, R.R.; Garry, P.J.; Lindeman, R.D. Epidemiology of sarcopenia among the elderly in new mexico. *Am. J. Epidemiol.* **1998**, *147*, 755–763. [CrossRef] [PubMed]
15. Roberts, H.C.; Denison, H.J.; Martin, H.J.; Patel, H.P.; Syddall, H.; Cooper, C.; Sayer, A.A. A review of the measurement of grip strength in clinical and epidemiological studies: Towards a standardised approach. *Age Ageing* **2011**, *40*, 423–429. [CrossRef] [PubMed]
16. Mathiowetz, V.; Kashman, N.; Volland, G.; Weber, K.; Dowe, M.; Rogers, S. Grip and pinch strength: Normative data for adults. *Arch. Phys. Med. Rehabil.* **1985**, *66*, 69–74. [PubMed]
17. Shon, O.-J.; Kim, G.B.; Cho, S.J. Does sarcopenia accompanying end-stage knee osteoarthritis affect the outcomes following total knee arthroplasty? *Medicina* **2023**, *59*, 1078. [CrossRef] [PubMed]
18. Austin, P.C. Statistical criteria for selecting the optimal number of untreated subjects matched to each treated subject when using many-to-one matching on the propensity score. *Am. J. Epidemiol.* **2010**, *172*, 1092–1097. [CrossRef] [PubMed]
19. Daines, B.K.; Dennis, D.A. Gap balancing vs. Measured resection technique in total knee arthroplasty. *Clin. Orthop. Surg.* **2014**, *6*, 1–8. [CrossRef]
20. Shon, O.-J.; Kim, G.B. Does the degree of intraoperatively identified cartilage loss affect the outcomes of primary total knee arthroplasty without patella resurfacing? A prospective comparative cohort study. *Knee Surg. Relat. Res.* **2022**, *34*, 36. [CrossRef]
21. Lakomkin, N.; Zuckerman, S.L.; Stannard, B.; Montejo, J.; Sussman, E.S.; Virojanapa, J.; Kuzmik, G.; Goz, V.; Hadjipanayis, C.G.; Cheng, J.S. Preoperative risk stratification in spine tumor surgery: A comparison of the modified charlson index, frailty index, and asa score. *Spine* **2019**, *44*, E782–E787. [CrossRef] [PubMed]

22. Lyman, S.; Lee, Y.-Y.; Franklin, P.D.; Li, W.; Cross, M.B.; Padgett, D.E. Validation of the koos, jr: A short-form knee arthroplasty outcomes survey. *Clin. Orthop. Relat. Res.* **2016**, *474*, 1461–1471. [CrossRef] [PubMed]
23. Bellamy, N.; Buchanan, W.W.; Goldsmith, C.H.; Campbell, J.; Stitt, L.W. Validation study of womac: A health status instrument for measuring clinically important patient relevant outcomes to antirheumatic drug therapy in patients with osteoarthritis of the hip or knee. *J. Rheumatol.* **1988**, *15*, 1833–1840. [PubMed]
24. Ware, J.E., Jr.; Kosinski, M.; Keller, S.D. A 12-item short-form health survey: Construction of scales and preliminary tests of reliability and validity. *Med. Care* **1996**, *34*, 220–233. [CrossRef]
25. Norkin, C.C.; White, D.J. *Measurement of Joint Motion: A Guide to Goniometry*; FA Davis: Philadelphia, PA, USA, 2016.
26. Song, S.J.; Kim, K.I.; Bae, D.K.; Park, C.H. Mid-term lifetime survivals of octogenarians following primary and revision total knee arthroplasties were satisfactory: A retrospective single center study in contemporary period. *Knee Surg. Relat. Res.* **2020**, *32*, 50. [CrossRef] [PubMed]
27. Parvizi, J.; Tan, T.L.; Goswami, K.; Higuera, C.; Della Valle, C.; Chen, A.F.; Shohat, N. The 2018 definition of periprosthetic hip and knee infection: An evidence-based and validated criteria. *J. Arthroplast.* **2018**, *33*, 1309–1314.e1302. [CrossRef] [PubMed]
28. Jo, C.; Ko, S.; Shin, W.C.; Han, H.-S.; Lee, M.C.; Ko, T.; Ro, D.H. Transfusion after total knee arthroplasty can be predicted using the machine learning algorithm. *Knee Surg. Sports Traumatol. Arthrosc.* **2020**, *28*, 1757–1764. [CrossRef]
29. Kemmler, W.; Teschler, M.; Goisser, S.; Bebenek, M.; von Stengel, S.; Bollheimer, L.C.; Sieber, C.C.; Freiberger, E. Prevalence of sarcopenia in germany and the corresponding effect of osteoarthritis in females 70 years and older living in the community: Results of the formosa study. *Clin. Interv. Aging* **2015**, *2015*, 1565–1573. [CrossRef]
30. Roh, Y.H.; Koh, Y.D.; Noh, J.H.; Gong, H.S.; Baek, G.H. Evaluation of sarcopenia in patients with distal radius fractures. *Arch. Osteoporos.* **2017**, *12*, 5. [CrossRef]
31. Ho, A.W.; Lee, M.M.; Chan, E.W.; Ng, H.M.; Lee, C.; Ng, W.; Wong, S. Prevalence of pre-sarcopenia and sarcopenia in hong kong chinese geriatric patients with hip fracture and its correlation with different factors. *Hong Kong Med. J.* **2016**, *22*, 23. [CrossRef]
32. Yoo, J.-I.; Ha, Y.-C.; Kwon, H.-B.; Lee, Y.-K.; Koo, K.-H.; Yoo, M.-J. High prevalence of sarcopenia in korean patients after hip fracture: A case-control study. *J. Korean Med. Sci.* **2016**, *31*, 1479–1484. [CrossRef]
33. Hashemi, R.; Shafiee, G.; Motlagh, A.D.; Pasalar, P.; Esmailzadeh, A.; Siassi, F.; Larijani, B.; Heshmat, R. Sarcopenia and its associated factors in iranian older individuals: Results of sarir study. *Arch. Gerontol. Geriatr.* **2016**, *66*, 18–22. [CrossRef]
34. Yamada, M.; Nishiguchi, S.; Fukutani, N.; Tanigawa, T.; Yukutake, T.; Kayama, H.; Aoyama, T.; Arai, H. Prevalence of sarcopenia in community-dwelling japanese older adults. *J. Am. Med. Dir. Assoc.* **2013**, *14*, 911–915. [CrossRef]
35. Boot, A.M.; de Ridder, M.A.; van der Sluis, I.M.; van Slobbe, I.; Krenning, E.P.; de Muinck Keizer-Schrama, S.M. Peak bone mineral density, lean body mass and fractures. *Bone* **2010**, *46*, 336–341. [CrossRef] [PubMed]
36. Dodds, R.M.; Syddall, H.E.; Cooper, R.; Benzeval, M.; Deary, I.J.; Dennison, E.M.; Der, G.; Gale, C.R.; Inskip, H.M.; Jagger, C. Grip strength across the life course: Normative data from twelve british studies. *PLoS ONE* **2014**, *9*, e113637. [CrossRef] [PubMed]
37. Schultz, K.A.; Westcott, B.A.; Barber, K.R.; Sandrock, T.A. Elevated 1-year mortality rate in males sustaining low-energy proximal femur fractures and subgroup analysis utilizing age-adjusted charlson comorbidity index. *Geriatr. Orthop. Surg. Rehabil.* **2020**, *11*, 2151459319898644. [CrossRef] [PubMed]
38. Schnell, S.; Friedman, S.M.; Mendelson, D.A.; Bingham, K.W.; Kates, S.L. The 1-year mortality of patients treated in a hip fracture program for elders. *Geriatr. Orthop. Surg. Rehabil.* **2010**, *1*, 6–14. [CrossRef] [PubMed]
39. Clark, D.J.; Patten, C.; Reid, K.F.; Carabello, R.J.; Phillips, E.M.; Fielding, R.A. Impaired voluntary neuromuscular activation limits muscle power in mobility-limited older adults. *J. Gerontol. A Biol. Sci. Med. Sci.* **2010**, *65*, 495–502. [CrossRef] [PubMed]
40. Zhai, J.; Ma, B.; Qin, J.; Lyu, Q.; Khatun, P.; Liang, R.; Cong, M.; Guo, L.; Kong, Y. Alcohol consumption patterns and the risk of sarcopenia: A population-based cross-sectional study among chinese women and men from henan province. *BMC Public Health* **2022**, *22*, 1894. [CrossRef] [PubMed]
41. Li, Y.; Wang, J.; Zhao, L.; Wang, Z.; Yu, D.; He, Y.; Ding, G. The drinking status and associated factors in adults in china. *Zhonghua Liu Xing Bing Xue Za Zhi* **2018**, *39*, 898–903. [PubMed]
42. World Health Organization. *World Health Organization (WHO) Report on the Global Tobacco Epidemic 2017-Country Profile Portugal*; World Health Organization: Geneva, Switzerland, 2017; Volume 10, p. 9781410610348.
43. Park, H.-R.; Cho, S.-K.; Im, S.G.; Jung, S.-Y.; Kim, D.; Jang, E.J.; Sung, Y.-K. Treatment patterns of knee osteoarthritis patients in korea. *Korean J. Intern. Med.* **2019**, *34*, 1145. [CrossRef] [PubMed]

medicina

MDPI

Article

Preoperative Central Sensitization Worsens Pain and Dissatisfaction Following Unicompartmental Knee Arthroplasty

Man-Soo Kim , Keun-Young Choi and Yong In *

Department of Orthopaedic Surgery, Seoul St. Mary's Hospital, College of Medicine, The Catholic University of Korea, 222, Banpo-daero, Seocho-gu, Seoul 06591, Republic of Korea; kms3779@naver.com (M.-S.K.); heaxagon@hanmail.net (K.-Y.C.)

* Correspondence: iy1000@catholic.ac.kr

Abstract: *Background and Objectives*: Central sensitization (CS) has been identified as a significant factor influencing persistent pain and dissatisfaction following total knee arthroplasty (TKA). However, its effect on unicompartmental knee arthroplasty (UKA) remains largely unexplored. Unlike TKA, UKA preserves most native knee structures, with less bone cut, leading to different postoperative pain mechanisms. Nevertheless, the revision rate for unexplained pain following UKA is higher than after TKA. This study investigates the influence of preoperative CS on pain and dissatisfaction after UKA. *Materials and Methods*: This retrospective cohort study included 121 patients who underwent primary UKA for medial compartment osteoarthritis of the knee. Patients were screened for CS preoperatively using the Central Sensitization Inventory (CSI) and categorized into a CS group (CSI $\geq$ 40; n = 26) and a non-CS group (CSI < 40; n = 95). Clinical outcomes, including the Western Ontario and McMaster Universities Osteoarthritis Index (WOMAC), Forgotten Joint Score (FJS), and patient satisfaction, were assessed at the 2-year postoperative follow-up visit. A multivariate regression analysis was used to determine the risk factors for postoperative dissatisfaction. *Results*: The CS group reported significantly worse postoperative WOMAC pain, function, and total scores than the non-CS group (all $p < 0.05$). FJS was also significantly worse in the CS group than in the non-CS group (64.4 vs. 72.7, respectively, $p = 0.005$). Patient satisfaction was significantly lower in the CS group than in the non-CS group (65.4% vs. 95.8%, respectively, $p < 0.001$). The multivariate logistic regression analysis demonstrated that patients with a CSI score $\geq$ 40 had an 11.349-fold increased likelihood of dissatisfaction after UKA (95% CI: 2.315–55.626, $p = 0.003$). *Conclusions*: This study underscores the importance of recognizing CS as a critical determinant of postoperative pain and functional recovery following UKA. Patients with high CSI scores experience greater pain, increased joint awareness, and overall poorer satisfaction despite technically successful surgeries.

Keywords: central sensitization; pain; dissatisfaction; unicomparmental knee arthroplasty

1. Introduction

Unicompartmental knee arthroplasty (UKA) is a well-established surgical procedure for treating unicompartmental osteoarthritis (OA), offering a less invasive alternative to total knee arthroplasty (TKA) with generally favorable outcomes [1–4]. However, a certain proportion of UKA patients experience persistent postoperative pain and discomfort, even in the absence of clear radiographic abnormalities or mechanical complications [5–7].

Among all revision cases, the proportion of revisions performed due to unexplained pain was higher after UKA (23%) than TKA (9%), raising concerns about factors influencing postoperative pain perception [5].

Persistent postoperative pain after knee arthroplasty has traditionally been attributed to peripheral mechanisms such as residual inflammation, tissue damage, or prosthetic malalignment, which activate peripheral nociceptors and lead to peripheral sensitization [8,9]. However, recent evidence suggests that in many chronic pain cases, particularly without clear anatomical abnormalities, central sensitization (CS) may play a key role. CS is a maladaptive response of the central nervous system marked by heightened pain sensitivity, reduced inhibitory control, and glial activation, often leading to allodynia and hyperalgesia [9,10]. This central amplification of pain signals—also referred to as "centralized pain," "central augmentation," or "pain hypersensitivity"—can persist long after the initial surgical insult has resolved [9,10]. In such cases, the brain and spinal cord essentially 'turn up the volume' of pain processing, independent of ongoing peripheral input [9,10]. This phenomenon helps explain why some patients report severe pain after knee arthroplasty despite good surgical outcomes and the absence of detectable complications [9,10].

Recent research has explored the role of CS in persistent pain following joint arthroplasty [8–10]. CS is a condition characterized by an exaggerated pain response due to alterations in central nervous system processing [8–10]. It is mediated by neurotransmitters such as serotonin and norepinephrine and leads to increased sensitivity to pain stimuli, lowered pain thresholds, and prolonged pain perception even after the initial source of pain has been resolved [8–10]. Patients with CS often report widespread pain, hyperalgesia, and allodynia, which can significantly affect their recovery following orthopedic procedures [8–10].

Previous studies have established a link between CS and poor outcomes following TKA [11–16]. Patients with high preoperative pain levels and low pain thresholds are more likely than others to experience severe postoperative pain and dissatisfaction, despite successful surgical intervention [11–16]. However, the role of CS in UKA remains relatively underexplored. Given that UKA is a less invasive procedure that preserves the surrounding soft tissues, it might be assumed that patients would experience less postoperative pain than TKA patients [3]. Persistent pain in a subset of UKA patients suggests that factors beyond structural abnormalities could be contributing to suboptimal outcomes [7].

Understanding the association between CS and postoperative pain in UKA patients is crucial for improving patient outcomes. Identifying patients with preoperative CS could allow for the implementation of targeted perioperative strategies to mitigate its effects. The purpose of this study was to investigate whether preoperative CS is associated with worse postoperative outcomes, including pain, function, and satisfaction, in patients undergoing UKA. We hypothesized that patients with preoperative CS would report inferior clinical outcomes and lower satisfaction following UKA compared to those without CS.

2. Materials and Methods

2.1. Study Design

This study used a retrospective cohort design to evaluate the effects of CS on postoperative outcomes following UKA. The study was conducted at a single tertiary medical center, and all procedures were performed by a single experienced orthopedic surgeon to minimize variability in surgical technique. Ethical approval for this study was obtained from the institutional review board, and informed consent was obtained from all patients prior to participation.

2.2. Patient Selection

Data from 131 patients who underwent unilateral UKA between 2014 and 2022 were initially included in the study. The inclusion criteria were as follows: (1) isolated medial compartment OA with an intact anterior cruciate ligament, (2) correctable varus deformity (less than 10 degrees), (3) minimum two-year follow-up period, and (4) no history of prior knee surgery on the affected side. Patients were excluded if they had: inflammatory arthritis (e.g., rheumatoid arthritis), osteonecrosis affecting the knee joint (1 patient), post-traumatic OA (1 patient), a history of knee infection, a documented history of CS-related conditions such as irritable bowel syndrome (1 patient) and chronic low back pain (2 patients), prior use of centrally acting agents or patients with diagnosed psychiatric conditions known to affect CS, such as anxiety or depressive disorders (2 patients), incomplete clinical outcome data (2 patients), or a subsequent operation on either knee during the follow-up period (1 patient). All patients were clinically screened for signs of peripheral neuropathy, including diabetic neuropathy, through neurologic examination and medical history review. Patients with confirmed or suspected peripheral neuropathy were excluded from the study. Notably, none of the enrolled participants exhibited clinical evidence of peripheral neuropathy. Following the application of those criteria, 10 patients were excluded from the study, resulting in a final cohort of 121 patients (Figure 1). All analyses were limited to patients who met the criteria for medial UKA, stratified by CS status. Patient demographics and baseline characteristics, including body mass index (BMI), comorbidities, and preoperative functional status, were collected through medical records and patient-reported questionnaires.

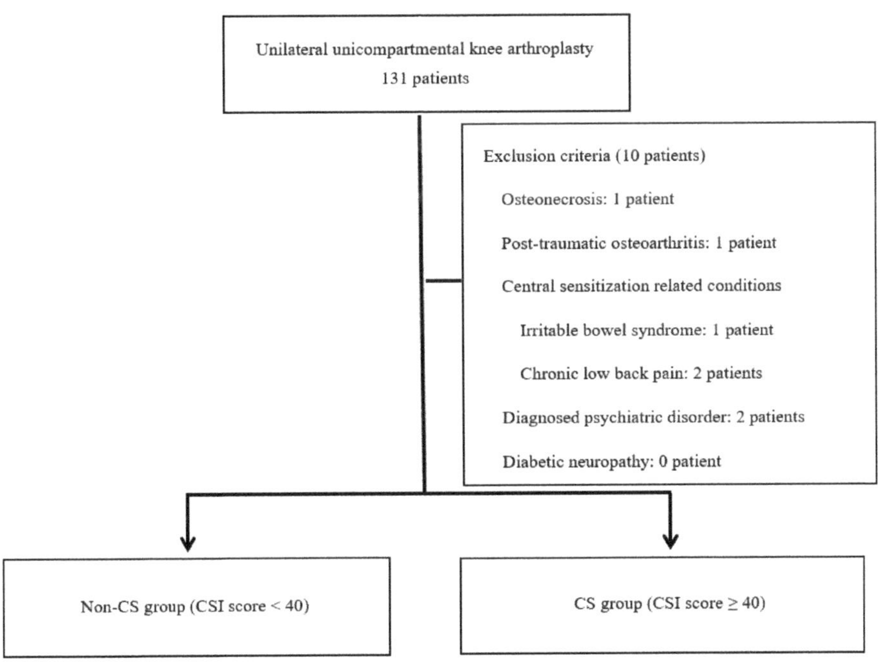

Figure 1. Participant flow diagram. CS: Central Sensitization, CSI: Central Sensitization Inventory.

CS is influenced by both non-modifiable factors, such as female sex [17] and genetic predisposition [18], and modifiable factors, including poor sleep, psychological distress, and CS-related conditions like restless leg syndrome or chronic fatigue syndrome [19,20]. To minimize confounding, we excluded patients with major psychiatric disorders, pain catastrophizing tendencies, or clinical features of CS-related diseases through thorough medical record reviews and preoperative interviews. This approach aimed to enhance the specificity of our findings on the impact of CS [19,20].

2.3. Assessment of Central Sensitization

The Central Sensitization Inventory (CSI) is commonly used to assess CS and offers significant practical benefits in clinical settings [17,18]. The CSI is a validated self-reported questionnaire designed to evaluate symptoms associated with CS. Unlike quantitative sensory testing (QST), which objectively measures sensory responses to external stimuli, the CSI focuses on subjective symptom assessment [17,18].

The CSI questionnaire consists of 25 items that capture a broad spectrum of somatic and emotional symptoms frequently observed in individuals with CS [17,18]. These include headaches, fatigue, sleep disturbances, cognitive difficulties, and psychological distress, as well as heightened pain sensitivity that can interfere with daily life. The CSI specifically evaluates the presence of unrefreshing sleep, muscle stiffness and pain, anxiety attacks, bruxism, gastrointestinal disturbances (diarrhea/constipation), difficulty daily activities, light sensitivity, physical fatigue, widespread pain, urinary discomfort, poor sleep quality, concentration issues, skin problems, stress-related physical symptoms, depression, low energy, muscle tension in the neck and shoulders, jaw pain, dizziness or nausea triggered by certain smells, frequent urination, restless legs, memory impairment, childhood trauma, and pelvic pain [17,18].

Each item is rated on a 5-point Likert scale ranging from 0 (never) to 4 (always), with a total possible score of 0 to 100. According to Neblett et al. [18], a score of 40 or higher suggests the presence of CS. The CSI is easy to administer, takes less than 10 min to complete, and does not require specialized equipment. Additionally, because it incorporates non-painful and hypothetical scenarios, it avoids ethical concerns associated with other assessment methods. These advantages make the CSI a highly useful tool for evaluating the severity of CS-related symptoms. It is widely recognized as a reliable and validated measure for quantifying CS symptom severity [17,18] (Supplementary Figure S1).

2.4. Surgical Procedure and Postoperative Management

All UKA procedures were performed by a single surgeon using a standardized minimally invasive approach. The same cemented, mobile-bearing (MB) UKA system (Microplasty Oxford MB UKA, Zimmer Biomet, Warsaw, IN, USA) was used in all cases to ensure consistency across patients. All operations were performed under general anesthesia through the mini-medial parapatellar approach. A pneumatic tourniquet that inflated to 300 mmHg was applied. The medial meniscus was resected, and the osteophytes of the medial femoral condyle and tibial plateau were carefully removed. With the Microplasty Oxford MB UKA system, the femoral gap-sizing spoons and G-clamp were used to assess the femoral component size, tibial cutting depth, and orientation. After determining the size of the medial femoral condyle and evaluating the gap between the femur and tibia using a series of femoral sizing spoons, the most suitable spoon was selected and positioned on the MFC. After securing the gap-sizing spoon to the tibial resection guide with the G-clamp, the guide was aligned parallel to the long axis of the tibia in both the coronal and sagittal planes. The tibia was then resected, and an intramedullary rod with a distal linking feature was inserted into the femoral canal until fully seated. With the IM link engaged, the femoral drill guide was positioned on the tibial cut surface to determine the femoral component position. A posterior femoral condylar cut was performed along the femoral cutting guide. Subsequently, distal femoral milling was carefully performed to balance the flexion and extension gaps without ligament release. Cement fixation was used for all femoral and tibial components. A compressive bandage was applied postoperatively.

Patients were allowed full weight-bearing on postoperative day 1 with the assistance of a walker, and a structured physical therapy program was initiated to optimize range of motion and quadriceps strengthening. The same preemptive multimodal analgesic regimen was applied to all patients. Postoperatively, intravenous patient-controlled analgesia, programmed to deliver 1 mL of a 100-mL solution containing 2000 μg of fentanyl, was used. Once the patients restarted oral intake, they received 10 mg of oxycodone every 12 h for one week, along with 200 mg of celecoxib, 37.5 mg of tramadol, and 650 mg of acetaminophen every 12 h for six weeks. Subsequent visits were scheduled at two weeks, six weeks, three months, six months, and one year, with yearly visits thereafter.

2.5. Outcome Measures

Postoperative outcomes were assessed at baseline and two years using validated patient-reported outcome measures (PROMs). Pain, stiffness, and function were evaluated using the Western Ontario and McMaster Universities Osteoarthritis Index (WOMAC), a well-established tool for assessing clinically relevant outcomes in patients undergoing treatment for OA of the hip or knee [19]. Additionally, joint awareness during daily activities was measured using the Forgotten Joint Score (FJS), which has been validated as a key indicator of successful joint arthroplasty [20]. To assess patient satisfaction, the new Knee Society Satisfaction (KSS) score, a five-item questionnaire designed to evaluate satisfaction with daily activities, was used. Patients were categorized as satisfied (total score 21–40) or dissatisfied (0–20), following the scoring system developed by Noble et al. [21] In addition to PROMs, postoperative complications—infection, implant loosening, and the need for revision surgery—were systematically recorded to provide a comprehensive evaluation of surgical outcomes.

3. Statistical Analysis

All data are presented as the mean and standard deviation. Data were compared between the non-CS group (preoperative CSI score < 40) and the CS group (preoperative CSI score $\geq$ 40). Continuous variables were analyzed using independent *t*-tests, and categorical variables were compared using chi-square tests. Patient demographics and surgical characteristics were collected as dependent variables to identify risk factors for patient dissatisfaction. A multivariable logistic regression analysis was conducted to evaluate associated factors, using a backward elimination approach to retain significant predictors of postoperative dissatisfaction following UKA. Odds ratios were calculated with 95% confidence intervals (CIs). Statistical analysis was performed using SPSS® for Windows v21.0, with $p < 0.05$ indicating statistical significance.

4. Results

The final cohort comprised 121 patients who underwent UKA and met the inclusion criteria. Participants included individuals aged 42 to 82 years who met the inclusion criteria for UKA. Patients were stratified into two groups based on their preoperative CSI scores: 95 patients (78.5%) had CSI scores below 40 (non-CS group), and 26 patients (21.5%) had CSI scores of 40 or higher (CS group). The two groups did not differ significantly in demographic characteristics or surgical factors, except for CSI scores (Table 1).

Preoperative WOMAC subscores differed significantly between the groups ($p < 0.05$). Before surgery, WOMAC pain, function, and total scores were significantly worse in the CS group than in the non-CS group, indicating worse baseline symptoms (all $p < 0.05$).

Table 1. Comparison of demographic characteristics and surgical factors in the central sensitization and non–central sensitization groups.

Variables	Non-CS Group (CSI < 40) (n = 95)	CS Group (CSI ≥ 40) (n = 26)	Cohen's d Effect Size	*p*-Value
Demographics				
Age (years)	61.5 ± 5.9	60.2 ± 7.4	0.21	0.366
Gender (Female, %)	84 (88.4%)	24 (22.2%)		0.732
BMI (kg/m^2)	25.6 ± 3.0	26.7 ± 3.3	−0.36	0.114
CSI score	22.7 ± 9.8	45.2 ± 4.2	−2.52	<0.001
ASA grade				
1	6 (6.3%)	2 (7.7%)		0.681
2	89 (93.7%)	24 (92.3%)		
Operation side (Right, %)	41 (43.2)	14 (53.8%)		0.514
Specific comorbidities				
Hypertension	29 (30.5%)	7 (19.4%)		0.812
Diabetes	16 (16.8%)	3 (11.5%)		0.762
Cardiac disease	12 (12.6%)	4 (15.4%)		0.746
Cerebrovascular event	5 (5.3%)	0 (0%)		0.584
Kidney disease	2 (2.1%)	0 (0%)		0.615
Thyroid disease	5 (5.3%)	1 (3.8%)		0.618
Pulmonary disease	10 (10.5%)	1 (3.8%)		0.453
Liver disease	3 (3.2%)	0 (0%)		0.481
Preoperative FTA (°)	Valgus 5.5 ± 2.7	Valgus 5.5 ± 3.2	0.0	0.970
Preoperative HKA (°)	Varus 0.6 ± 3.4	Varus 1.2 ± 3.8	−0.17	0.441
Postoperative FTA (°)	Valgus 1.8 ± 3.2	Valgus 2.3 ± 2.6	−0.16	0.454
Postoperative HKA (°)	Varus 4.7 ± 3.4	Varus 4.4 ± 3.2	0.09	0.664
Preoperative FC	3.4 ± 5.4	3.1 ± 5.3	0.06	0.774
Preoperative FF	127.7 ± 11.7	126.2 ± 15.4	0.12	0.583
Postoperative FC	0.3 ± 1.2	0.8 ± 2.7	−0.31	0.209
Postoperative FF	129.7 ± 3.8	129.0 ± 3.0	0.19	0.361

Values are presented as means and standard deviations or n (%). BMI, Body Mass Index; CSI, Central Sensitization Inventory; ASA, American Society of Anesthesiologists; FTA, Femorotibial Angle; HKA, Hip/Knee/Ankle Angle; FC, Flexion Contracture; FF, Further Flexion.

In both groups, all WOMAC subscores (pain, function, and total scores) showed significant improvements postoperatively, compared with the preoperative values (all $p < 0.05$) (Table 2). However, the mean postoperative WOMAC pain score was still higher in the CS group than the non-CS group (7.8 vs. 1.8, respectively, $p < 0.001$) 2 years postoperatively. Similarly, the postoperative total WOMAC score was significantly higher in the CS group than in the non-CS group (30.5 vs. 12.8, respectively, $p < 0.001$). The improvement in preoperative to postoperative WOMAC subscores (pain, function, and total) was significantly greater in the non-CS group than in the CS group (all $p < 0.05$) (Table 2).

The FJS, which evaluates joint awareness during daily activities, was significantly lower in the CS group than in the non-CS group (64.4 vs. 72.7, respectively, $p = 0.005$). This finding suggests that patients with CS were more likely than those without CS to be aware of their knee joint postoperatively (Table 3).

The new KSS score was 33.1 in the non-CS group and 25.5 in the CS group ($p < 0.001$). Among non-CS group patients, 91 (95.8%) were satisfied with their UKAs, whereas only 17 (65.4%) patients in the CS group reported satisfaction with the surgery ($p < 0.001$). Satisfaction in the CS group was, thus, significantly lower than in the non-CS group, not only for light daily activities such as sitting, lying in bed, and getting out of bed, but also for physically demanding tasks such as household chores and recreational or leisure activities (all $p < 0.05$) (Table 4).

The multivariate logistic regression analysis demonstrated that patients with a CSI score ≥ 40 had a 6.526-fold increased likelihood of dissatisfaction after UKA (95% CI: 2.298–18.531, $p < 0.001$), compared with patients with a CSI score < 40. The associations remained statistically significant after adjusting for age, gender, BMI, American Society of Anesthesiologists grade, preoperative flexion contracture and further flexion, preoperative hip/knee/ankle angle, and preoperative WOMAC total scores (Table 5). No patient in either group experienced complications requiring additional surgery or revision during the follow-up period.

Table 2. Preoperative and postoperative patient-reported outcomes.

Variables	Non-CS Group (CSI < 40) (n = 95)	CS Group (CSI ≥ 40) (n = 26)	Cohen's d Effect Size	*p*-Value
Preoperative				
WOMAC Total	54.4 ± 11.6	63.7 ± 12.0	−0.80	0.001
WOMAC Pain	14.5 ± 4.2	17.5 ± 4.1	−0.72	0.001
WOMAC Stiffness	4.4 ± 2.9	4.8 ± 2.0	−0.15	0.509
WOMAC Function	36.1 ± 9.6	41.8 ± 8.2	−0.61	0.006
Postoperative				
WOMAC Total	12.8 ± 7.1	30.5 ± 12.0	−2.11	<0.001
WOMAC Pain	1.8 ± 1.4	7.8 ± 4.1	−2.67	<0.001
WOMAC Stiffness	1.2 ± 1.3	1.8 ± 1.7	−0.43	0.030
WOMAC Function	9.6 ± 5.4	20.8 ± 7.7	−1.88	<0.001
WOMAC Change				
WOMAC Total	41.6 ± 12.7	33.1 ± 16.7	0.62	0.006
WOMAC Pain	12.7 ± 4.5	9.7 ± 5.6	0.63	0.005
WOMAC Stiffness	3.2 ± 2.7	3.0 ± 2.2	0.08	0.632
WOMAC Function	26.5 ± 10.3	21.0 ± 10.8	0.53	0.019

Values are presented as means and standard deviations. CS, Central Sensitization; CSI, Central Sensitization Inventory; WOMAC, Western Ontario and McMaster Universities Osteoarthritis Index.

Table 3. Postoperative Forgotten Joint Score (FJS) results.

Variables	Non-CS Group (CSI < 40) (n = 95)	CS Group (CSI ≥ 40) (n = 26)	Cohen's d Effect Size	*p*-Value
FJS conditions	72.7 ± 12.1	64.4 ± 16.3	0.63	0.005
1. In bed at night	1.1 ± 0.7	1.6 ± 0.9	−0.67	0.004
2. When sitting on a chair for more than 1 h	1.0 ± 0.8	1.5 ± 0.8	−0.63	0.006
3. When walking for more than 15 min	1.1 ± 0.8	1.5 ± 0.8	−0.50	0.187
4. When taking a bath/shower	1.2 ± 0.8	1.6 ± 1.1	−0.46	0.054
5. When traveling in a car	1.0 ± 0.7	1.2 ± 1.0	−0.26	0.166
6. When climbing stairs	1.1 ± 0.9	1.2 ± 1.0	−0.11	0.576
7. When walking on uneven ground	1.4 ± 0.9	1.5 ± 0.8	−0.11	0.541
8. When standing up from a low-sitting position	1.2 ± 0.8	1.6 ± 1.1	−0.46	0.042
9. When standing for long periods of time	0.8 ± 0.8	1.2 ± 1.0	−0.47	0.051
10. When doing housework or gardening	1.0 ± 0.8	1.5 ± 1.0	−0.59	0.003
11. When taking a walk or hiking	1.1 ± 0.9	1.5 ± 0.7	−0.47	0.087
12. When doing a favorite sport	0.9 ± 0.6	1.3 ± 0.8	−0.62	0.007

Values are presented as means and standard deviations. CS, Central Sensitization; CSI, Central Sensitization Inventory; FJS, Forgotten Joint Score.

Table 4. Comparison of satisfaction scores and proportions.

Variables	Non-CS Group (CSI < 40) (n = 95)	CS Group (CSI ≥ 40) (n = 26)	Cohen's d Effect Size	*p*-Value
Satisfaction score				
Sitting	7.2 ± 1.3	6.3 ± 1.9	0.62	0.004
Lying in bed	7.3 ± 1.2	6.4 ± 1.7	0.68	0.002
Getting out of bed	6.8 ± 1.5	5.8 ± 2.0	0.62	0.013
Light household duties	6.2 ± 1.6	5.4 ± 1.8	0.49	0.027
Leisure recreational activities	5.5 ± 1.8	3.5 ± 1.7	1.12	<0.001
Total	33.1 ± 6.1	25.5 ± 8.8	1.12	<0.001
Proportion				
Satisfied	91 (95.8%)	17 (65.4%)		<0.001
Dissatisfied	4 (4.2%)	9 (34.6%)		

Values are presented as means and standard deviations or n (%). CS, Central Sensitization; CSI, Central Sensitization Inventory.

Table 5. Results of multivariate analysis of risk factors predicting dissatisfaction.

Preoperative Variables	Univariate Regression Coefficient	95% CI	*p*-Value	Multivariate Regression Coefficient †	95% CI	*p*-Value
Age	1.008	0.945–1.075	0.816	0.982	0.912–1.057	0.620
Sex (male vs. female)	1.282	0.330–4.981	0.720	0.989	0.212–4.626	0.989
BMI (kg/m^2)	0.955	0.840–1.086	0.483	0.976	0.842–1.131	0.747
Preoperative HKA (°)	1.072	0.957–1.201	0.232	1.114	0.982–1.265	0.094
ASA grade (grade 2 vs. 1)	1.134	0.217–5.922	0.881	1.308	0.201–8.532	0.779
Preoperative FC (°)	1.016	0.939–1.099	0.691	1.018	0.921–1.126	0.722
Preoperative FF (°)	0.998	0.966–1.031	0.905	0.997	0.958–1.039	0.899
Preoperative WOMAC total score	0.977	0.944–1.012	0.192	0.999	0.960–1.039	0.960
CSI score (≥40)	5.833	2.297–14.814	<0.001	6.526	2.298–18.531	<0.001

BMI, Body Mass Index; HKA, Hip/Knee/Ankle angle; ASA, American Society of Anestheologists; FC, Flexion Contracture; FF, Further Flexion; WOMAC, Western Ontario and McMaster Universities Osteoarthritis Index; CSI, Central Sensitization Inventory. † Multivariate regression coefficient analyses were adjusted for age, gender, BMI, American Society of Anesthesiologists grade, preoperative flexion contracture and further flexion, preoperative hip/knee/ankle angle, and preoperative WOMAC total scores.

To assess whether the sample size was sufficient to detect the observed difference in satisfaction between the groups, we conducted a post-hoc power analysis using the observed satisfaction rates (95.8% in the non-CS group vs. 65.4% in the CS group). Based on a two-sided α of 0.05 and group sizes of 92 and 26, the power to detect a statistically significant difference was calculated to be 95.7% using a two-proportion z-test. This suggests that despite the unequal group sizes, the study was adequately powered to detect the observed effect.

5. Discussion

The findings of this study highlight the significant role that CS plays in postoperative pain and dissatisfaction following UKA. Patients with preoperative CS, identified as a CSI score of 40 or higher, demonstrated significantly worse postoperative pain scores, increased joint awareness, and inferior functional outcomes compared with those without CS. These results provide valuable insights into the influence of preoperative pain processing mechanisms on surgical recovery and patient satisfaction.

Several tools are available to assess CS, including QST and advanced imaging modalities such as functional magnetic resonance imaging (fMRI). QST objectively measures pain and sensory thresholds to external stimuli at local or remote sites, and has been widely used to detect abnormal pain processing suggestive of CS [21,22]. fMRI has also provided insights into altered brain structure and neurochemical activity in CS, such as decreased cortical thickness and elevated glutamate levels [23,24]. In this study, we chose to use the CSI, a validated self-reported questionnaire specifically designed to identify symptoms associated with CS [13,19,20,25,26]. While CSI is a self-reported measure and inherently subject to potential response bias, it offers several advantages that help mitigate these concerns. First, the CSI has been shown to have high internal consistency and reliability, and a cutoff score of 40 has been validated to identify patients with clinically significant central sensitization [19,20,25]. It is composed of items that assess not only pain but also other non-painful characteristic symptoms of CS, such as fatigue, poor sleep, and concentration difficulties, reducing the likelihood of misclassification due to isolated pain complaints [13,19,20,25,26]. Second, to minimize confounding factors, we excluded patients with known CS-related conditions (e.g., fibromyalgia, irritable bowel syndrome) and psychiatric disorders, both of which are known to influence CSI scores [19,20,25]. This allowed for a more specific assessment of CS-related symptoms within the context of knee OA [19,20,25]. Finally, although objective methods such as QST can provide valuable information about the sensory nervous system and local/distant hyperalgesia, they require specialized equipment and training, and are not always feasible in a retrospective design [19,20,25]. The CSI, in contrast, is efficient (<10 min), easy to administer, and ethically unproblematic, making it an appropriate tool for screening CS in clinical populations when used with appropriate exclusion criteria [13,19,20,25,26]. Given these benefits and considering the retrospective nature of our study, CSI provided an efficient and robust tool to stratify patients based on their CS status [19,20,25].

Patients with preoperative CS experienced significantly worse postoperative pain and functional outcomes than those without CS, despite the theoretical advantages of UKA over TKA, such as a smaller incision, preservation of most soft tissues, and less bone resection [3]. Our findings reveal that the CS group reported notably higher pain scores two years postoperatively. No previous studies investigated the effects of preoperative CS on UKA outcomes. However, numerous studies have examined the relationship between preoperative CS and clinical outcomes following TKA [11–16,27,28], and the evidence suggests that patients with preoperative CS are at greater risk than those without CS for chronic postoperative pain [11–16,27,28]. Martinez et al. [28] found that TKA patients with heat hyperalgesia reported greater pain both before and after surgery and required higher doses of postoperative morphine. Similarly, Lundblad et al. [27] followed 69 patients for 18 months after TKA and noted that persistent pain was more prevalent among those with high preoperative pain levels and a lower pain threshold—both indicative of CS-related mechanisms. In another study, Kim et al. [13] reported that patients with a high CSI score ($\geq$40) experienced more intense postoperative pain and required greater analgesic use during the first three months postoperatively. Their study also demonstrated that higher CSI scores were associated with more severe preoperative pain, persistent postoperative pain, and lower satisfaction with pain relief three months after surgery. Interestingly, although UKA is designed to preserve native ligaments and provide more natural knee kinematics, patients with CS did not appear to benefit from those advantages [3]. Instead, they continued to experience significant pain and functional limitations. This suggests that in CS patients, abnormalities in pain processing play a more important role in postoperative recovery than the specific surgical technique used. These findings further support the hypothesis that postoperative pain perception is not solely dictated by structural changes but is also influenced by alterations in central nervous system pain processing.

Preoperative CS not only contributes to persistent pain following surgery but also significantly affects functional outcomes and overall patient satisfaction. In our study, the CS group exhibited poorer WOMAC function and total scores than the non-CS group at the two-year follow-up visit. Additionally, the FJS scores were notably lower in the CS group, indicating a greater level of functional impairment. These findings align with previous studies of TKA [12,14]. Kim et al. [12] reported that the CS group showed significantly inferior preoperative and postoperative WOMAC function and total scores than the non-CS group. Similarly, Koh et al. [14] found that the CS group experienced worse quality of life and greater functional disability than the non-CS group after TKA. In addition, one of the most striking findings of our study is the significant effect of CS on patient satisfaction following UKA. Whereas 88% of patients in the non-CS group reported being satisfied with their surgical outcomes, only 62% of those in the CS group expressed satisfaction ($p < 0.01$). Sasaki et al. [16] demonstrated that preoperative CS was also negatively associated with postoperative EQ-5D scores in TKA patients. Moreover, Koh et al. [14], using the same new KSS score as in our study, showed that patients in the CS group were significantly more dissatisfied than those in the non-CS group. Further supporting this, our multivariate regression analysis identified CS as a significant predictor of dissatisfaction. The preoperative CSI score (adjust odds ratio = 11.349, $p = 0.003$) was independently associated with lower satisfaction rates. These findings underscore the importance of preoperative CS assessment, which may help screen high-risk patients and enable tailored interventions, including education and preemptive medication, to improve postoperative satisfaction.

CS is strongly associated with poor clinical outcomes following UKA for several reasons. First, patients with CS often have higher preoperative expectations than those without CS. Specifically, they anticipate greater pain relief and psychological well-being after surgery [29]. Although high expectations can sometimes contribute to favorable postoperative outcomes [30], excessively high expectations are closely linked to dissatisfaction and poor clinical results [31]. Second, the heightened pain sensitivity of CS patients negatively affects their postoperative outcomes [29]. Individuals with CS experience increased pain perception, often presenting with hyperalgesia and allodynia as characteristic symptoms [9]. This heightened sensitivity can play a crucial role in difficulties with post-surgical pain and recovery, further contributing to suboptimal clinical results [29]. Third, CS patients tend to have higher minimal clinically important difference (MCID) thresholds than non-CS patients. As a result, their overall postoperative outcomes tend to be worse, and the likelihood of achieving the MCID is significantly lower [12]. For those reasons, patients with CS are more prone than those without CS to experience persistent pain and inferior outcomes following UKA.

Effective management of CS, particularly in patients undergoing knee arthroplasty, requires a multidimensional approach that extends beyond conventional surgical intervention [14,32–34]. First, preoperative education and expectation setting play a crucial role. Numerous studies have demonstrated that preoperative expectations are closely linked to postoperative satisfaction and clinical outcomes [33,34]. For patients with CS, it is especially important to provide detailed explanations about the potential impact of CS on pain perception and recovery trajectory [33,34]. By aligning patient expectations with realistic outcomes, clinicians can mitigate dissatisfaction and enhance shared decision-making [33,34]. Furthermore, specific education on the nature of CS and its role in persistent postoperative pain should be incorporated into preoperative counseling sessions for patients with knee OA scheduled for UKA [33,34]. Second, pharmacologic treatment targeting central pain mechanisms can be an effective adjunct. Among the available agents, the serotonin-norepinephrine reuptake inhibitor (SNRI) duloxetine has shown particular promise in CS-associated pain [32]. In a randomized controlled trial by Koh et al., patients with CS undergoing TKA who received duloxetine experienced not only significant pain reduction starting two weeks postoperatively, but also notable improvements in mood, mental health, sleep quality, and social functioning [14]. These findings suggest that targeting descending pain modulation pathways may alleviate both sensory and affective components of CS-related pain [14]. Taken together, these strategies—preoperative patient-centered education and targeted pharmacotherapy—represent critical components in the perioperative management of patients with CS to improve both subjective and objective surgical outcomes [14,32–34]. Although UKA is widely regarded as a minimally invasive and function-preserving procedure, patients with CS may not fully experience its expected clinical benefits due to persistent central pain mechanisms [14,32–34]. This does not imply that UKA is counterproductive in CS patients, but rather highlights the need for realistic expectation-setting, individualized pain management, and possibly multimodal interventions to support postoperative recovery in this subgroup.

This study has several strengths, including a well-defined patient cohort, a standardized surgical technique performed by a single surgeon, and the use of validated outcome measures such as the WOMAC and FJS. These factors minimize variability and enhance the reliability of our findings. However, there are also limitations to consider. First, most of the patients who underwent UKAs were female (108 of 131, 89%). Although this demographic trend is well-documented in the Korean population, the underlying reasons remain unclear [35–41]. Second, although the data were collected prospectively, this study was conducted as a retrospective review using a single-institution database. As a result, inherent limitations such as selection bias might have influenced the findings. Third, various tools exist for assessing patient satisfaction after surgery [42]. In this study, we used the new KSS system, a validated tool designed to minimize the evaluation burden [43]. Although the KSS is widely accepted, incorporating additional assessment methods could provide a more comprehensive evaluation of patient satisfaction. Fourth, the follow-up period was limited to two years, and patient satisfaction was assessed only at the two-year postoperative mark. Longer-term studies are needed to better understand how postoperative satisfaction and its relationship with CS evolve over time. Fifth, the study might be underpowered, increasing the risk of type II errors and potentially limiting the ability to detect all relevant associations. Larger prospective studies with a broader and more diverse patient population are needed to strengthen these findings. Sixth, we used the CSI as the primary tool for assessing CS. Although the CSI is a validated and widely used screening measure [19,20], it is based on self-reported data and might not fully capture the neurophysiological aspects of CS. Future studies incorporating QST or functional neuroimaging could provide a more comprehensive understanding of CS in patients undergoing UKA [44]. Seventh, all surgeries were performed at a single institution by a single surgeon, which might limit the generalizability of the findings to other surgical settings. A multicenter study would help validate these results across different patient populations. Eighth, although we aimed to isolate the impact of CS on UKA outcomes by excluding patients with major psychiatric disorders and CS-related conditions through predefined exclusion criteria [19,20], it is important to acknowledge that completely eliminating all potential CS-associated factors is inherently challenging. Subclinical symptoms or undiagnosed comorbidities, such as mild sleep disturbances or psychological stress, may have persisted and influenced outcomes, representing a limitation of this study. Additionally, although patients with peripheral neuropathy were excluded based on clinical screening, we did not conduct formal neurologic or electrophysiological evaluations. Future studies may benefit from incorporating objective neuropathy assessments and stratifying patients by metabolic comorbidities to better isolate the effects of CS [45]. Lastly, anxiety and depression were excluded based on preoperative evaluation; we did not assess subclinical levels of anxiety or depressive symptoms postoperatively. Considering the established relationship between CS and mood disturbances, this remains a relevant limitation that may have influenced subjective outcome measures [14]. Despite those limitations, this study provides valuable insights into the relationship between CS and both pain and dissatisfaction following UKA.

6. Conclusions

This study underscores the importance of recognizing CS as a critical determinant of postoperative pain and dissatisfaction following UKA. Patients with high CSI scores experience greater pain, increased joint awareness, and overall poorer outcomes despite technically successful surgeries. Patients with CS should be closely monitored postoperatively and provided with appropriate pain management strategies to optimize their surgical outcomes. Future research should focus on refining these strategies and exploring innovative approaches to pain modulation in this patient population.

Supplementary Materials: The following supporting information can be downloaded at: https://www.mdpi.com/article/10.3390/medicina61050912/s1, Figure S1: Central Sensitization Inventory.

Author Contributions: Y.I. had full access to all the data in the study and takes responsibility for the integrity of the data and the accuracy of the data analysis. Concept and design: M.-S.K. and Y.I.; Acquisition, analysis, or interpretation of data: M.-S.K. and K.-Y.C.; Drafting of the manuscript: M.-S.K. and Y.I.; Critical revision of the manuscript for important intellectual content: All authors; Administrative, technical, or material support: M.-S.K. and K.-Y.C.; Supervision: Y.I. All authors have read and agreed to the published version of the manuscript.

Funding: This work was supported by the National Research Foundation of Korea (NRF) grant funded by the Korean Government (MSIT) (RS-2023-00215891) and Research Fund of Seoul St. Mary's Hospital, The Catholic University of Korea (ZC25CISI0102).

Institutional Review Board Statement: The study was conducted in accordance with the Declaration of Helsinki, and approved by the Institutional Review Board of Seoul St. Mary's Hospital (KC22RISI0506).

Informed Consent Statement: Informed consent was obtained from all subjects involved in the study.

Data Availability Statement: The data published in this research are available on request from the corresponding author (Y.I.).

Conflicts of Interest: The authors declare no conflict of interest.

Abbreviations

CS	Central Sensitization
UKA	Unicompartmental Knee Arthroplasty
TKA	Total Knee Arthroplasty
CSI	Central Sensitization Inventory
WOMAC	Western Ontario and McMaster Universities Osteoarthritis Index
FJS	Forgotten Joint Score
OA	Osteoarthritis
CNS	Central Nervous System
QST	Quantitative Sensory Testing
MB	Mobile-Bearing
PROMs	Patient-Reported Outcome Measures
KSS	Knee Society Satisfaction

References

1. Digennaro, V.; Ferri, R.; Panciera, A.; Bordini, B.; Cecchin, D.; Benvenuti, L.; Traina, F.; Faldini, C. Coronal plane alignment of the knee (CPAK) classification and its impact on medial unicompartmental knee arthroplasty: Exposing a unexpected external shift of limb mechanical axis in case of prearthritic constitutional valgus alignment: A retrospective radiographic study. *Knee Surg. Relat. Res.* **2024**, *36*, 14. [CrossRef] [PubMed]
2. Koshino, T.; Sato, K.; Umemoto, Y.; Akamatsu, Y.; Kumagai, K.; Saito, T. Clinical results of unicompartmental arthroplasty for knee osteoarthritis using a tibial component with screw fixation. *Int. Orthop.* **2015**, *39*, 1085–1091. [CrossRef] [PubMed]
3. Vasso, M.; Antoniadis, A.; Helmy, N. Update on unicompartmental knee arthroplasty: Current indications and failure modes. *EFORT Open Rev.* **2018**, *3*, 442–448. [CrossRef]
4. Vasso, M.; Del Regno, C.; Perisano, C.; D'Amelio, A.; Corona, K.; Schiavone Panni, A. Unicompartmental knee arthroplasty is effective: Ten year results. *Int. Orthop.* **2015**, *39*, 2341–2346. [CrossRef]
5. Baker, P.N.; Petheram, T.; Avery, P.J.; Gregg, P.J.; Deehan, D.J. Revision for unexplained pain following unicompartmental and total knee replacement. *J. Bone Jt. Surg. Am.* **2012**, *94*, e126. [CrossRef]
6. Calkins, T.E.; Hannon, C.P.; Fillingham, Y.A.; Culvern, C.C.; Berger, R.A.; Della Valle, C.J. Fixed-Bearing Medial Unicompartmental Knee Arthroplasty in Patients Younger Than 55 Years of Age at 4–19 Years of Follow-Up: A Concise Follow-Up of a Previous Report. *J. Arthroplasty* **2021**, *36*, 917–921. [CrossRef]
7. Walsh, J.M.; Burnett, R.A.; Serino, J.; Gerlinger, T.L. Painful Unicompartmental Knee Arthroplasty: Etiology, Diagnosis and Management. *Arch. Bone Jt. Surg.* **2024**, *12*, 546–557. [CrossRef]
8. Clauw, D.J.; Hassett, A.L. The role of centralised pain in osteoarthritis. *Clin. Exp. Rheumatol.* **2017**, *107*, 79–84.
9. Woolf, C.J. Central sensitization: Implications for the diagnosis and treatment of pain. *Pain* **2011**, *152*, S2–S15. [CrossRef]
10. Nijs, J.; Leysen, L.; Vanlauwe, J.; Logghe, T.; Ickmans, K.; Polli, A.; Malfliet, A.; Coppieters, I.; Huysmans, E. Treatment of central sensitization in patients with chronic pain: Time for change? *Expert Opin. Pharmacother.* **2019**, *20*, 1961–1970. [CrossRef]
11. Dave, A.J.; Selzer, F.; Losina, E.; Usiskin, I.; Collins, J.E.; Lee, Y.C.; Band, P.; Dalury, D.F.; Iorio, R.; Kindsfater, K.; et al. The association of pre-operative body pain diagram scores with pain outcomes following total knee arthroplasty. *Osteoarthr. Cartil.* **2017**, *25*, 667–675. [CrossRef] [PubMed]
12. Kim, M.S.; Koh, I.J.; Choi, K.Y.; Seo, J.Y.; In, Y. Minimal Clinically Important Differences for Patient-Reported Outcomes After TKA Depend on Central Sensitization. *J. Bone Jt. Surg. Am.* **2021**, *103*, 1374–1382. [CrossRef] [PubMed]
13. Kim, S.H.; Yoon, K.B.; Yoon, D.M.; Yoo, J.H.; Ahn, K.R. Influence of Centrally Mediated Symptoms on Postoperative Pain in Osteoarthritis Patients Undergoing Total Knee Arthroplasty: A Prospective Observational Evaluation. *Pain Pract.* **2015**, *15*, E46–E53. [CrossRef]
14. Koh, I.J.; Kang, B.M.; Kim, M.S.; Choi, K.Y.; Sohn, S.; In, Y. How Does Preoperative Central Sensitization Affect Quality of Life Following Total Knee Arthroplasty? *J. Arthroplasty* **2020**, *35*, 2044–2049. [CrossRef]
15. Lape, E.C.; Selzer, F.; Collins, J.E.; Losina, E.; Katz, J.N. Stability of Measures of Pain Catastrophizing and Widespread Pain Following Total Knee Replacement. *Arthritis Care Res.* **2020**, *72*, 1096–1103. [CrossRef]
16. Sasaki, E.; Kasai, T.; Araki, R.; Sasaki, T.; Wakai, Y.; Akaishi, K.; Chiba, D.; Kimura, Y.; Yamamoto, Y.; Tsuda, E.; et al. Central Sensitization and Postoperative Improvement of Quality of Life in Total Knee and Total Hip Arthroplasty: A Prospective Observational Study. *Prog. Rehabil. Med.* **2022**, *7*, 20220009. [CrossRef] [PubMed]
17. Iio, R.; Manaka, T.; Nakazawa, K.; Hirakawa, Y.; Ito, Y.; Ogura, A.; Nakamura, H. Assessment of Prevalence and Risk Factors for Central Sensitization Related to Shoulder Osteoarthritis and Rotator Cuff Tears Using the Central Sensitization Inventory: A Cross-Sectional Study in Shoulder Surgery Patients. *J. Clin. Med.* **2023**, *12*, 5633. [CrossRef]
18. Buskila, D. Genetics of chronic pain states. *Best Pract. Res. Clin. Rheumatol.* **2007**, *21*, 535–547. [CrossRef]
19. Mayer, T.G.; Neblett, R.; Cohen, H.; Howard, K.J.; Choi, Y.H.; Williams, M.J.; Perez, Y.; Gatchel, R.J. The development and psychometric validation of the central sensitization inventory. *Pain Pract.* **2012**, *12*, 276–285. [CrossRef]
20. Neblett, R.; Cohen, H.; Choi, Y.; Hartzell, M.M.; Williams, M.; Mayer, T.G.; Gatchel, R.J. The Central Sensitization Inventory (CSI): Establishing clinically significant values for identifying central sensitivity syndromes in an outpatient chronic pain sample. *J. Pain* **2013**, *14*, 438–445. [CrossRef]
21. Lluch, E.; Torres, R.; Nijs, J.; Van Oosterwijck, J. Evidence for central sensitization in patients with osteoarthritis pain: A systematic literature review. *Eur. J. Pain* **2014**, *18*, 1367–1375. [CrossRef] [PubMed]
22. Staud, R.; Robinson, M.E.; Price, D.D. Temporal summation of second pain and its maintenance are useful for characterizing widespread central sensitization of fibromyalgia patients. *J. Pain* **2007**, *8*, 893–901. [CrossRef] [PubMed]
23. Jensen, K.B.; Srinivasan, P.; Spaeth, R.; Tan, Y.; Kosek, E.; Petzke, F.; Carville, S.; Fransson, P.; Marcus, H.; Williams, S.C.; et al. Overlapping structural and functional brain changes in patients with long-term exposure to fibromyalgia pain. *Arthritis Rheum.* **2013**, *65*, 3293–3303. [CrossRef]
24. Napadow, V.; Kim, J.; Clauw, D.J.; Harris, R.E. Decreased intrinsic brain connectivity is associated with reduced clinical pain in fibromyalgia. *Arthritis Rheum.* **2012**, *64*, 2398–2403. [CrossRef]

25. Akinci, A.; Al Shaker, M.; Chang, M.H.; Cheung, C.W.; Danilov, A.; José Dueñas, H.; Kim, Y.C.; Guillen, R.; Tassanawipas, W.; Treuer, T.; et al. Predictive factors and clinical biomarkers for treatment in patients with chronic pain caused by osteoarthritis with a central sensitisation component. *Int. J. Clin. Pract.* **2016**, *70*, 31–44. [CrossRef]
26. Kim, M.S.; Koh, I.J.; Kim, C.K.; Choi, K.Y.; Kim, C.Y.; In, Y. Cross-cultural adaptation and validation of the Korean version of the Central Sensitization Inventory in patients undergoing total knee arthroplasty for knee osteoarthritis. *PLoS ONE* **2020**, *15*, e0242912. [CrossRef]
27. Lundblad, H.; Kreicbergs, A.; Jansson, K.A. Prediction of persistent pain after total knee replacement for osteoarthritis. *J. Bone Jt. Surg. Br.* **2008**, *90*, 166–171. [CrossRef]
28. Martinez, V.; Fletcher, D.; Bouhassira, D.; Sessler, D.I.; Chauvin, M. The evolution of primary hyperalgesia in orthopedic surgery: Quantitative sensory testing and clinical evaluation before and after total knee arthroplasty. *Anesth. Analg.* **2007**, *105*, 815–821. [CrossRef]
29. Kim, M.S.; Koh, I.J.; Sung, Y.G.; Park, D.C.; Yoon, E.J.; In, Y. Influence of increased pain sensitivity on patient-reported outcomes following total knee arthroplasty. *Knee Surg. Sports Traumatol. Arthrosc.* **2022**, *30*, 782–790. [CrossRef]
30. Flood, A.B.; Lorence, D.P.; Ding, J.; McPherson, K.; Black, N.A. The role of expectations in patients' reports of post-operative outcomes and improvement following therapy. *Med. Care* **1993**, *31*, 1043–1056. [CrossRef]
31. Mancuso, C.A.; Reid, M.C.; Duculan, R.; Girardi, F.P. Improvement in Pain After Lumbar Spine Surgery: The Role of Preoperative Expectations of Pain Relief. *Clin. J. Pain* **2017**, *33*, 93–98. [CrossRef] [PubMed]
32. Itoh, N.; Tsuji, T.; Ishida, M.; Ochiai, T.; Konno, S.; Uchio, Y. Efficacy of duloxetine for multisite pain in patients with knee pain due to osteoarthritis: An exploratory post hoc analysis of a Japanese phase 3 randomized study. *J. Orthop. Sci.* **2021**, *26*, 141–148. [CrossRef] [PubMed]
33. Louw, A.; Diener, I.; Butler, D.S.; Puentedura, E.J. The effect of neuroscience education on pain, disability, anxiety, and stress in chronic musculoskeletal pain. *Arch. Phys. Med. Rehabil.* **2011**, *92*, 2041–2056. [CrossRef] [PubMed]
34. Watson, J.A.; Ryan, C.G.; Cooper, L.; Ellington, D.; Whittle, R.; Lavender, M.; Dixon, J.; Atkinson, G.; Cooper, K.; Martin, D.J. Pain Neuroscience Education for Adults with Chronic Musculoskeletal Pain: A Mixed-Methods Systematic Review and Meta-Analysis. *J. Pain* **2019**, *20*, 1140.e1–1140.e22. [CrossRef]
35. Kim, D.H.; Jeong, S.Y.; Yang, J.H.; Choi, C.H. Evaluation of Appropriateness of the Reimbursement Criteria of Korean Health Insurance Review and Assessment Service for Total Knee Arthroplasty. *Clin. Orthop. Surg.* **2023**, *15*, 241–248. [CrossRef]
36. Kim, K.I.; Kim, J.H.; Min, K. Does the clinical and radiologic outcomes following total knee arthroplasty using a new design cobalt-chrome tibial plate or predecessor different? *Knee Surg. Relat. Res.* **2024**, *36*, 34. [CrossRef]
37. Kim, S.E.; Ro, D.H.; Lee, M.C.; Han, H.S. Can individual functional improvements be predicted in osteoarthritic patients after total knee arthroplasty? *Knee Surg. Relat. Res.* **2024**, *36*, 31. [CrossRef]
38. Ko, K.; Kim, K.H.; Ko, S.; Jo, C.; Han, H.S.; Lee, M.C.; Ro, D.H. Total Knee Arthroplasty: Is It Safe? A Single-Center Study of 4124 Patients in South Korea. *Clin. Orthop. Surg.* **2023**, *15*, 935–941. [CrossRef]
39. Lee, Y.M.; Kim, G.W.; Lee, C.Y.; Song, E.K.; Seon, J.K. No Difference in Clinical Outcomes and Survivorship for Robotic, Navigational, and Conventional Primary Total Knee Arthroplasty with a Minimum Follow-up of 10 Years. *Clin. Orthop. Surg.* **2023**, *15*, 82–91. [CrossRef]
40. Nagata, N.; Hiranaka, T.; Okamoto, K.; Fujishiro, T.; Tanaka, T.; Kensuke, A.; Kitazawa, D.; Kotoura, K. Is simultaneous bilateral unicompartmental knee arthroplasty and total knee arthroplasty better than simultaneous bilateral total knee arthroplasty? *Knee Surg. Relat. Res.* **2023**, *35*, 12. [CrossRef]
41. Park, J.; Chang, M.J.; Kim, T.W.; D'Lima, D.D.; Kim, H.; Han, H.S. Serial changes in patient-reported outcome measures and satisfaction rate during long-term follow-up after total knee arthroplasty: A systematic review and meta-analysis. *Knee Surg. Relat. Res.* **2024**, *36*, 43. [CrossRef]
42. Webster, K.E.; Feller, J.A. Comparison of the short form-12 (SF-12) health status questionnaire with the SF-36 in patients with knee osteoarthritis who have replacement surgery. *Knee Surg. Sports Traumatol. Arthrosc.* **2016**, *24*, 2620–2626. [CrossRef] [PubMed]
43. Noble, P.C.; Scuderi, G.R.; Brekke, A.C.; Sikorskii, A.; Benjamin, J.B.; Lonner, J.H.; Chadha, P.; Daylamani, D.A.; Scott, W.N.; Bourne, R.B. Development of a new Knee Society scoring system. *Clin. Orthop. Relat. Res.* **2012**, *470*, 20–32. [CrossRef]
44. Wylde, V.; Palmer, S.; Learmonth, I.D.; Dieppe, P. The association between pre-operative pain sensitisation and chronic pain after knee replacement: An exploratory study. *Osteoarthr. Cartil.* **2013**, *21*, 1253–1256. [CrossRef]
45. Currado, D.; Berardicurti, O.; Saracino, F.; Trunfio, F.; Kun, L.; Marino, A.; Corberi, E.; Lamberti, L.; Ruscitti, P.; Liakouli, V.; et al. The Relationship Between Metabolic Syndrome and Pain Catastrophizing in Psoriatic Arthritis. *Rheumatol. Ther.* **2025**, *12*, 581–592. [CrossRef]

medicina

MDPI

Article

Assessment of Quadriceps Muscle in Advanced Knee Osteoarthritis and Correlation with Lower Limb Alignment

Ki-Cheor Bae †, Eun-Seok Son †, Chang-Jin Yon, Jubin Park and Du-Han Kim *

Department of Orthopedic Surgery, Keimyung University Dongsan Hospital, Keimyung University School of Medicine, Daegu 42601, Republic of Korea; bkc@dsmc.or.kr (K.-C.B.); esson@dsmc.or.kr (E.-S.S.); poweryon@dsmc.or.kr (C.-J.Y.); 230514@dsmc.or.kr (J.P.)

* Correspondence: osmdkdh@gmail.com; Tel.: +82-53-258-7930

† These authors contributed equally to this work.

Abstract: *Background and Objectives*: Despite extensive studies of the role of quadriceps and quadriceps/hamstring balance in knee osteoarthritis (OA), the roles of the vastus intermedius, medialis, and lateralis in OA remain unclear. The purpose of this study was to investigate the relationship of lower limb alignment and the ratio of the quadriceps femoris muscle to the knee extensor muscle. *Materials and Methods*: This study included 50 patients with advanced knee OA (Kellgren/Lawrence grade of 3 or 4) and 25 healthy control persons between June 2021 and May 2022. The osteoarthritis grade and anatomical tibiofemoral angle were measured based on plain radiography and scanography. All participants were divided into normal (0~5°), mild varus (5°~10°), and severe varus (>10°) groups. Using MRI, muscle size was determined by calculating the cross-sectional area (CSA) of the total quadriceps (rectus femoris, vastus intermedius, vastus medialis, and vastus lateralis) and its components. *Results*: The CSA ratio of the vastus lateralis was significantly smaller in the severe varus group than in the normal or mild varus groups. There was a significant positive correlation between the mechanical tibiofemoral angle and vastus lateralis CSA ($\rho = 0.282$, $p = 0.014$) and between the anatomical tibiofemoral angle and vastus lateralis CSA ($\rho = 0.294$, $p = 0.011$). There was a significant negative correlation between the mechanical tibiofemoral angle and vastus intermedius CSA ($\rho = -0.263$, $p = 0.023$) and between the anatomical tibiofemoral angle and vastus intermedius CSA ($\rho = -0.243$, $p = 0.036$). *Conclusions*: Patients with severe varus alignment exhibited vastus lateralis atrophy. This study highlights vastus lateralis atrophy in severe varus alignment, though causality between atrophy and varus knee OA remains uncertain. We think that patients with severe varus may require strengthening exercises focused on the vastus lateralis before and after surgery for alignment correction.

Keywords: knee; osteoarthritis; quadriceps; varus deformity; muscle atrophy

1. Introduction

Quadriceps muscle dysfunction is a common feature in knee osteoarthritis (OA) and is associated with functional decline and disease progression. However, patient satisfaction rates lower than 80% after conventional total knee arthroplasty have been reported in the literature [1–4]. A typical feature of knee osteoarthritis (OA) is knee extensor weakness, which is associated with the development of symptomatic knee OA as well as functional decline over time in people with knee OA [5]. Knee extensor muscle condition has been studied in patients with knee osteoarthritis to determine its association with varying degrees of functional impairment and disease progression. Several studies have suggested that the quadriceps muscle seems to be related to lower risk of symptomatic OA, but not radiographic OA [5]. While quadriceps muscles have been studied, their specific contributions to OA pathogenesis, particularly in relation to lower limb alignment, remain less established.

In particular, the vastus medialis (VM) is being studied in various ways in knee-related conditions such as patellofemoral pain syndrome and knee osteoarthritis [6,7]. Patients exhibited atrophy of the VM in patellofemoral pain syndrome. Pattyn et al. found that the cross-sectional area (CSA) of VM was significantly smaller in the patients' group. A tendency was also noted for the patellofemoral pain syndrome group toward a smaller CSA of the total quadriceps at the midthigh level [6]. While VM has been associated with patellofemoral pain syndrome, its role in knee OA, particularly in conjunction with other quadriceps components, warrants further investigation. According to the knee OA study, increased VM size was associated with reduced knee pain and structural improvements in knee OA [3,4,7,8]. Conversely, Pan et al. suggested that the ratio between vastus lateralis (VL) and VM cross-sectional area may influence the progression of OA [9].

However, there are few studies of the relationship between lower limb alignment and knee extensor muscle volume in knee OA. The purpose of this study was to investigate the relationship between lower limb alignment and the ratio of the quadriceps femoris muscle to the knee extensor muscle using magnetic resonance imaging (MRI). We hypothesize that lower limb alignment would be correlated with the ratio of the quadriceps femoris muscle.

2. Materials and Methods

2.1. Participants

We performed a retrospective review of medical records for patients with knee OA from June 2021 and May 2022. The diagnosis of knee OA was established using patient medical history, plain radiographs, and MRI. This study included a total of 75 patients, comprising 50 patients with knee OA and 25 healthy individuals who had never had knee pain before.

Patients who met the following criteria were included in the study: (1) >20 years old, and (2) patients with confirmed symptomatic knee OA with a Kellgren/Lawrence (KL) grade of 3 or 4 [10]. Exclusion criteria included patients who (1) had no preoperative MRI or a poor-quality image that was difficult to measure, (2) had concomitant fractures, or (3) had a previous history of knee surgery or trauma.

2.2. Radiographic Evaluations

Radiographic images were acquired using an SH3 system (DK Medical, Seoul, Republic of Korea). Knee OA was confirmed through anterior–posterior and lateral weight-bearing radiographs, as well as non-weight-bearing skyline radiographs. An experienced orthopedic surgeon utilized these images to grade bilateral tibiofemoral OA based on the KL criteria. Participants were included in the knee OA group if they were classified as grade III or IV (unilateral or bilateral) on the KL scale and exhibited clinical symptoms. Participants were included in the control group if their knees were classified as grade 0 or I on the KL scale and were asymptomatic.

All participants underwent conventional scanography. Patients were positioned to stand with equal weight distribution on both lower extremities without an assistive device, with both patellae pointing anteriorly and feet straight, parallel to each other. The patient-to-tube distance was typically 101 cm. Three separate $35 \times 9 \times 43$ cm cassettes were used to obtain three separate images centered over the hip, knee, and ankle joints. Based on scanography alignment, the hip–knee–ankle (HKA) angle was measured and defined as the angle between the mechanical axes of the femur and tibia. All participants were divided into normal (Group I), mild varus (Group II), and severe varus (Group III) groups. Group I was defined as between 5 degrees of valgus and 5 degrees of varus, Group II was defined as between 5 and 10 degrees of varus, and Group III was defined as >10 degrees of varus [11].

2.3. Thigh Muscle Cross-Sectional Area Measurement

A consecutive series of MRI scans of each patient's thighs was acquired using a 1.5T MRI system (Siemens Magnetom Avanto System; Siemens Medical, Erlangen, Germany). Close collaboration with the radiology department was maintained throughout the study to ensure precise measurements. Oblique sagittal T2 TSE MRI scans, perpendicular to the long axis of the scapular body, were obtained with a slice thickness of 3 mm. The contours of the rectus femoris (RF), vastus intermedius (VI), vastus medialis (VM), and vastus lateralis (VL) muscles were manually traced using PACS software (Picture Archiving and Communication System, DICOM version 3.0 INFINITT, Infinitt Healthcare, Seoul, Republic of Korea). As illustrated in Figure 1, the borders of the four muscle groups were delineated in the mid-thigh view on the axial plane. The software then automatically calculated the cross-sectional area (CSA) for each muscle. Subsequently, the percentage of each muscle relative to the total quadriceps muscles (rCSA) was determined. Two knee-specializing orthopedic surgeons, who worked in the territory university hospital (*** and ***), independently performed the image measurements. Interobserver reliability was reassessed through a randomized analysis conducted three months later.

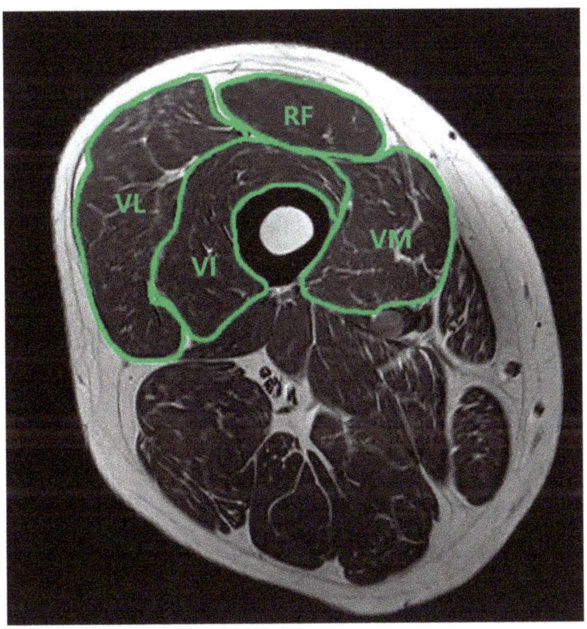

Figure 1. Axial T2 TSE MRI. Measurement of the cross-sectional area of the quadriceps muscle in mid-thigh view. Rectus femoris (RF), vastus intermedius (VI), vastus medialis (VM), and vastus lateralis (VL).

2.4. Statistical Analysis

Statistical analysis was performed using SPSS 24.0 software. Two methods were used to assess the measurement reliability. The Mann–Whitney test was used to evaluate the difference in rCSA between the OA patients and the control group. The mean difference of the rCSA between each alignment group was estimated using the Kruskal–Wallis test. Furthermore, the Spearman correlation coefficient was used to examine the correlation between the lower limb alignment and CSA. The test–retest reliability was evaluated initially; subsequently, internal consistency reliability was assessed using the Bland and Altman method for calculating inter- and intraclass correlation (ICC). A threshold for statistical significance was established at $p < 0.05$. Results with p-values below this threshold were deemed statistically significant, whereas those with p-values above this threshold were not.

3. Results

Participant characteristics are shown in Table 1. Age and BMI (mean ± SD) were 69.3 ± 6.7 years and 26.4 ± 3.2 kg/m^2 in the OA group, and 44.8 ± 15.1 years and 27.6 ± 4.7 in control group, respectively.

Table 1. Demographic data of participants classified according to OA status.

	OA Group (n = 50)	Control Group (n = 25)	p-Value
Age (years)			0.000 *
Mean ± SD	69.3 ± 6.7	44.8 ± 15.1	
Gender			0.008 *
Male, n (%)	9 (18.0%)	13 (52.0%)	
Female, n (%)	41 (82.0%)	12 (48.0%)	
Height (cm)			0.000 *
Mean ± SD	154.9 ± 9.6	165.9 ± 8.4	
Weight (kg)			0.000 *
Mean ± SD	63.3 ± 9.0	76.3 ± 16.1	
BMI (kg/m^2)			0.247
Mean ± SD	26.4 ± 3.2	27.6 ± 4.7	
Side			0.624
Right, n (%)	23 (46.0%)	13 (52.0%)	
Left, n (%)	27 (54.0%)	12 (48.0%)	
Alignment classification			0.000 *
Normal, n (%)	13 (26.0%)	23 (92.0%)	
Mild varus, n (%)	15 (30.0%)	2 (8.0%)	
Severe varus, n (%)	22 (44.0%)	0 (0%)	
OA grade (KL)			0.000 *
KL 0, n (%)	0 (0%)	4 (16.0%)	
KL 1, n (%)	0 (0%)	11 (44.0%)	
KL 2, n (%)	0 (0%)	10 (40.0%)	
KL 3, n (%)	5 (10.0%)	0 (0%)	
KL 4, n (%)	45 (90.0%)	0 (0%)	

OA: osteoarthritis, SD: standard deviation, BMI: body mass index, KL: Kellgren/Lawrence. * statistically significant.

3.1. OA Grade Differences in Thigh Muscle CSA Measurements

The CSA of the total quadriceps and each component was significantly smaller in the OA group than in the control group. Additionally, we analyzed the ratio of percentages between each component. As a result, no significant differences of the CSA ratio between the knee OA patients and the control group were found (Table 2).

Table 2. CSA ratio of the quadriceps components.

	OA Group (n = 50)	Control Group (n = 25)	p-Value
RF	10.52 ± 2.15	10.94 ± 1.92	0.408
VI	33.14 ± 3.48	32.26 ± 4.27	0.338
VM	22.39 ± 2.77	21.67 ± 3.39	0.327
VL	33.94 ± 2.65	35.13 ± 4.17	0.203

CSA: cross-sectional area, RF: rectus femoris, VI: vastus intermedius, VM: vastus medialis, VL: vastus lateralis.

3.2. Muscle CSA in Relation to Knee Alignment

Table 3 shows participant characteristic data classified according to mechanical alignment. The CSA ratio of the vastus lateralis was significantly smaller in the severe varus group than in the normal ($Z = -2.452$, $p = 0.014$) or mild varus groups ($Z = -2.251$, $p = 0.011$) (Table 4). There was a significant positive correlation between the mechanical tibiofemoral angle and vastus lateralis CSA ($\rho = 0.282$, $p = 0.014$), and between the anatomical tibiofemoral angle and vastus lateralis CSA ($\rho = 0.294$, $p = 0.011$). There was a significant negative correlation between the mechanical tibiofemoral angle and vastus intermedius CSA ($\rho = -0.263$, $p = 0.023$), and between the anatomical tibiofemoral angle and vastus intermedius CSA ($\rho = -0.243$, $p = 0.036$).

Table 3. Demographic data of participants classified according to mechanical alignment.

	Group I (*n* = 36) **Normal Alignment**	**Group II (*n* = 17)** **Mild Varus Alignment**	**Group III (*n* = 22)** **Severe Varus Alignment**	***p*-Value**	
Age (years)				0.000 *	I < II, III
Mean ± SD	51.2 ± 17.4	66.4 ± 10.5	69.3 ± 7.7		
Gender				0.247	
Male, *n* (%)	14 (38.9%)	3 (17.6%)	5 (22.7%)		
Female, *n* (%)	22 (61.1%)	14 (82.4%)	17 (77.3%)		
Height (cm)				0.008 *	I < III
Mean ± SD	163.5 ± 9.8	155.4 ± 8.9	154.6 ± 10.6		
Weight (kg)				0.028 *	I < III
Mean ± SD	73.2 ± 14.6	65.5 ± 12.8	62.1 ± 10.6		
BMI (kg/m^2)				0.564	
Mean ± SD	27.3 ± 4.1	27.1 ± 4.0	26.0 ± 3.7		
Side				0.594	
Right, *n* (%)	20 (55.6%)	5 (29.4%)	11 (50.0%)		
Left, *n* (%)	16 (44.4%)	12 (70.6%)	11 (50.0%)		
OA grade (KL)				0.000 *	
KL 0, *n* (%)	4 (11.1%)	0 (0%)	0 (0%)		
KL 1, *n* (%)	10 (27.8%)	1 (5.9%)	0 (0%)		
KL 2, *n* (%)	9 (25.0%)	1 (5.9%)	0 (0%)		
KL 3, *n* (%)	2 (5.6%)	1 (5.9%)	2 (9.1%)		
KL 4, *n* (%)	11 (30.6%)	14 (82.4%)	20 (90.9%)		

OA: osteoarthritis, SD: standard deviation, BMI: body mass index, KL: Kellgren/Lawrence. * statistically significant.

Table 4. CSA ratio of the quadriceps components in each alignment group.

	Group I (*n* = 36) **Normal Alignment**	**Group II (*n* = 17)** **Mild Varus Alignment**	**Group III (*n* = 22)** **Severe Varus Alignment**	***p*-Value**	
RF	10.86 ± 2.12	9.92 ± 2.17	10.90 ± 1.86	0.251	
VI	31.88 ± 3.71	33.05 ± 2.62	34.27 ± 4.21	0.058	
VM	22.31 ± 3.22	21.96 ± 3.00	22.04 ± 2.70	0.907	
VL	34.94 ± 3.67	35.06 ± 3.00	32.78 ± 2.14	0.027 *	I, II > III

RF: rectus femoris, VI: vastus intermedius, VM: vastus medialis, VL: vastus lateralis. * statistically significant.

4. Discussion

Our study examined differences in thigh muscle CSA among participants with knee OA and a control group. While overall quadriceps CSA was reduced in OA patients, the disproportionate atrophy of the vastus lateralis in the severe varus group suggests a targeted impact of knee alignment on muscle morphology.

Notably, the CSA ratio of the vastus lateralis was considerably smaller in the severe varus group compared to the normal or mild varus groups. Additionally, there were significant correlations found between knee alignment and CSA. There was a positive correlation with the vastus lateralis and a negative correlation with the vastus intermedius, highlighting how changes in knee mechanics are associated with muscle morphology in knee OA.

The quadriceps femoris muscle is commonly associated with tibiofemoral OA and is a critical factor in determining disability [12]. Thomas et al. found that women with radiographic OA had 22% less quadriceps strength compared to women without OA, aligning with various reports of isometric and isokinetic knee extension torque deficits ranging from 20% to 40% [13–15]. Adequate quadriceps strength in knee OA patients is essential for performing daily activities, and strengthening this muscle has been shown to improve physical function in those affected by the disease [12,16,17]. Pietrosimone et al. reported that individuals with high physical activity levels had significantly greater quadriceps strength compared to those with lower activity levels, indicating a positive association between quadriceps strength and physical activity [18]. Greater quadriceps muscle strength is also linked to a lower risk of developing symptomatic knee OA [19]. However, evidence supporting the quadriceps muscle's significant role in the incidence of radiographic knee OA remains limited.

There are several methods used to evaluate the quadriceps muscle change in patients with osteoarthritis [20–22]. Using ultrasonography to measure muscle thickness and echo intensity in various lower extremity muscles, Taniguchi et al. measured muscle quantity and quality in 21 women with knee OA and 23 healthy individuals. Their results indicated that muscle changes associated with OA, such as decreased muscle thickness and increased echo intensity, are more pronounced as OA severity increases and vary among different muscles, particularly in the vastus medialis and intermedius [21]. Segal et al. conducted their study using dual-energy X-ray absorptiometry. They found that, contrary to previous beliefs about the protective role of quadriceps strength, greater thigh muscle mass does not protect against the development or worsening of knee OA or joint space narrowing. Instead, higher specific strength in the knee extensors significantly lowers the risk for symptomatic knee OA and joint space narrowing. This result suggests that neuromuscular activation and muscle physiology may be more crucial factors to consider than muscle mass alone [23].

Research suggests that muscle atrophy and fatty infiltration are common in the quadriceps of knee OA patients, often with disproportionate atrophy in the vastus medialis [7,8,11,24]. Van der Noort et al. found that a higher percentage of non-contractile tissue in the VM muscle is linked to weaker muscle strength and longer performance times in mobility tests in patients with knee OA measured by MRI. Their results also showed that women with a high BMI were more at risk for having a high amount of non-contractile tissue [24]. Fink et al. performed histopathological examination of the vastus medialis muscle. In their study, patients with end-stage OA revealed widespread atrophy and changes indicative of neurogenic muscular atrophy and pain-associated disuse, highlighting the multifactorial nature of muscle deterioration in osteoarthritis. Their findings suggest a complex interaction between structural muscle changes and clinical symptoms like leg axis deviation [11]. Our findings of targeted vastus lateralis atrophy in severe varus alignment complement previous studies showing muscle-specific changes in OA, suggesting that muscle morphology may be influenced by joint mechanics. We are also not sure which came first. However, we think that this group of patients may require strengthening exercises focused on the vastus lateralis before and after surgery for alignment correction.

Our study had several limitations. First, the retrospective nature of this study limited the ability to establish causality between muscle cross-sectional area changes and knee osteoarthritis progression. The second limitation was measurement bias. While muscle CSA measurements were performed by experienced orthopedic surgeons, manual tracing and reliance on clinical MRI may have introduced variability that could affect the precision and repeatability of the measurements. If automated three-dimensional reconstruction had been used as a measurement method, accuracy may have been even higher. Third, this study sample was comprised only of patients with advanced knee osteoarthritis and a control group, which may not be representative of all stages of the disease or broader demographic characteristics. We also did not perform an age- and sex-matched study because we wanted to compare an old-age OA group with a young healthy group.

5. Conclusions

When compared to healthy individuals, patients with advanced knee OA had extensor muscle atrophy. However, there was no difference in the ratio of each component. Patients with severe varus alignment exhibited vastus lateralis atrophy. Although it is not clear whether this unbalanced atrophy is a result or a cause of varus knee OA, our results suggest that vastus lateralis atrophy may contribute to the severity of varus knee OA. To establish the cause–effect relation of vastus lateralis atrophy and varus knee OA, longitudinal and prospective studies on the causal relationship between muscle atrophy and knee alignment are needed.

Author Contributions: Conceptualization, K.-C.B. and D.-H.K.; methodology, J.P.; software, C.-J.Y.; validation, C.-J.Y. and D.-H.K.; formal analysis, E.-S.S. and C.-J.Y.; investigation, C.-J.Y.; resources, J.P.; data curation, J.P.; writing—original draft preparation, D.-H.K.; writing—review and editing, E.-S.S. and D.-H.K.; visualization, K.-C.B. and E.-S.S.; supervision, K.-C.B. and E.-S.S.; project administration, D.-H.K. All authors have read and agreed to the published version of the manuscript.

Funding: This research received no external funding.

Institutional Review Board Statement: The study was conducted in accordance with the Declaration of Helsinki, and approved by the Institutional Review Board (or Ethics Committee) of Keimyung University Dongsan Hospital. (IRB No. 2024-09-030), approval number: 26 September 2024.

Informed Consent Statement: Informed consent was obtained from all subjects involved in the study.

Data Availability Statement: The data presented in this study are available on request from the corresponding author due to privacy concerns.

Acknowledgments: The authors thank Eun-Ji Jeon, and Ye-Ji Kim for their support. This research was supported by the Bisa Research Grant of Keimyung University in 20220357.

Conflicts of Interest: The authors declare no conflicts of interest.

References

1. Lawrence, K.W.; Link, L.; Lavin, P.; Schwarzkopf, R.; Rozell, J.C. Characterizing patient factors, perioperative interventions, and outcomes associated with inpatients falls after total knee arthroplasty. *Knee. Surg. Relat. Res.* **2024**, *36*, 11. [CrossRef] [PubMed]
2. Kim, C.H.; Park, Y.B.; Baek, S.H. Clinical and Radiological Outcomes of Computer-Assisted Navigation in Primary Total Knee Arthroplasty for Patients with Extra-articular Deformity: Systematic Review and Meta-Analysis. *Clin. Orthop. Surg.* **2024**, *16*, 430–440. [CrossRef] [PubMed]
3. Li, G.; Zhou, C.; Li, S.; Yu, J.; Foster, T.; Bedair, H. Tibiofemoral articulation and axial tibial rotation of the knee after a cruciate retaining total knee arthroplasty. *Knee. Surg. Relat. Res.* **2024**, *36*, 20. [CrossRef]
4. Yang, H.Y.; Yoon, T.W.; Kim, J.Y.; Seon, J.K. Radiologic Assessment of Knee Phenotypes Based on the Coronal Plane Alignment of the Knee Classification in a Korean Population. *Clin. Orthop. Surg.* **2024**, *16*, 422–429. [CrossRef]
5. Øiestad, B.E.; Juhl, C.B.; Eitzen, I.; Thorlund, J.B. Knee extensor muscle weakness is a risk factor for development of knee osteoarthritis. A systematic review and meta-analysis. *Osteoarthr. Cartilage.* **2015**, *23*, 171–177. [CrossRef] [PubMed]
6. Pattyn, E.; Verdonk, P.; Steyaert, A.; Vanden Bossche, L.; Van den Broecke, W.; Thijs, Y.; Witvrouw, E. Vastus medialis obliquus atrophy: Does it exist in patellofemoral pain syndrome? *Am. J. Sports Med.* **2011**, *39*, 1450–1455. [CrossRef]

7. Wang, Y.; Wluka, A.E.; Berry, P.A.; Siew, T.; Teichtahl, A.J.; Urquhart, D.M.; Lloyd, D.G.; Jones, G.; Cicuttini, F.M. Increase in vastus medialis cross-sectional area is associated with reduced pain, cartilage loss, and joint replacement risk in knee osteoarthritis. *Arthritis. Rheum.* **2012**, *64*, 3917–3925. [CrossRef]
8. Raynauld, J.P.; Pelletier, J.P.; Roubille, C.; Dorais, M.; Abram, F.; Li, W.; Wang, Y.; Fairley, J.; Cicuttini, F.M.; Martel-Pelletier, J. Magnetic Resonance Imaging-Assessed Vastus Medialis Muscle Fat Content and Risk for Knee Osteoarthritis Progression: Relevance From a Clinical Trial. *Arthritis. Care. Res.* **2015**, *67*, 1406–1415. [CrossRef]
9. Pan, J.; Stehling, C.; Muller-Hocker, C.; Schwaiger, B.J.; Lynch, J.; McCulloch, C.E.; Nevitt, M.C.; Link, T.M. Vastus lateralis/vastus medialis cross-sectional area ratio impacts presence and degree of knee joint abnormalities and cartilage T2 determined with 3T MRI—An analysis from the incidence cohort of the Osteoarthritis Initiative. *Osteoarthr. Cartilage.* **2011**, *19*, 65–73. [CrossRef]
10. Kellgren, J.H.; Lawrence, J.S. Radiological assessment of osteo-arthrosis. *Ann Rheum Dis.* **1957**, *16*, 494–502. [CrossRef]
11. Fink, B.; Egl, M.; Singer, J.; Fuerst, M.; Bubenheim, M.; Neuen-Jacob, E. Morphologic changes in the vastus medialis muscle in patients with osteoarthritis of the knee. *Arthritis Rheum.* **2007**, *56*, 3626–3633. [CrossRef] [PubMed]
12. Palmieri-Smith, R.M.; Thomas, A.C.; Karvonen-Gutierrez, C.; Sowers, M.F. Isometric quadriceps strength in women with mild, moderate, and severe knee osteoarthritis. *Am. J. Phys. Med. Rehabil.* **2010**, *89*, 541–548. [CrossRef]
13. Murray, A.M.; Thomas, A.C.; Armstrong, C.W.; Pietrosimone, B.G.; Tevald, M.A. The associations between quadriceps muscle strength, power, and knee joint mechanics in knee osteoarthritis: A cross-sectional study. *Clin. Biomech.* **2015**, *30*, 1140–1145. [CrossRef]
14. Slemenda, C.; Brandt, K.D.; Heilman, D.K.; Mazzuca, S.; Braunstein, E.M.; Katz, B.P.; Wolinsky, F.D. Quadriceps weakness and osteoarthritis of the knee. *Ann Intern. Med.* **1997**, *127*, 97–104. [CrossRef]
15. Liikavainio, T.; Lyytinen, T.; Tyrväinen, E.; Sipilä, S.; Arokoski, J.P. Physical function and properties of quadriceps femoris muscle in men with knee osteoarthritis. *Arch. Phys. Med. Rehabil.* **2008**, *89*, 2185–2194. [CrossRef]
16. Segal, N.A.; Torner, J.C.; Felson, D.; Niu, J.; Sharma, L.; Lewis, C.E.; Nevitt, M. Effect of thigh strength on incident radiographic and symptomatic knee osteoarthritis in a longitudinal cohort. *Arthritis Rheum.* **2009**, *61*, 1210–1217. [CrossRef]
17. Omori, G.; Koga, Y.; Tanaka, M.; Nawata, A.; Watanabe, H.; Narumi, K.; Endoh, K. Quadriceps muscle strength and its relationship to radiographic knee osteoarthritis in Japanese elderly. *J. Orthop. Sci.* **2013**, *18*, 536–542. [CrossRef]
18. Pietrosimone, B.; Thomas, A.C.; Saliba, S.A.; Ingersoll, C.D. Association between quadriceps strength and self-reported physical activity in people with knee osteoarthritis. *Int. J. Sports Phys. Ther.* **2014**, *9*, 320–328.
19. Segal, N.A.; Glass, N.A. Is quadriceps muscle weakness a risk factor for incident or progressive knee osteoarthritis? *Phys. Sportsmed.* **2011**, *39*, 44–50. [CrossRef] [PubMed]
20. Alnahdi, A.H.; Zeni, J.A.; Snyder-Mackler, L. Muscle impairments in patients with knee osteoarthritis. *Sports Health* **2012**, *4*, 284–292. [CrossRef] [PubMed]
21. Taniguchi, M.; Fukumoto, Y.; Kobayashi, M.; Kawasaki, T.; Maegawa, S.; Ibuki, S.; Ichihashi, N. Quantity and Quality of the Lower Extremity Muscles in Women with Knee Osteoarthritis. *Ultrasound Med. Biol.* **2015**, *41*, 2567–2574. [CrossRef]
22. Berger, M.J.; Chess, D.G.; Doherty, T.J. Vastus medialis motor unit properties in knee osteoarthritis. *BMC Musculoskelet Disord.* **2011**, *12*, 199. [CrossRef]
23. Segal, N.A.; Findlay, C.; Wang, K.; Torner, J.C.; Nevitt, M.C. The longitudinal relationship between thigh muscle mass and the development of knee osteoarthritis. *Osteoarthr. Cartilage.* **2012**, *20*, 1534–1540. [CrossRef]
24. van den Noort, J.C.; van der Leeden, M.; Stapper, G.; Wirth, W.; Maas, M.; Roorda, L.D.; Lems, W.F.; Dekker, J.; van der Esch, M. Muscle weakness is associated with non-contractile muscle tissue of the vastus medialis muscle in knee osteoarthritis. *BMC Musculoskelet Disord.* **2022**, *23*, 91. [CrossRef]

medicina

MDPI

Article

The Association between the Extent of the Osteoarthritic Meniscus Degeneration and Cigarette Smoking—A Pilot Study

Maria Zabrzyńska [1,*], Maciej Pasiński [2], Maciej Gagat [3,4], Michał Kułakowski [5], Łukasz Woźniak [6], Karol Elster [5], Paulina Antosik [7] and Jan Zabrzyński [2]

1 Faculty of Medicine, Collegium Medicum in Bydgoszcz, Nicolaus Copernicus University in Toruń, 85-067 Bydgoszcz, Poland
2 Department of Orthopaedics and Traumatology, Faculty of Medicine, Collegium Medicum in Bydgoszcz, Nicolaus Copernicus University in Toruń, 85-067 Bydgoszcz, Poland; pamacos2014@gmail.com (M.P.); zabrzynski@gmail.com (J.Z.)
3 Department of Histology and Embryology, Faculty of Medicine, Collegium Medicum in Bydgoszcz, Nicolaus Copernicus University in Toruń, 85-067 Bydgoszcz, Poland; mgagat@cm.umk.pl
4 Faculty of Medicine, Collegium Medicum, Mazovian Academy in Płock, 09-402 Płock, Poland
5 Independent Public Healthcare Center in Rypin, 87-500 Rypin, Poland; mkulakowski@poczta.fm (M.K.); karol.elster@gmail.com (K.E.)
6 Department of Orthopaedics and Traumatology, University of Medical Sciences, 61-701 Poznan, Poland
7 Department of Clinical Pathology, Faculty of Medicine, Collegium Medicum in Bydgoszcz, Nicolaus Copernicus University in Toruń, 85-067 Bydgoszcz, Poland; paulina.antosik@cm.umk.pl
* Correspondence: maria.zabrzynska@gmail.com

Abstract: *Background and Objectives*: The negative effects of smoking on the musculoskeletal system were presented by many authors, although the relationship between smoking and osteoarthritis remains unclear. The aim of this paper was to investigate the negative effects of smoking on meniscal tissue in osteoarthritic knees by microscopic examination, by adapting the Bonar scoring system and its modifications. *Materials and Methods*: The study involved 34 patients with varus knees, from whom 65 samples of knee menisci were obtained. The mean age in the studied group was 65.385 years. The smoking status of the patients concluded that there were 13 smokers and 21 nonsmokers. *Results*: Among smokers, the mean classical Bonar score was 8.42 and the mean modified Bonar score was 6.65, while nonsmokers were characterized by scores of 8.51 and 7.35, respectively. There was a statistically significant negative correlation between the number of cigarettes and the collagen in the medial meniscus ($p = 0.0197$). Moreover, in the medial meniscus, the modified Bonar score correlated negatively with the number of cigarettes ($p = 0.0180$). Similarly, such a correlation was observed between the number of cigarettes and the modified Bonar score in the lateral meniscus ($p = 0.04571$). Furthermore, no correlation was identified between the number of cigarettes and the classical Bonar score in the lateral meniscus. There was a statistically significant difference in the collagen variable value between the smokers and nonsmokers groups ($p = 0.04525$). *Conclusions*: The microscopic investigation showed no differences in the menisci of smokers and nonsmokers, except for the collagen, which was more organized in smokers. Moreover, the modified Bonar score was correlated negatively with the number of cigarettes, which supports the role of neovascularization in meniscus pathology under the influence of tobacco smoking.

Keywords: meniscus; meniscus tear; osteoarthritis; smoking; Bonar score system; varus knees

1. Introduction

Nowadays, there is a growing interest and understanding of the knee menisci and their crucial role in maintaining proper knee joint congruence and kinematics, despite the fact that in the past they were considered to be functionless, vestigial structures and were often excised with an open total meniscectomy [1–3]. The menisci can be described as a fibrocartilaginous, crescent-shaped wedge structure located between the condyles of the femur and tibia [2,4]. They cover 75% to 93% of the articular surface of the corresponding tibial plateau, forming the acetabulum of the knee joint [1,5]. Their function allows them to maintain proper knee joint performance and biomechanical functions. They are mainly involved in load-bearing, load transmission, and shock absorption. Moreover, they participate in proprioception, articular cartilage nutrition, lubrication, and protection. They are also important passive joint stabilizers (Figure 1) [2,6,7].

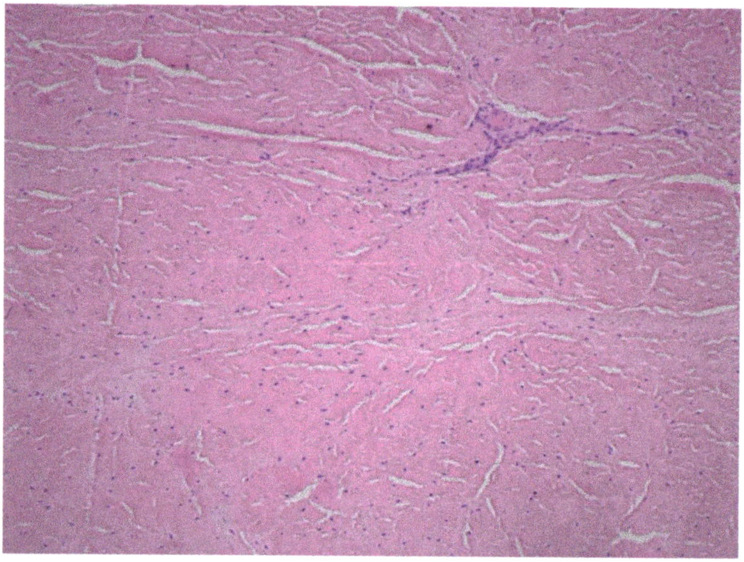

Figure 1. Microscopic evaluation of the meniscal sample stained with H&E showed a red–white zone of the menisci.

The Bonar score system is the most common and established scale to assess the microscopic evaluation of tendon pathology. This semiquantitative scoring system has been modified many times in order to improve diagnostic and microscopic evaluation [8–14]. Thus, it can be modified to quantify the pathological changes in meniscal tissue. Park et al. were the first to present the use of the Bonar score in meniscus root pathology in knee osteoarthritis (OA). Their study presented the similarity between meniscus root fibrous connective tissue, and tendons connective tissue microstructure [15].

Osteoarthritis is characterized by knee cartilage volume loss and structural modification of cartilage, subchondral bone, Hoffa's fat pad, synovial membrane, ligaments, and muscles. All of these features distinguish OA as a whole-joint disease [16,17]. Meniscal damage or meniscal excision are known as primary risk factors for rapid cartilage loss [18,19]. Both the excision of the meniscus and meniscal tears are factors resulting in cartilage lesions leading to knee joint OA [20]. Meniscal tears can easily lead to OA, and, on the other hand, osteoarthritis knees may develop meniscal tears. However, healthy menisci rarely occur in knees with OA [21]. Early knee OA is associated with either meniscal tears or symptoms such as synovial inflammation. Synovial inflammation is known as a major risk factor for OA's rapid progression. Meniscal tissue with synovial inflammation differs with an enhanced level of metalloproteinase-13, which plays a major role in the degeneration of cartilage tissue in OA [22]. Menisci in OA knees display signs of pathological changes. They are often torn, macerated with cracks, have structural disorganization and fractures, or are even completely damaged, rather than without signs of degeneration [21]. Awareness of their importance prompts people to avoid meniscectomy and encourages the evolution of modern treatment methods for meniscal repair in order to save meniscal tissue [23,24].

Even though meniscal injuries are the second most common trauma to the knee, the data are still lacking in epidemiology and prognostic factors [23]. Blackwell et al. observed that current smokers were significantly more likely to undergo meniscectomy shortly after meniscus repair [25]. The negative association of smoking and pack-years with knee joint cartilage suggests that cartilage loss and defect may be inducted by smoking [26–29]. On the other hand, a few authors showed no negative association between smoking habits and meniscal tissue [30–33]. Nevertheless, smoking is commonly known as an important negative factor in orthopedics. Tobacco smoking results in decreased healing, complications, and poor postoperative outcomes in orthopedic surgery [23,34]. The relationship between smoking and OA remains unclear. Tobacco users may have an enhanced risk of OA due to cartilage damage and the ongoing inflammation process [35]. Nicotine, one of the constituents of tobacco smoke, promotes chondrocyte proliferation, migration, capillary formation, and decreased collagen synthesis [36,37]. Moreover, it stimulates the neovascularization process, which is known to take part in OA [38]. However, the effects of smoking on meniscal tissue have not been well explored yet. However, many authors present the negative effects of smoking on the musculoskeletal system, although there are still papers that undermine these outcomes. We hypothesized that the known negative effects of nicotine, such as neovascularization and stimulating inflammation, may negatively affect meniscal tissue healing. It would lead to the degeneration of meniscal tissue, which could be quantified using the Bonar scoring system. Thus, the aim of this study was to assess degeneration of the meniscal tissue in OA knees in correlation with smoking using the Bonar score in microscopic examination. Smoking may turn out to be an important negative factor in the degeneration of meniscal tissue in the OA knees. In this study, we attempted to investigate the negative association between smoking and meniscal tissue.

2. Materials and Methods

The study followed the principles outlined in the Declaration of Helsinki for experiments involving human subjects. Before the commencement of the study, approval was obtained from the local institutional Bioethics Committee (approval number KB 131/2022). The study included consecutive patients who underwent total knee arthroplasty for symptomatic OA between 2022 and 2023. All participants included in the survey were preoperatively diagnosed with gonarthrosis based on a clinical examination, as well as imaging modalities such as X-rays or magnetic resonance.

Inclusion criteria included the presence of severe unilateral OA with varus knee deformity (Kellgren–Lawrence score II or more), rheumatological diseases, and informed consent from the patient. Genu varum malalignment is characterized by $<4^{\circ}$ valgus knee axis or mechanical axis falling medial to the center of the knee. The following exclusion criteria were selected: secondary OA, previous surgical procedures within the affected knee, valgus deformity of the knee joint, severe deformity (>20 degrees varus), advanced OA in other joints, diabetes, advanced atherosclerosis of the lower limbs, cancer, and immunological diseases.

Patient demographic data, preoperative ROM, and preoperative X-rays (a long leg standing X-ray and an AP, lateral X-ray of both knee joints) were recorded. Written informed consent was obtained from all patients before they participated in the study.

The patient population was categorized as smokers or nonsmokers (those who had never used any nicotine supplement, such as nicotine gum or patch, oral snuff or moist snuff, cigars, or cigarettes). Also, dose-dependent and time-dependent data about smoking habits were collected, including the period of cigarette smoking (smoking years), the mean number of cigarettes smoked per day, and the pack-years index (one pack contains 20 cigarettes in Poland. The surgeons were blinded to the smoking status of the patients.

2.1. Surgical Technique

Total knee arthroplasty was performed in each case. All procedures were performed using an anteromedial approach; a tourniquet was applied in each case. In patients, the infrapatellar fat pad was bluntly divided from the patellar ligament and resected using electrocautery. However, surgeons incised it at the medial border of the patellar ligament to gain exposure to the knee joint. In all cases, the anteromedial joint capsule was routinely released from the tibia. The surgeries were performed following the concept of mechanical alignment; femoral components were implanted using the posterior referencing technique, while the rotation of tibial components was established parallel to a line drawn from the posterior cruciate ligament to the medial third of the tibial tuberosity. In all cases, the patella was neither resurfaced nor denervated, although large patellar osteophytes were removed if present. During the surgery, the menisci (both lateral and medial in each case) were dissected totally to preserve their original shape.

2.2. Histopathological Assessment

The menisci samples were fixed in 10% buffered formalin that was fresh and sterile. The samples were prepared using the hematoxylin and eosin (H&E) staining method, as well as the Alcian blue protocol. They were examined under light microscopy (Olympus BX46, Tokyo, Japan) using 5 μm sections. Alcian blue staining was explicitly employed to inspect the presence of ground substance glycosaminoglycans. It was carried out in accordance with the alcian blue protocol, respectively: deparaffinization of slides and hydrating to distilled water, staining in alcian blue solution for 30 min, washing in running tap water for 2 min, rinsing in distilled water, counterstaining in nuclear fast red solution for 5 min, washing in running tap water for 1 min, dehydrating through 95% alcohol, 2 times changing of absolute alcohol for 3 min each, clearing in xylene, and, in the end, mounting with resinous mounting medium.

The microscopic evaluation was carried out by two experienced observers who specialized in connective tissue. They were blinded to the identity of the samples. The extent of histopathological changes was assessed based on the classical Bonar score assumptions and their modifications. The classical Bonar scoring system evaluates four main variables: fibroblast/chondrocyte morphology, accumulation of ground substance elements, neovascularity, and collagen architecture. A scoring range of 0 to 3 points was assigned to each variable, with 0 indicating normal tissue and 3 representing extreme pathology. An utterly normal tissue would score 0, while a severely degenerated tendon would score 12.

In the second step of the examination, meniscal samples were evaluated using the modified Bonar scores developed by Zabrzyński et al. [14]. In this modified scoring system, a new Bonar score, the attributes of the neovascularization variable in the original Bonar scale were reversed. A score of three points was assigned to normal tissue with minimal occurrence of blood vessels (absent neovascularization), two points for the incidental presence of capillary clusters of less than one per 10 high-power fields (HPFs; mild neovascularization), one point for 1–2 clusters per 10 HPFs (moderate neovascularization), and zero points for more than two clusters per 10 HPFs (abundant neovascularization).

2.3. Statistical Analysis

Group comparisons and statistical analyses were conducted by two independent investigators using GraphPad Prism version 8.0.1 for Windows, GraphPad Software, Dotmatics, UK, www.graphpad.com (accessed on 24 December 2023). A p-value less than 0.05 was considered statistically significant. The normality of the variables was assessed using the Shapiro–Wilk test. Relationships between the studied parameters were evaluated using Spearman's rank correlation coefficient. According to the nonnormal distribution of the data, intergroup comparisons were performed using nonparametric tests, specifically the Mann–Whitney U-test, for comparing two groups.

Correlation Analyses

The results of the Bonar and new Bonar scores were correlated with smoking indexes such as smoking years, the mean number of cigarettes smoked per day, and the pack-years index.

3. Results

The study involved 34 patients with varus knees, from whom 65 samples of knee menisci were obtained. The mean age in the studied group was 65.385 years (range: 54–81; SD = 6.88) at enrollment; the gender distribution was 21 women to 13 men. The demographic data are presented in Table 1.

Table 1. Summary of demographic and clinical characteristics of patients.

Characteristics	Total	Smokers	Nonsmokers
No. of patients	34	13	21
Female	21	7	14
Male	13	6	7
Age	65.385 (54–81)	64.231 (54–72)	66.154 (55–81)
Classical Bonar score	8.4462 (4–12)	8.4231 (6–12)	8.5128 (4–11)
Modified Bonar score	7.0462 (3–11)	6.6538 (3–10)	7.3590 (4–11)

By smoking status, there were 13 smokers (including 14 women and 7 men) and 21 nonsmokers (including 7 women and 6 men). No patients changed their smoking habits during the follow-up. Specifically, the mean age in the smoker group was 64.231 (range 54–72, SD = 6.0286) and 66.154 (range 55–81, SD = 7.3683) in the nonsmokers group (Table 1).

The mean classical Bonar score was 8.4462 (range 4–12, SD=1.5715). The mean modified Bonar score, which includes the reversed neovascularization variable, was 7.0462 (range 3–11, SD = 1.7804). Among smokers, the mean classical Bonar score was 8.4231 (range 6–12, SD = 1.6775) and the mean modified Bonar score was 6.6538 (range 3–10, SD = 1.8318), while among nonsmokers it was 8.5128 (range 4–11, SD = 1.5706) and 7.3590 (range 4–11, SD = 1.7089), respectively (Table 1).

The mean classical Bonar score for the medial menisci was 8.5000 (range 4–11, SD=1.5240), and for the lateral menisci, it was 8.3939 (range 6–12, SD = 1.6382). Regarding the modified Bonar score, the mean score for the medial menisci was 6.9375 (range 3–10, SD = 1.7586), and for the lateral menisci, it was 7.1515 (range 3–11, SD = 1.8221) (Table 2).

Table 2. Summary of meniscus characteristics.

Characteristic	Total	Meniscus	
		Medial	Lateral
No. of samples	65	32	33
No. of cigarettes	5.2308 (0–25)	7.5000 (0–25)	3.0303 (0–25)
Classical Bonar score	8.4462 (4–12)	8.5000(4–11)	8.3939(6–12)
Modified Bonar score	7.0462 (3–11)	6.9375 (3–10)	7.1515 (3–11)

The mean number of cigarettes smoked per day was 5.2308 (range 0–25); for the medial menisci group it was 7.5 (range 0–25, SD = 9.5883), and for the lateral menisci group it was 3.0303 (range 0–25, SD = 6.9529) (Table 2).

Macroscopically, all examined menisci displayed signs of degeneration, including cracks, structural disorganization, and fractures. Histological examination of the meniscal specimens under a light microscope revealed tissue degeneration in all cases, both in the medial and lateral menisci (Figure 2).

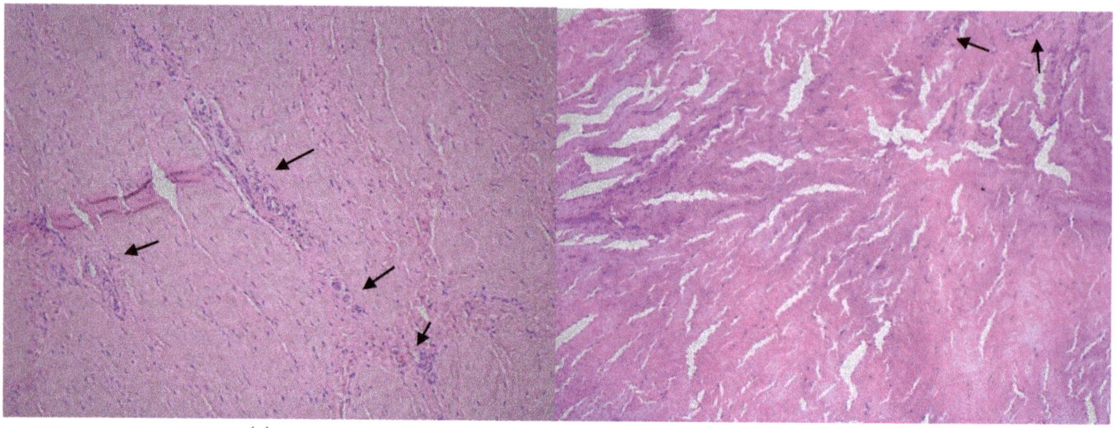

(**a**) (**b**)

Figure 2. Microscopic evaluation of the meniscal sample stained with H&E. (**a**) Red–white zone in smokers groups with randomly scattered clusters of vessels (arrows). (**b**) Red–white zone in nonsmokers group with randomly scattered clusters of vessels (arrows).

The three variables of the classical Bonar score (chondrocyte morphology, ground substance, and vascularity) and modified neovascularization variable [14] showed no association with the number of cigarettes in medial menisci (p = 0.3072, p = 0.3052, p = 0.1910, p = 0.1910) (Figure 3A,B,D,E). However, there was a statistically significant negative correlation between the number of cigarettes and collagen in the medial menisci (p = 0.0197) (Figure 3C).

Additionally, we noted that the modified Bonar score correlated negatively with the number of cigarettes (p = 0.0180), but the classical Bonar score showed no association with the daily number of cigarettes smoked, in the medial menisci (p = 0.0635) (Figure 4).

Furthermore, no correlation was identified between the number of cigarettes and all four variables of the classical Bonar score in the lateral menisci (p = 0.06078, p = 0.3060, p = 0.4067, p = 0.09576) (Figure 5A–D). The number of cigarettes did not exhibit a correlation with the modified neovascularization variable [14] as well (p = 0.09576) (Figure 5E).

On the other hand, we observed a statistically significant correlation between the number of cigarettes and the modified Bonar score (p = 0.04571), but no correlation with the classical Bonar score in the lateral menisci (p = 0.3959) (Figure 6A, B).

Chondrocyte morphology, accumulation of ground substance, vascularity, collagen, age, and modified neovascularization variables did not show any significant difference between the smokers and nonsmokers groups in the lateral menisci (p = 0.3416, p = 0.9561, p = 0.1681, p = 0.6394, p = 0.7777, p = 0.1681) (Figure 7A–F).

Moreover, there were no statistically significant differences, either in the classical Bonar score or the modified Bonar score, between smokers and nonsmokers for the lateral menisci (p = 0.8314, p = 0.4636) (Figure 8).

Similarly, between smokers and nonsmokers, no statistically significant differences were observed in the chondrocyte morphology (p = 0.5267), ground substance (p = 0.5827), vascularity (p = 0.4326), reversed vascularity (p = 0.4326), and age (p = 0.7834), assessing medial menisci (Figure 9A–C,E,F). Regarding the collagen variable, there was a statistically significant difference between the smokers and nonsmokers groups, as presented in Figure 9D (p = 0.04525).

When comparing the classical Bonar score and modified Bonar score in the medial menisci in terms of smoking status, no statistically significant differences were found (p = 0.3433 and p = 0.2062) (Figure 10A,B).

Furthermore, there were no statistically significant differences between the smokers and nonsmokers group when comparing the chondrocyte morphology (p = 0.2214), ground substance (p = 0.8215), vascularity (p = 0.1063), collagen (p = 0.2964), reversed vascularity (p = 0.1063), and age (p = 0.6816) in both medial and lateral menisci, as presented in Figure 11A–F.

Moreover, the classical Bonar score and modified Bonar score variables exhibited no differences based on smoking status in both the lateral and medial menisci (p = 0.6763, p = 0.1511) (Figure 12A,B).

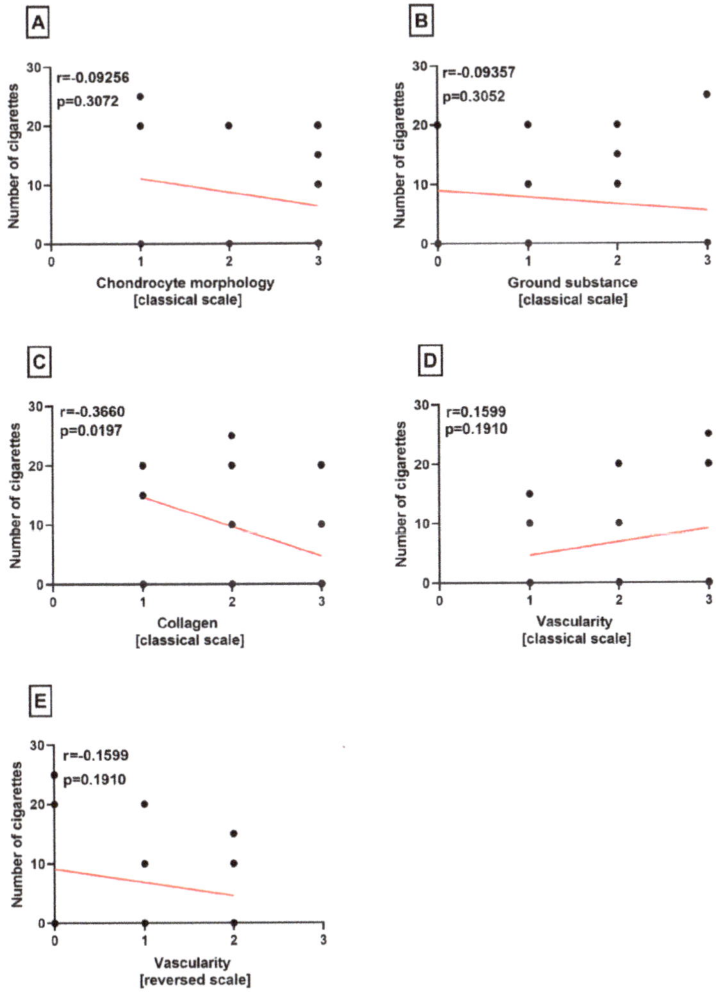

Figure 3. Summarized statistical analysis based on the chondrocyte morphology, ground substance, collagen, vascularity, and reversed vascularity in the **medial menisci**. (**A**) Correlation between the **chondrocyte morphology and number of cigarettes** smoked per day. (**B**) Correlation between the **ground substance and number of cigarettes** smoked per day. (**C**) Correlation between the **collagen composition and number of cigarettes** smoked per day. (**D**) Correlation between the **vascularity and number of cigarettes** smoked per day. (**E**) Correlation between the **reversed vascularity and number of cigarettes** smoked per day.

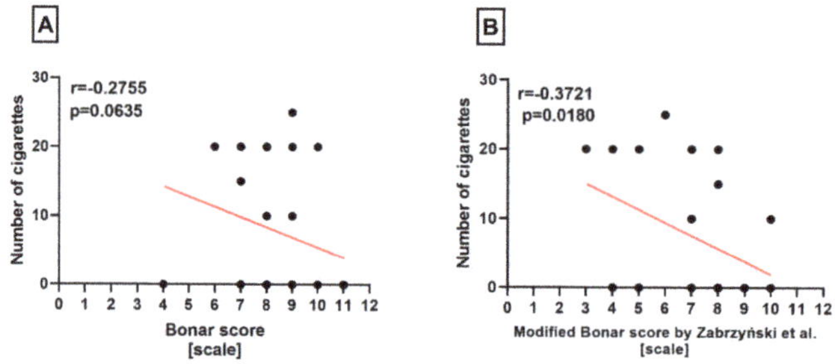

Figure 4. Summarized statistical analysis based on the classical Bonar score and modified Bonar score in the **medial menisci**. (**A**) Correlation between the **classical Bonar score and the number of cigarettes** smoked per day. (**B**) Correlation between the **modified Bonar score [14] and the number of cigarettes** smoked per day.

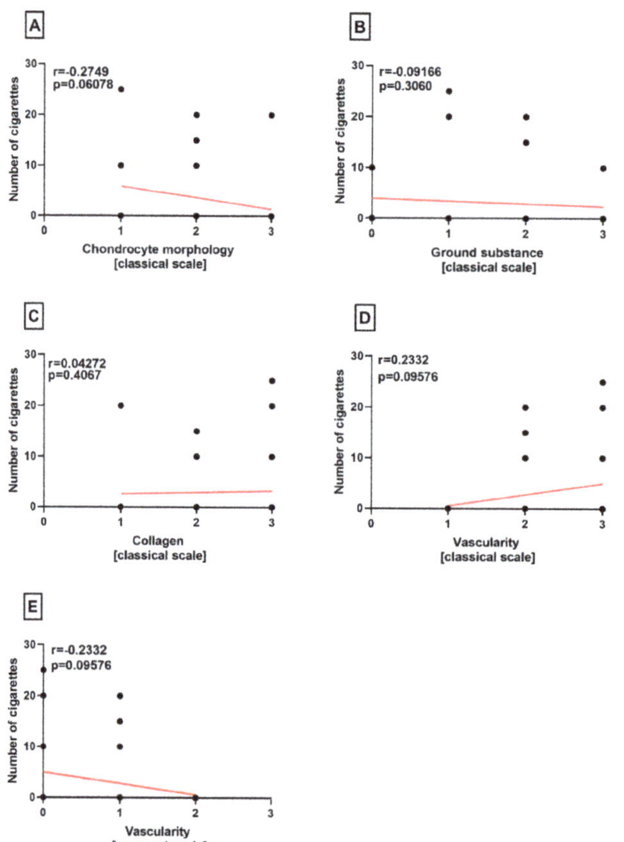

Figure 5. Summarized statistical analysis based on the chondrocyte morphology, ground substance, collagen, vascularity, and reversed vascularity in the **lateral menisci**. (**A**) Correlation between the **chondrocyte morphology and the number of cigarettes** smoked per day. (**B**) Correlation between the **ground substance and the number of cigarettes** smoked per day. (**C**) Correlation between the **collagen composition and the number of cigarettes** smoked per day. (**D**) Correlation between the **vascularity and the number of cigarettes** smoked per day;(**E**) Correlation between the **reversed vascularity and the number of cigarettes** smoked per day.

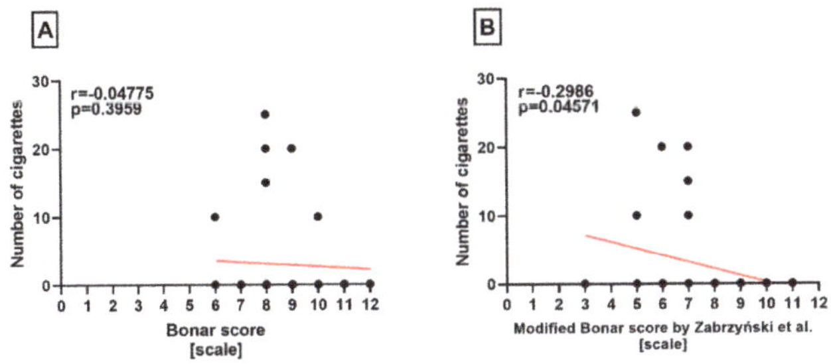

Figure 6. Summarized statistical analysis based on the classical Bonar score and the modified Bonar score in the **lateral menisci**. (**A**) Correlation between the **classical Bonar score and the number of cigarettes** smoked per day. (**B**) Correlation between the **modified Bonar score [14] and the number of cigarettes** smoked per day.

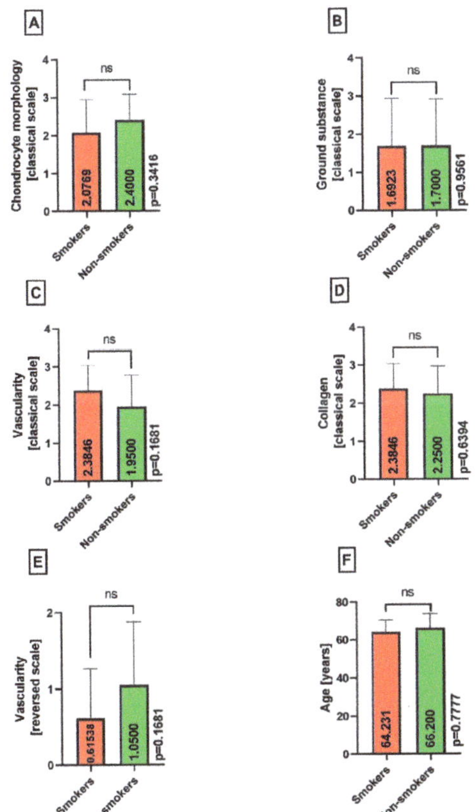

Figure 7. Summarized statistical analysis based on the chondrocyte morphology, ground substance, vascularity, collagen, reversed vascularity, and age in the **lateral menisci** (ns meaning not statistically significant). (**A**) Comparison of the **chondrocyte morphology between the smokers and nonsmokers** groups. (**B**) Comparison of the **ground substance between the smokers and nonsmokers** groups. (**C**) Comparison of the **vascularity between the smokers and nonsmokers** groups. (**D**) Comparison of the **collagen composition between the smokers and nonsmokers** groups. (**E**) Comparison of the reversed **vascularity between the smokers and nonsmokers** groups. (**F**) Comparison of the **age between the smokers and nonsmokers** groups.

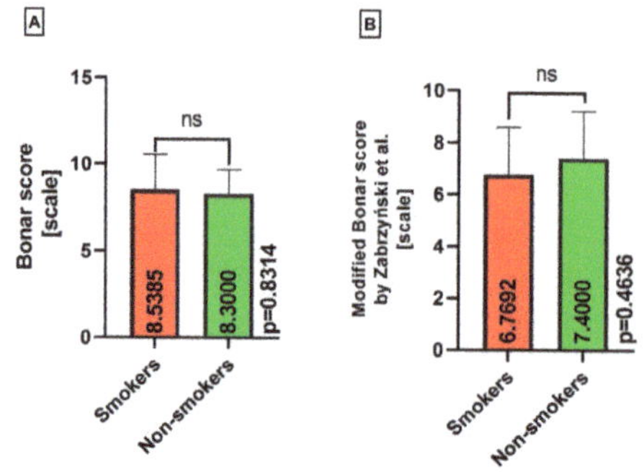

Figure 8. Summarized statistical analysis based on the classical Bonar score and the modified Bonar score in the **lateral menisci** (ns meaning not statistically significant). (**A**) Comparison of the **classical Bonar score between the smokers and nonsmokers** groups. (**B**) Comparison of the **modified Bonar score [14] between the smokers and nonsmokers** groups.

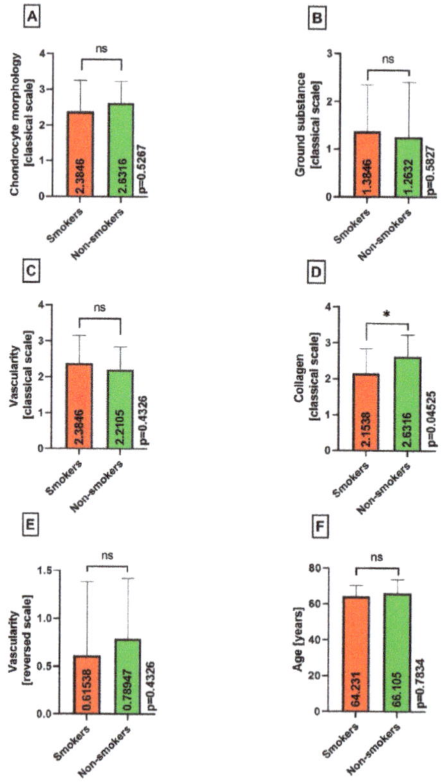

Figure 9. Summarized statistical analysis based on the chondrocyte morphology, ground substance, vascularity, collagen, reversed vascularity, and age in the **medial menisci** (ns meaning not statistically significant and * meaning statistically significant). (**A**) Comparison of the **chondrocyte morphology between the smokers and nonsmokers** groups. (**B**) Comparison of the **ground substance between the smokers and nonsmokers** groups. (**C**) Comparison of the **vascularity between the smokers and nonsmokers** groups. (**D**) Comparison of the **collagen composition between the smokers and nonsmokers** groups. (**E**) Comparison of the reversed **vascularity between the smokers and nonsmokers** groups. (**F**) Comparison of the **age between the smokers and nonsmokers** groups.

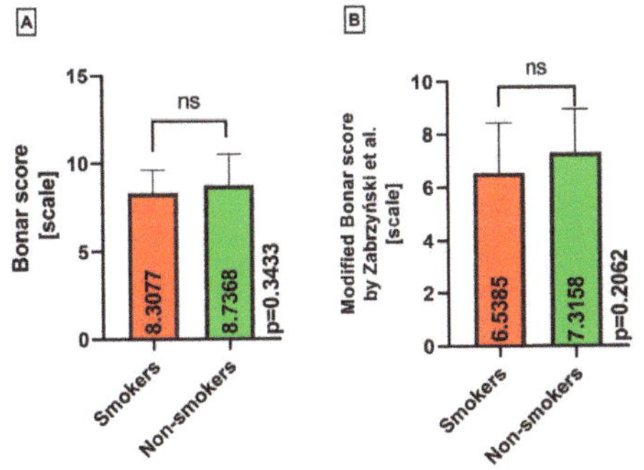

Figure 10. Summarized statistical analysis based on the classical Bonar score and modified Bonar score in the **medial menisci** (ns meaning not statistically significant). (**A**) Comparison of the **classical Bonar score between the smokers and nonsmokers** groups. (**B**) Comparison of the **modified Bonar score [14] between the smokers and nonsmokers** groups.

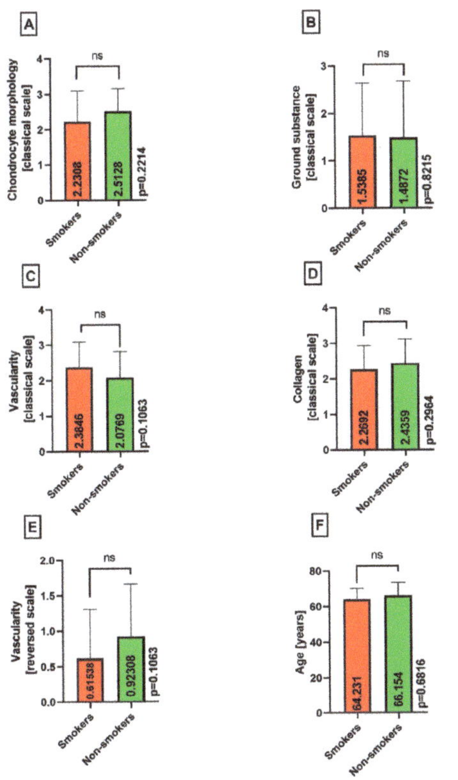

Figure 11. Summarized statistical analysis based on the chondrocyte morphology, ground substance, vascularity, collagen, reversed vascularity, and age **in both menisci** (ns meaning not statistically significant). (**A**) Comparison of the **chondrocyte morphology between the smokers and nonsmokers** groups. (**B**) Comparison of the **ground substance between the smokers and nonsmokers** groups. (**C**) Comparison of the **vascularity between the smokers and nonsmokers** groups. (**D**) Comparison of the **collagen composition between the smokers and nonsmokers** groups. (**E**) Comparison of the **reversed vascularity between the smokers and nonsmokers** groups. (**F**) Comparison of the **age between the smokers and nonsmokers** groups.

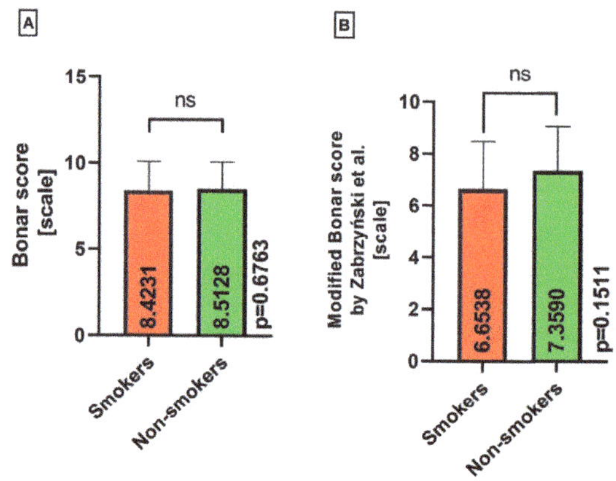

Figure 12. Summarized statistical analysis based on the classical Bonar score and modified Bonar score in **both menisci** (ns meaning not statistically significant). (**A**) Comparison of the **classical Bonar score between the smokers and nonsmokers** groups. (**B**) Comparison of the **modified Bonar score [14] between the smokers and nonsmokers** groups.

4. Discussion

In our study, we found no evidence of an association between nicotine and the degeneration of meniscal tissue using the Bonar score system. The effect of nicotine on meniscal tissue was quantified using the Bonar scoring system and its modifications in microscopic examination. The most important finding of this study was the negative correlation between the modified Bonar score and the number of cigarettes. To the best of our knowledge, this is the first study aimed at assessing the differences in human meniscal tissue histopathology between smokers and nonsmokers. This study is also another attempt to explore the use of the Bonar score in meniscus pathology.

Nicotine product use has doubtless adverse effects on human health. Numerous studies confirm that tobacco smoking is the main contributor to lung and upper respiratory tract cancer and a significant risk factor for cardiovascular diseases, prostate, and bladder cancers [39–41]. It makes tobacco use the leading avoidable cause of death worldwide [39]. The advent of tobacco use associated with e-cigarette vaping seems to postpone the perspective of a nicotine-free society [42–44].

The effect of nicotine's use on the musculoskeletal system is well established, too. It directly toxifies osteoblast and osteoclast activity and indirectly negatively regulates sex and adrenocortical hormones, vitamin D, intestinal calcium absorption, vessels, and oxygen supply [45]. It leads to lower bone mineral density, increased fracture risk, impaired fracture or soft tissue healing, and increased joint disease activity. Moreover, it adversely affects muscles, tendons, cartilage, and ligaments [26,46]. Rose et al. proved that secondhand smoke caused more severe OA in medial meniscus destabilized mice models compared to room-air-exposed mice when assessed by the histopathological Mankin score because of increased expression of proinflammatory molecules [47].

Despite the well-known adverse effects of smoking on soft tissues, few papers have focused on the impact of tobacco on meniscal tissue, providing inconclusive outcomes. Domzalski et al. proved that smokers used to have a lower KOOS score and prolonged time to return to activities of daily living and sport when compared to nonsmokers after outside-in meniscal repair [48]. Blackwell et al. documented the failure rate after meniscal repairs in smokers to be 27%, compared to 7% in nonsmokers [25]. In Uzun et al.'s material, there was a higher failure rate in medial and lateral menisci repairs in smokers than in nonsmokers in the follow-up of 51.2 and 63.2 months, respectively [28,29]. Haklar et al. observed that smoking significantly affected meniscal healing [49]. Overall, many authors highlight the negative effect of smoking on meniscal surgery postoperative outcomes [25,28,29,48,49].

Franovic et al. noted that active smoking not only has an impact on patients' postoperative outcomes but also their smoking history [50]. On the other hand, Astur et al. found no difference in the quality of life of nicotine users and nonsmokers six months after anterior cruciate or meniscal surgery [51]. Moses et al.'s evaluation proved no association between smoking and failed meniscus repair in bucket-handle tears [32]. Also, Zabrzyński et al. [14] found no connection between smoking indices (smoking years, number of cigarettes per day, pack-year index) and functional outcomes after all-inside repair of chronic medial meniscus tears [23]. Moreover, smoking was not associated with failure after all-inside meniscus repair in Laurendon et al.'s material [31]. What is interesting, on the other hand, is that the literature is quite univocal when it comes to the detrimental effect of cigarette smoking on ligament and tendon health and the results of their reconstructions and repairs [34,52–59].

In this study, we aimed to assess the differences in human meniscal tissue histopathology between smokers and nonsmokers. The comparison did not prove significant differences in the total Bonar score and the new Bonar score in the medial and lateral menisci between both groups. No differences existed in every variable assessed (chondrocyte morphology, ground substance, collagen composition, vascularity score, and reversed vascularity score) in the lateral menisci groups. The only difference in scores was in the collagen organization of medial menisci, which was, surprisingly, more organized in the smoker group. Unexpectedly, the present study showed a weak negative correlation between the number of cigarettes per day and the new Bonar score result. This might suggest that the higher the number of cigarettes smoked daily, the less severe the negative involvement of meniscal histology. It should be pointed out that the correlation is weak, and enrolling more patients in the study could strengthen this correlation.

Park et al. introduced the use of the Bonar score for the first time in assessing meniscus root pathology in knee osteoarthritis. In their study, the mean Bonar score for patients with degeneration was higher (8.5 and 13.5) than those without degeneration (4) [15]. Quite the opposite was true in our study, in which smokers should have a higher Bonar score, although they had an 8.42 and nonsmokers had an 8.51. On the other hand, in our study, the modified Bonar score was lower in smokers than in nonsmokers. This can indicate the much more advanced pathological process of neovascularization, implying that the degeneration process is developed to a lesser extent. However, compared to Park et al.'s results, the more advanced the process of meniscal degeneration, the higher the degree of neovascularization. Moreover, Zabrzyński et al. [14] observed that neovascularization occurs in pathological conditions such as OA in tendons [14]. Noting similarities in the microstructure of fibrous connective tissue between meniscus roots and tendons, it can also confirm that neovascularization is related to a higher degree of degeneration. As mentioned above, our study results showed the opposite.

Nevertheless, this finding, interpreted with caution, might be hypothetically explained by the fact that low-metabolism tissues like menisci may paradoxically benefit from transient ischemia caused by cigarette smoking. Hypoxia caused by tobacco smoke triggers vascular endothelial growth factor (VEGF) synthesis, which is responsible for capillary expansion and stimulates the angiogenesis process in tissues. Many disorders related to smoking: OA, retinopathy, inflammation, tumors, and advanced tendinopathy, are associated with neovascularization. Nicotine plays a major role in the neovascularization process, stimulating endothelial growth, migration, survival, tube formation, and nitric oxide production. This process is described as the pathological formation process of new capillaries with abnormal permeability [38,60–63], which can be the reason for lower modified Bonar score in smokers group.

Even though pathological, the more significant number of vessels might be attributed to the higher blood flow and partially explain the contraindicatory results in studies that examined the effects of meniscal repair in smokers and nonsmokers. What supports this hypothesis is the relatively low number of cigarettes smoked per day in our groups (the mean of 5.2308), which might be considered a factor contributing to interrupted hypoxia events.

Several limitations were noted in this study. We recommend interpreting our findings cautiously because one of the paper's limitations is the relatively low menisci in the smokers' group. If true, these "benefits" are not to overrule the disastrous effect of tobacco smoking on the cardiovascular system and its neoplastic potential. Furthermore, the sample size was modest, with a predominance of female participants and nonsmokers. To create a more homogeneous population, strict exclusion criteria were applied to enhance the statistical power. Additionally, the Bonar score system was developed primarily for tendon pathology instead of meniscus. This could potentially introduce bias in our results.

5. Conclusions

The microscopic investigation showed no differences in the menisci of smokers and nonsmokers, except for the collagen, which was more organized in smokers. Moreover, the modified Bonar score was negatively correlated with the number of cigarettes, which supports the role of neovascularization in meniscus pathology under the influence of tobacco smoking.

We want to examine a more extended group, such as 200 patients, as this paper is only the pilot study. Also, the neovascularization issue is very interesting, suggesting that vascularization could be a game changer in meniscus histopathology, as we observed that smokers had an abundant neovascularization process.

Author Contributions: Conceptualization, M.Z. and M.P.; methodology, M.Z., P.A., M.P. and M.G.; software, P.A. and M.G.; validation, J.Z.; formal analysis, M.Z., M.P., M.G. and Ł.W.; investigation, M.Z., M.P. and P.A.; resources, M.P. and K.E.; data curation, K.E, M.Z. and M.K.; writing original draft preparation, M.Z. and M.P.; writing—review and editing, M.K, M.G., Ł.W. and J.Z.; visualization, M.Z. and M.P.; supervision, J.Z. and M.G.; project administration, M.Z. All authors have read and agreed to the published version of the manuscript.

Funding: This research received no external funding.

Institutional Review Board Statement: The study was conducted in accordance with the Declaration of Helsinki, and approved by the local institutional Bioethics Committee of Collegium Medicum in Bydgoszcz, Poland (protocol code KB131/2022 and date of approval: 15 February 2022).

Informed Consent Statement: Informed consent was obtained from all subjects involved in the study. Written informed consent has been obtained from the patient(s) to publish this paper.

Data Availability Statement: Data are contained within the article.

Conflicts of Interest: The authors declare no conflicts of interest.

References

1. Pasiński, M.; Zabrzyńska, M.; Adamczyk, M.; Sokołowski, M.; Głos, T.; Ziejka, M.; Augustynowicz, P.; Boguszewski, K.; Piotrowski, W.; Michał, B.; et al. A Current Insight into Human Knee Menisci. *Transl. Res. Anat.* **2023**, *32*, 100259. [CrossRef]
2. Mordecai, S.C. Treatment of Meniscal Tears: An Evidence Based Approach. *World J. Orthop.* **2014**, *5*, 233. [CrossRef] [PubMed]
3. Maffulli, N.; Tarantino, D.; Aicale, R. Meniscal Tears. In *Evidence-Based Orthopedics*; Bhandari, M., Ed.; Wiley: New York, NY, USA, 2021; pp. 787–791, ISBN 978-1-119-41400-1.
4. Fox, A.J.S.; Bedi, A.; Rodeo, S.A. The Basic Science of Human Knee Menisci: Structure, Composition, and Function. *Sports Health* **2012**, *4*, 340–351. [CrossRef] [PubMed]
5. Bryceland, J.K.; Powell, A.J.; Nunn, T. Knee Menisci: Structure, Function, and Management of Pathology. *Cartilage* **2017**, *8*, 99–104. [CrossRef] [PubMed]
6. Hutchinson, I.D.; Moran, C.J.; Potter, H.G.; Warren, R.F.; Rodeo, S.A. Restoration of the Meniscus: Form and Function. *Am. J. Sports Med.* **2014**, *42*, 987–998. [CrossRef]
7. Makris, E.A.; Hadidi, P.; Athanasiou, K.A. The Knee Meniscus: Structure–Function, Pathophysiology, Current Repair Techniques, and Prospects for Regeneration. *Biomaterials* **2011**, *32*, 7411–7431. [CrossRef]
8. Zabrzyńska, M.; Grzanka, D.; Zielińska, W.; Jaworski, Ł.; Pękala, P.; Gagat, M. The Bonar Score in the Histopathological Assessment of Tendinopathy and Its Clinical Relevance—A Systematic Review. *Medicina* **2021**, *57*, 367. [CrossRef]

9. Fearon, A.; Dahlstrom, J.E.; Twin, J.; Cook, J.; Scott, A. The Bonar Score Revisited: Region of Evaluation Significantly Influences the Standardized Assessment of Tendon Degeneration. *J. Sci. Med. Sport* **2014**, *17*, 346–350. [CrossRef] [PubMed]
10. Lundgreen, K.; Lian, Ø.; Scott, A.; Engebretsen, L. Increased Levels of Apoptosis and P53 in Partial-Thickness Supraspinatus Tendon Tears. *Knee Surg. Sports Traumatol. Arthrosc.* **2013**, *21*, 1636–1641. [CrossRef] [PubMed]
11. Fearon, A.M.; Twin, J.; Dahlstrom, J.E.; Cook, J.L.; Cormick, W.; Smith, P.N.; Scott, A. Increased Substance P Expression in the Trochanteric Bursa of Patients with Greater Trochanteric Pain Syndrome. *Rheumatol. Int.* **2014**, *34*, 1441–1448. [CrossRef]
12. Docking, S.I.; Cook, J.; Chen, S.; Scarvell, J.; Cormick, W.; Smith, P.; Fearon, A. Identification and Differentiation of Gluteus Medius Tendon Pathology Using Ultrasound and Magnetic Resonance Imaging. *Musculoskelet. Sci. Pract.* **2019**, *41*, 1–5. [CrossRef] [PubMed]
13. Okazaki, Y.; Furumatsu, T.; Maehara, A.; Miyazawa, S.; Kamatsuki, Y.; Hino, T.; Ozaki, T. Histological Alterations to the Hamstring Tendon Caused by Cleaning during Autograft Preparation. *Muscle Ligaments Tendons J.* **2019**, *09*, 217. [CrossRef]
14. Zabrzyński, J.; Paczesny, Ł.; Łapaj, Ł.; Grzanka, D.; Szukalski, J. Process of Neovascularisation Compared with Pain Intensity in Tendinopathy of the Long Head of the Biceps Brachii Tendon Associated with Concomitant Shoulder Disorders, after Arthroscopic Treatment. Microscopic Evaluation Supported by Immunohistochemical. *Folia Morphol.* **2018**, *77*, 378–385. [CrossRef] [PubMed]
15. Park, D.Y.; Min, B.-H.; Choi, B.H.; Kim, Y.J.; Kim, M.; Suh-Kim, H.; Kim, J.H. The Degeneration of Meniscus Roots Is Accompanied by Fibrocartilage Formation, Which May Precede Meniscus Root Tears in Osteoarthritic Knees. *Am. J. Sports Med.* **2015**, *43*, 3034–3044. [CrossRef]
16. Giorgino, R.; Albano, D.; Fusco, S.; Peretti, G.M.; Mangiavini, L.; Messina, C. Knee Osteoarthritis: Epidemiology, Pathogenesis, and Mesenchymal Stem Cells: What Else Is New? An Update. *Int. J. Mol. Sci.* **2023**, *24*, 6405. [CrossRef] [PubMed]
17. Primorac, D.; Molnar, V.; Rod, E.; Jeleč, Ž.; Čukelj, F.; Matišić, V.; Vrdoljak, T.; Hudetz, D.; Hajsok, H.; Borić, I. Knee Osteoarthritis: A Review of Pathogenesis and State-Of-The-Art Non-Operative Therapeutic Considerations. *Genes* **2020**, *11*, 854. [CrossRef]
18. Jarraya, M.; Roemer, F.W.; Englund, M.; Crema, M.D.; Gale, H.I.; Hayashi, D.; Katz, J.N.; Guermazi, A. Meniscus Morphology: Does Tear Type Matter? A Narrative Review with Focus on Relevance for Osteoarthritis Research. *Semin. Arthritis Rheum.* **2017**, *46*, 552–561. [CrossRef] [PubMed]
19. Roemer, F.W.; Zhang, Y.; Niu, J.; Lynch, J.A.; Crema, M.D.; Marra, M.D.; Nevitt, M.C.; Felson, D.T.; Hughes, L.B.; El-Khoury, G.Y.; et al. Tibiofemoral Joint Osteoarthritis: Risk Factors for MR-Depicted Fast Cartilage Loss over a 30-Month Period in the Multicenter Osteoarthritis Study. *Radiology* **2009**, *252*, 772–780. [CrossRef]
20. Lamplot, J.D.; Tompkins, W.P.; Friedman, M.V.; Nguyen, J.T.; Rai, M.F.; Brophy, R.H. Radiographic and Clinical Evidence for Osteoarthritis at Medium-Term Follow-up after Arthroscopic Partial Medial Meniscectomy. *Cartilage* **2021**, *13*, 588S–594S. [CrossRef]
21. Englund, M.; Guermazi, A.; Lohmander, L.S. The Meniscus in Knee Osteoarthritis. *Rheum. Dis. Clin. N. Am.* **2009**, *35*, 579–590. [CrossRef]
22. Olivotto, E.; Trisolino, G.; Belluzzi, E.; Lazzaro, A.; Strazzari, A.; Pozzuoli, A.; Cigolotti, A.; Ruggieri, P.; Evangelista, A.; Ometto, F.; et al. Macroscopic Synovial Inflammation Correlates with Symptoms and Cartilage Lesions in Patients Undergoing Arthroscopic Partial Meniscectomy: A Clinical Study. *J. Clin. Med.* **2022**, *11*, 4330. [CrossRef] [PubMed]
23. Zabrzyński, J.; Paczesny, Ł.; Zabrzyńska, A.; Huri, G.; Graboń, K.; Pielak, T.; Kruczyński, J.; Łapaj, Ł. Smoking Has No Influence on Outcomes after Repair of the Medial Meniscus in the Hypo and Avascular Zones—A Pilot Study. *Int. J. Environ. Res. Public Health* **2022**, *19*, 16127. [CrossRef] [PubMed]
24. Doral, M.N.; Bilge, O.; Huri, G.; Turhan, E.; Verdonk, R. Modern Treatment of Meniscal Tears. *EFORT Open Rev.* **2018**, *3*, 260–268. [CrossRef] [PubMed]
25. Blackwell, R.; Schmitt, L.; Flanigan, D.C.; Magnussen, R.A. Smoking Increases the Risk of Early Meniscus Repair Failure. *Orthop. J. Sports Med.* **2014**, *2*, 2325967114S0011. [CrossRef]
26. AL-Bashaireh, A.M.; Haddad, L.G.; Weaver, M.; Kelly, D.L.; Chengguo, X.; Yoon, S. The Effect of Tobacco Smoking on Musculoskeletal Health: A Systematic Review. *J. Environ. Public Health* **2018**, *2018*, 4184190. [CrossRef] [PubMed]
27. Davies-Tuck, M.L.; Wluka, A.E.; Forbes, A.; Wang, Y.; English, D.R.; Giles, G.G.; Cicuttini, F. Smoking Is Associated with Increased Cartilage Loss and Persistence of Bone Marrow Lesions over 2 Years in Community-Based Individuals. *Rheumatology* **2009**, *48*, 1227–1231. [CrossRef] [PubMed]
28. Uzun, E.; Misir, A.; Kizkapan, T.B.; Ozcamdalli, M.; Akkurt, S.; Guney, A. Factors Affecting the Outcomes of Arthroscopically Repaired Traumatic Vertical Longitudinal Medial Meniscal Tears. *Orthop. J. Sports Med.* **2017**, *5*, 232596711771244. [CrossRef]
29. Uzun, E.; Misir, A.; Kizkapan, T.B.; Ozcamdalli, M.; Akkurt, S.; Guney, A. Evaluation of Midterm Clinical and Radiographic Outcomes of Arthroscopically Repaired Vertical Longitudinal and Bucket-Handle Lateral Meniscal Tears. *Orthop. J. Sports Med.* **2019**, *7*, 232596711984320. [CrossRef]
30. Snoeker, B.A.M.; Bakker, E.W.P.; Kegel, C.A.T.; Lucas, C. Risk Factors for Meniscal Tears: A Systematic Review Including Meta-Analysis. *J. Orthop. Sports Phys. Ther.* **2013**, *43*, 352–367. [CrossRef]
31. Laurendon, L.; Neri, T.; Farizon, F.; Philippot, R. Prognostic Factors for All-inside Meniscal Repair. A 87-Case Series. *Orthop. Traumatol. Surg. Res.* **2017**, *103*, 1017–1020. [CrossRef]
32. Moses, M.J.; Wang, D.E.; Weinberg, M.; Strauss, E.J. Clinical Outcomes Following Surgically Repaired Bucket-Handle Meniscus Tears. *Physician Sportsmed.* **2017**, *45*, 329–336. [CrossRef] [PubMed]

33. Johnsen, M.B.; Pihl, K.; Nissen, N.; Sørensen, R.R.; Jørgensen, U.; Englund, M.; Thorlund, J.B. The Association between Smoking and Knee Osteoarthritis in a Cohort of Danish Patients Undergoing Knee Arthroscopy. *BMC Musculoskelet. Disord.* **2019**, *20*, 141. [CrossRef]
34. Kanneganti, P.; Harris, J.D.; Brophy, R.H.; Carey, J.L.; Lattermann, C.; Flanigan, D.C. The Effect of Smoking on Ligament and Cartilage Surgery in the Knee: A Systematic Review. *Am. J. Sports Med.* **2012**, *40*, 2872–2878. [CrossRef] [PubMed]
35. Haugen, I.K.; Magnusson, K.; Turkiewicz, A.; Englund, M. The Prevalence, Incidence, and Progression of Hand Osteoarthritis in Relation to Body Mass Index, Smoking, and Alcohol Consumption. *J. Rheumatol.* **2017**, *44*, 1402–1409. [CrossRef] [PubMed]
36. Zabrzyński, J.; Szukalski, J.; Paczesny, Ł.; Szwedowski, D.; Grzanka, D. Cigarette Smoking Intensifies Tendinopathy of the LHBT. A Microscopic Study after Arthroscopic Treatment. *Pol. J. Pathol.* **2019**, *70*, 134–138. [CrossRef] [PubMed]
37. Ying, X.; Cheng, S.; Shen, Y.; Cheng, X.; An Rompis, F.; Wang, W.; Lin, Z.; Chen, Q.; Zhang, W.; Kou, D.; et al. Nicotine Promotes Proliferation and Collagen Synthesis of Chondrocytes Isolated from Normal Human and Osteoarthritis Patients. *Mol. Cell. Biochem.* **2012**, *359*, 263–269. [CrossRef] [PubMed]
38. Cooke, J.; Bitterman, H. Nicotine and Angiogenesis: A New Paradigm for Tobacco-related Diseases. *Ann. Med.* **2004**, *36*, 33–40. [CrossRef]
39. Kondo, T.; Nakano, Y.; Adachi, S.; Murohara, T. Effects of Tobacco Smoking on Cardiovascular Disease. *Circ. J.* **2019**, *83*, 1980–1985. [CrossRef]
40. Salehi, N.; Janjani, P.; Tadbiri, H.; Rozbahani, M.; Jalilian, M. Effect of Cigarette Smoking on Coronary Arteries and Pattern and Severity of Coronary Artery Disease: A Review. *J. Int. Med. Res.* **2021**, *49*, 030006052110598. [CrossRef]
41. Darcey, E.; Boyle, T. Tobacco Smoking and Survival after a Prostate Cancer Diagnosis: A Systematic Review and Meta-Analysis. *Cancer Treat. Rev.* **2018**, *70*, 30–40. [CrossRef]
42. Neczypor, E.W.; Mears, M.J.; Ghosh, A.; Sassano, M.F.; Gumina, R.J.; Wold, L.E.; Tarran, R. E-Cigarettes and Cardiopulmonary Health: Review for Clinicians. *Circulation* **2022**, *145*, 219–232. [CrossRef] [PubMed]
43. Banks, E.; Yazidjoglou, A.; Brown, S.; Nguyen, M.; Martin, M.; Beckwith, K.; Daluwatta, A.; Campbell, S.; Joshy, G. Electronic Cigarettes and Health Outcomes: Umbrella and Systematic Review of the Global Evidence. *Med. J. Aust.* **2023**, *218*, 267–275. [CrossRef]
44. Gordon, T.; Karey, E.; Rebuli, M.E.; Escobar, Y.-N.H.; Jaspers, I.; Chen, L.C. E-Cigarette Toxicology. *Annu. Rev. Pharmacol. Toxicol.* **2022**, *62*, 301–322. [CrossRef] [PubMed]
45. Abate, M.; Silbernagel, K.G.; Siljeholm, C.; Di Iorio, A.; De Amicis, D.; Salini, V.; Werner, S.; Paganelli, R. Pathogenesis of Tendinopathies: Inflammation or Degeneration? *Arthritis Res. Ther.* **2009**, *11*, 235. [CrossRef]
46. Abate, M.; Vanni, D.; Pantalone, A.; Salini, V. Cigarette Smoking and Musculoskeletal Disorders. *Muscles Ligaments Tendons J.* **2013**, *3*, 63–69. [CrossRef]
47. Rose, B.J.; Weyand, J.A.; Liu, B.; Smith, J.F.; Perez, B.R.; Clark, J.C.; Goodman, M.; Budge, K.M.H.; Eggett, D.L.; Arroyo, J.A.; et al. Exposure to Second-Hand Cigarette Smoke Exacerbates the Progression of Osteoarthritis in a Surgical Induced Murine Model. *Histol. Histopathol.* **2021**, *36*, 347–353. [CrossRef] [PubMed]
48. Domzalski, M.; Muszynski, K.; Mostowy, M.; Wojtowicz, J.; Garlinska, A. Smoking Is Associated with Prolonged Time of the Return to Daily and Sport Activities and Decreased Knee Function after Meniscus Repair with Outside-in Technique: Retrospective Cohort Study. *J. Orthop. Surg.* **2021**, *29*, 230949902110122. [CrossRef]
49. Haklar, U.; Donmez, F.; Basaran, S.H.; Canbora, M.K. Results of Arthroscopic Repair of Partial- or Full-Thickness Longitudinal Medial Meniscal Tears by Single or Double Vertical Sutures Using the Inside-Out Technique. *Am. J. Sports Med.* **2013**, *41*, 596–602. [CrossRef]
50. Franovic, S.; Kuhlmann, N.A.; Pietroski, A.; Schlosser, C.T.; Page, B.; Okoroha, K.R.; Moutzouros, V.; Makhni, E.C. Preoperative Patient-Centric Predictors of Postoperative Outcomes in Patients Undergoing Arthroscopic Meniscectomy. *Arthrosc. J. Arthrosc. Relat. Surg.* **2020**, *37*, 964–971. [CrossRef]
51. Astur, D.C.; Sbampato, I.N.; Arliani, G.G.; Franciozi, C.E.d.S.; Debieux, P.; Cohen, M. Association of Tobacco Dependence, Alcoholism and Anabolic Steroids with Meniscoligamentous Injuries. *Acta Ortop. Bras.* **2018**, *26*, 236–239. [CrossRef]
52. Gittings, D.; Riggin, C.; Boorman-Padgett, J.; Weiss, S.; Fryhofer, G.; Farber, D.; Steinberg, D.; Soslowsky, L.J. Chronic Nicotine Exposure Alters Uninjured Tendon Vascularity and Viscoelasticity. *Foot Ankle Orthop.* **2019**, *4*, 247301141984252. [CrossRef]
53. Ağladıoğlu, K.; Akkaya, N.; Güngör, H.R.; Akkaya, S.; Ök, N.; Özçakar, L. Effects of Cigarette Smoking on Elastographic Strain Ratio Measurements of Patellar and Achilles Tendons. *J. Ultrasound Med.* **2016**, *35*, 2431–2438. [CrossRef]
54. Baumgarten, K.M.; Gerlach, D.; Galatz, L.M.; Teefey, S.A.; Middleton, W.D.; Ditsios, K.; Yamaguchi, K. Cigarette Smoking Increases the Risk for Rotator Cuff Tears. *Clin. Orthop. Relat. Res.* **2010**, *468*, 1534–1541. [CrossRef]
55. Novikov, D.A.; Swensen, S.J.; Buza, J.A.; Gidumal, R.H.; Strauss, E.J. The Effect of Smoking on ACL Reconstruction: A Systematic Review. *Physician Sportsmed.* **2016**, *44*, 335–341. [CrossRef]
56. Jensen, A.R.; Taylor, A.J.; Sanchez-Sotelo, J. Factors Influencing the Reparability and Healing Rates of Rotator Cuff Tears. *Curr. Rev. Musculoskelet. Med.* **2020**, *13*, 572–583. [CrossRef]
57. Caughey, W.J.; Maher, A.; Leigh, W.B.; Brick, M.J.; Young, S.W.; Walker, C.G.; Caughey, M.A. Impact of Smoking on Pain and Function in Rotator Cuff Repair: A Prospective 5-year Cohort Follow-up of 1383 Patients. *ANZ J. Surg.* **2021**, *91*, 2153–2158. [CrossRef]

58. Livesey, M.G.; Bains, S.S.; Weir, T.B.; Kolakowski, L.; Rocca, M.S.; Remily, E.A.; Gilotra, M.N.; Hasan, S.A. Does Timing Matter? The Effect of Preoperative Smoking Cessation on the Risk of Infection or Revision Following Rotator Cuff Repair. *J. Shoulder Elb. Surg.* **2023**, *32*, 1937–1944. [CrossRef]
59. Carbone, S.; Gumina, S.; Arceri, V.; Campagna, V.; Fagnani, C.; Postacchini, F. The Impact of Preoperative Smoking Habit on Rotator Cuff Tear: Cigarette Smoking Influences Rotator Cuff Tear Sizes. *J. Shoulder Elb. Surg.* **2012**, *21*, 56–60. [CrossRef] [PubMed]
60. Cooke, J.P. New Insights into Tobacco-Induced Vascular Disease: Clinical Ramifications. *Methodist. DeBakey Cardiovasc. J.* **2015**, *11*, 156. [CrossRef] [PubMed]
61. Lee, J.; Cooke, J.P. Nicotine and Pathological Angiogenesis. *Life Sci.* **2012**, *91*, 1058–1064. [CrossRef] [PubMed]
62. Khodabandeh, Z.; Valilo, M.; Velaei, K.; Pirpour Tazehkand, A. The Potential Role of Nicotine in Breast Cancer Initiation, Development, Angiogenesis, Invasion, Metastasis, and Resistance to Therapy. *Breast Cancer* **2022**, *29*, 778–789. [CrossRef] [PubMed]
63. Zabrzynski, J.; Gagat, M.; Paczesny, L.; Grzanka, D.; Huri, G. Correlation between Smoking and Neovascularization in Biceps Tendinopathy—A Functional Preoperative and Immunohistochemical Study. *Ther. Adv. Chronic Dis.* **2020**, *11*, 2040622320956418. [CrossRef] [PubMed]

medicina MDPI

Technical Note

Posterior Medial Meniscus Root Repair Using Two Transtibial Tunnels with Modified Mason–Allen Stitches: A Technical Note

Du-Han Kim *, Ki-Cheor Bae, Chang-Jin Yon and Ji-Hoon Kim

Department of Orthopedic Surgery, Keimyung University Dongsan Hospital, Keimyung University School of Medicine, Daegu 42601, Republic of Korea
* Correspondence: osmdkdh@gmail.com; Tel.: +82-2-53-258-4771

Abstract: Complete tear of the posterior medial meniscus root can result in a loss of hoop tension and increased contact pressure. Thus, medial meniscus posterior root tear (MMPRT) is increasingly recognized as an important pathology. Although several surgical techniques for MMPRT have recently been introduced, the ideal technique is not yet established. This technical note is aimed at introducing a novel surgical technique using two transtibial tunnels with modified Mason–Allen stitches in the treatment of MMPRT.

Keywords: meniscus; meniscus root tear; repair; arthroscopy; knee

1. Introduction

A complete tear of the medial meniscus posterior root (MMPR) can cause a complete loss of hoop tension and increased contact pressure due to altered biomechanics of the normal knee joint, paralleling complete meniscectomy or radial tear [1,2]. As an aging society progresses, the incidence of medial meniscus posterior root tear (MMPRT) is increased. Furthermore, the high incidence in Asia (27.8%) has been attributed to squatting and sitting on the floor with folded legs [3].

No benefit in halting arthritic progression was obtained by use of nonoperative treatment or partial meniscectomy for the treatment of complete MMPRT [4,5]. Krych et al. reported the results of partial meniscectomy for MMPRT. They found that patients who undergo arthroscopic partial meniscectomy for MMPRTs still progress to significant arthritis and concluded that repair should be considered in select patients without degenerative changes [5]. Therefore, if possible, restoration of meniscal function by surgical repair is necessary.

Numerous surgical methods have recently been suggested for the repair of the MMPR. Among them, the popularity of a transtibial pullout technique has increased consequent to the idea that the contact pressure and contact are normalized [6]. Of the currently available stitches, the modified Mason–Allen (MA) stitch has been accepted as an effective technical approach [2,7].

In this study, we describe the procedure for the repair of MMPRT using two transtibial tunnels with modified MA stitches.

2. Methods and Results

2.1. Preoperative Evaluations and Indication

All included patients underwent plain radiography and MRI to confirm the MMPRT. We defined an MMPRT when two or more of the following signs appeared on MRI: the absence of an identifiable meniscus or a high signal that replaced the normal dark meniscus signal (i.e., the ghost sign) in the sagittal view, a vertical linear defect at the meniscus root in the coronal view, and/or a radial linear defect at the posterior insertion in the axial view [8].

The inclusion criteria were (1) an MMPRT on MRI in a patient with a Kellgren–Lawrence (K–L) grade 1 or less, (2) those willing to follow a rehabilitation process postoperatively, (3) a symmetric hip–knee–ankle angle less than 5°, (4) Outerbridge classification less than grade III, and (5) younger than 70 years of age.

2.2. Diagnostic Arthroscopy and Superficial Medial Collateral Ligament (sMCL) Release

General arthroscopic examination using anterolateral (AL) and anteromedial (AM) portals was performed according to routine. An arthroscope (ConMed Linvatec, Largo, FL, USA) was inserted through the AL portal, and working devices were inserted using the AM portal.

If MMPRT was confirmed, we performed sMCL release to provide ample working space. A ~3–4 cm vertical incision was made using a No. 15 blade at the anteromedial aspect of the proximal tibia (Figure 1). Then, we found the sMCL and sartorius fascia. To preserve deep MCL and proximal attachment of the sMCL, the sMCL was released more downward than the sartorius fascia using a periosteum elevator.

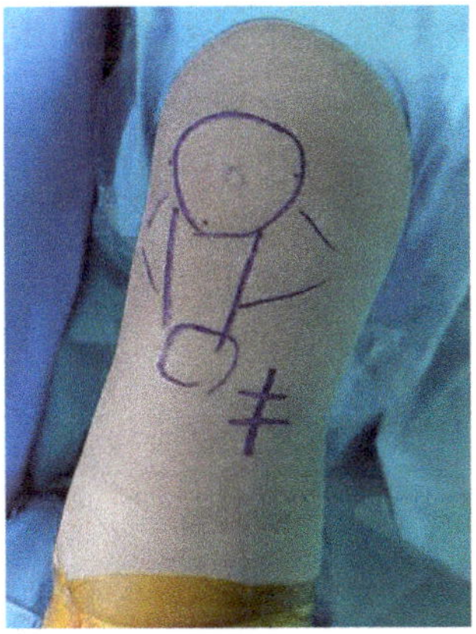

Figure 1. Vertical incision made at the anteromedial aspect of the proximal tibia.

2.3. Preparation for Root Repair

An arthroscopic PassPort cannula (Arthrex, Naples, FL, USA) was inserted for the performance of a convenient procedure and to prevent twisting of the stitch. Landmarks relevant to the insertion of the MMPH, including tibial attachment of the posterior cruciate ligament, tibial medial eminence, and articular surface of the tibial plateau, were then identified. Unhealthy tissue removal of the torn meniscus edge was conducted using an arthroscopic shaver (ConMed Linvatec, Largo, FL, USA). For the creation of a bony bed, a curette was inserted through the AM portal, and bony preparation was performed (Figure 2).

2.4. MMPR Stitches

Passage of the Knee Scorpion suture passer (Arthrex, Naples, FL, USA) loaded with a No. 2 Ultrabraid (Smith and Nephew, Andover, MA, USA) through the AM portal was then performed. The separated segment of the medial meniscus posterior horn (MMPH) was penetrated using a Scorpion needle at about 5 mm medial point to a detached margin. The second stitch was penetrated in the anterior location of the first stitch, using the same method. The upper two strands of the stitches were pulled out and tied. Using the shuttle relay technique, the first stitch was exchanged with the second stitch to make a horizontal loop (Figure 3).

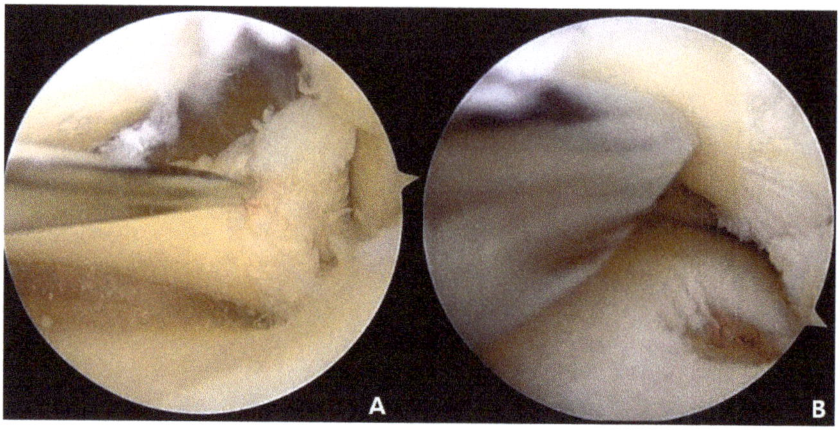

Figure 2. Arthroscopic findings: (**A**) arthroscopic view through the anterolateral portal of medial meniscus posterior horn in left knee; (**B**) bone bed decortication at the attachment site of the medial meniscus.

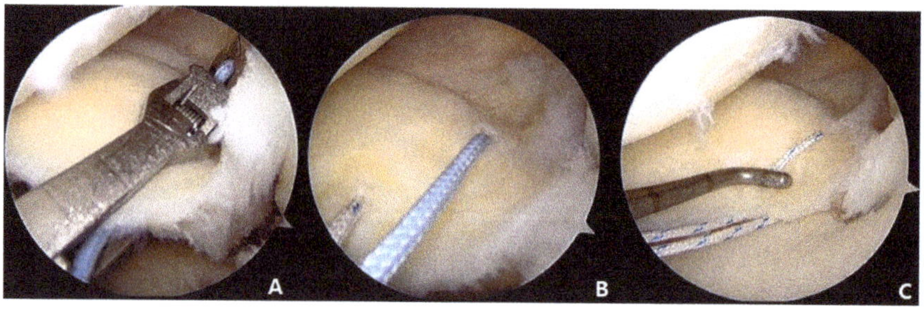

Figure 3. (**A**) The MMPH penetrated using a Knee Scorpion suture passer (Arthrex, Naples, FL, USA) at about 5 mm medial to the detached margin. (**B**) The second stitch located in the anterior position of the first stitch in the same manner. (**C**) Using the shuttle relay method, exchange of the first suture with the second suture to create a horizontal loop.

The Knee Scorpion suture passer (Arthrex, Naples, FL, USA) was reintroduced using the AM portal, and two vertical stitches penetrated just the medial side of the horizontal stitch.

2.5. Tibial Tunnel Making

Insertion of the Meniscus Root Repair System (Smith and Nephew, Andover, MA, USA) was conducted using the AM portal. The tip of the guide was placed in the most medial side of the decorticated site of MMPR. A 2.4 mm Kirschner wire (K-wire) was advanced through the guide system. The location of the K-wire was confirmed using an arthroscope via the AL portal. The second K-wire was placed parallel and about 5 mm laterally to the first tunnel (Figure 4). Once it was verified that the position of the K-wire was acceptable, the medial-side K-wire was removed first. A metal wire was inserted into the created tunnel, and then it was withdrawn through the AM portal using an arthroscopic grasper.

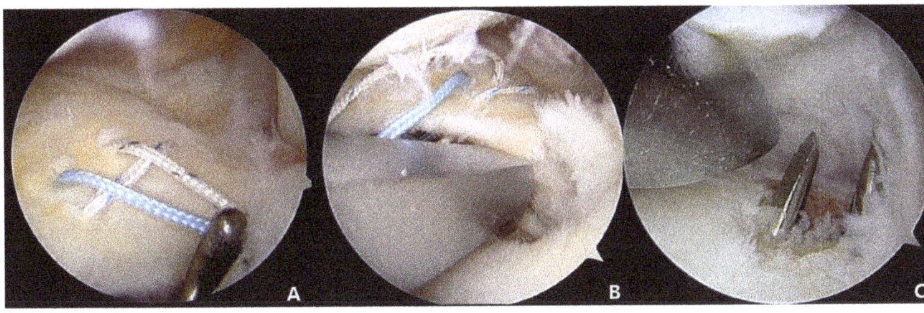

Figure 4. (**A**) Two vertical stitches overlaying and crossing the center of the horizontal suture. (**B**) Meniscus Root Repair System (Smith and Nephew, Andover, MA, USA) advanced using the AM portal, with the tip of the guide placed in the most medial side of the decorticated site of MMPR. (**C**) The second K-wire placed parallel and about 5 mm lateral to the first tunnel.

2.6. Repair of MMRT

The wire was pulled through the tibial tunnel. For the medial tunnel, two horizontal stitches and two inferior vertical stitches were passed, resulting in a total of four stitches. For the lateral tunnel, the two superior vertical stitches were passed. The sutures from both tunnels were tied over the anteromedial tibial cortex, with the knee at 30° flexion. An arthroscopic re-evaluation was conducted to check for repair of the torn posterior root and to restore tension within the entire medial meniscus (Figure 5).

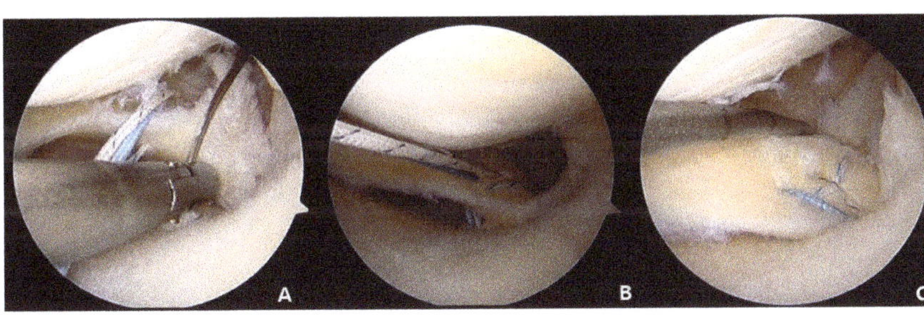

Figure 5. (**A**) Metal wire inserted into the tibial tunnel and pulled out through the AM portal using an arthroscopic grasper. (**B**) For the medial tunnel, passage of the two horizontal stitches and the two inferior vertical stitches, resulting in a total of 4 stitches. For the lateral tunnel, passage of the two superior vertical stitches. (**C**) An arthroscopic re-evaluation to confirm repair of the MMPH and to restore tension of the meniscus using arthroscopic probe device.

3. Case Series

A total of 20 patients were included. Their mean age was 61.5 years (range: 55–68) and their mean preoperative alignment was 2.0° (range: 0.6–4.4°).

The International Knee Documentation Committee (IKDC) score and Lysholm score were compared preoperatively and 1 year postoperatively; preoperative and postoperative mean IKDC scores were 40.9 ± 11.8 and 69.5 ± 11.9, and preoperative and postoperative Lysholom scores were 60.2 ± 11.0 and 88.3 ± 9.99, respectively. Both clinical scores were significantly improved 1 year postoperatively compared with baseline. Upon image evaluation, there was no significant difference in HKA angle at 1 year after surgery (2.0° versus 2.8°, p = 0.08). Four of 20 knees had progressed osteoarthritis from KL grade 0 to grade 1.

4. Discussion

Findings from several clinical studies have shown an association between nonoperative treatment or meniscectomy with poor outcomes for the prevention or delay of osteoarthritis in patients with MMPRT [4,5]. Instead, repair of MMPRT can result in restoration of the hoop tension biomechanically. According to a systematic review and long-term clinical study, repair of the MMRT showed better outcomes and survivorship than other treatments for long-term follow-up [9]. Chung et al. found that root repair showed better results than meniscectomy in functional scores and survivorship for more than 10 years of follow-up. According to their study, the survival rates of the repair and meniscectomy groups were 79.6% and 44.4% at 10 years, respectively [9].

Among several techniques, repair of the MMPR using a transtibial pullout technique was shown to restore contact pressures to the normal states and allow for the dispersal of hoop stresses across the meniscus [10]. However, there is still considerable debate regarding the number of tunnels.

The goal of the two-tunnel technique is to recover the normal anatomy of the MMPHR attachments. However, some authors have expressed concern that a problematic tunnel coalition may lead to a narrow attachment area for the meniscus, which could cause breakage. The single-tunnel technique reduces operation time and avoids these disadvantages [2].

There are few clinical or biomechanical comparative studies with one or two tunnels. According to LaPrade et al., similar biomechanical results for the transtibial pullout technique were shown using one- and two-tunnel techniques. They conducted a human cadaveric study that involved a transtibial pullout repair using one or two tunnels, and they found no significant difference in ultimate failure loads between both techniques [6]. Instead, similar studies are being actively conducted in the field of rotator cuffs [11,12]. Park conducted a biomechanical comparative study of single-point and double-point repairs. They found that double-point fixation (modified double row) had significantly more footprint contact than single-row repair [11]. Quigley et al. also reported that double fixation was superior to single fixation biomechanically.

Therefore, we thought that the two-tunnel technique might provide greater advantages than the one-tunnel technique in biomechanical and biological healing. In addition, as a result of development of arthroscopic instruments such as the Meniscus Root Repair System (Smith and Nephew) and the Knee Scorpion suture passer (Arthrex), the operation time can be gradually reduced.

The MA stitch leads to minimal slippage and elongation of the longitudinally oriented fibers of the meniscus or tendon and provides a greater holding power [2]. In a comparative study of MMPRT repair using MA or simple stitches, the MA stitch showed significantly superior outcomes with respect to postoperative extrusion and root healing. [13]. By using these devices, there is also room for passing the thread through the tunnel, providing easier use of the double Mason–Allen stitches.

5. Conclusions

Although several repair techniques for MMPRT have recently been introduced, the ideal technique has not yet been established. Our technique might be beneficial in the restoration of the function of the medial meniscus in patients who present MMPRT. However, further clinical and biomechanical studies are necessary to validate this technique.

Author Contributions: D.-H.K. contributed to the conceptualization of the approach, surgical procedures, data analysis, writing of article, and submission of article; D.-H.K. and C.-J.Y. contributed to the writing of the article; K.-C.B. and J.-H.K. contributed to the data collection and critical review of the article. All authors have read and agreed to the published version of the manuscript.

Funding: This research was supported by the Bisa Research Grant of Keimyung University in 2022(20220357).

Institutional Review Board Statement: Not applicable.

Informed Consent Statement: Written informed consent was obtained from the patients to publish this paper.

Data Availability Statement: Not applicable.

Conflicts of Interest: The authors declare no conflict of interest.

References

1. Hong, S.Y.; Han, W.; Jang, J.; Lee, J.; Ro, D.H.; Lee, M.C.; Han, H.-S. Prognostic Factors of Mid- to Long-term Clinical Outcomes after Arthroscopic Partial Meniscectomy for Medial Meniscal Tears. *Clin. Orthop. Surg.* **2022**, *14*, 227–235. [CrossRef] [PubMed]
2. Lee, D.W.; Jang, S.H.; Ha, J.K.; Kim, J.G.; Ahn, J.H. Meniscus root refixation technique using a modified Mason-Allen stitch. *Knee Surg. Sport. Traumatol. Arthrosc.* **2013**, *21*, 654–657. [CrossRef] [PubMed]
3. Bin, S.I.; Kim, J.M.; Shin, S.J. Radial tears of the posterior horn of the medial meniscus. *Arthroscopy* **2004**, *20*, 373–378. [CrossRef] [PubMed]
4. Krych, A.J.; Reardon, P.J.; Johnson, N.R.; Mohan, R.; Peter, L.; Levy, B.A.; Stuart, M.J. Non-operative management of medial meniscus posterior horn root tears is associated with worsening arthritis and poor clinical outcome at 5-year follow-up. *Knee Surg. Sport. Traumatol. Arthrosc.* **2017**, *25*, 383–389. [CrossRef] [PubMed]
5. Krych, A.J.; Johnson, N.R.; Mohan, R.; Dahm, D.L.; Levy, B.A.; Stuart, M.J. Partial meniscectomy provides no benefit for symptomatic degenerative medial meniscus posterior root tears. *Knee Surg. Sport. Traumatol. Arthrosc.* **2018**, *26*, 1117–1122. [CrossRef] [PubMed]
6. LaPrade, C.M.; LaPrade, M.D.; Turnbull, T.L.; Wijdicks, C.A.; LaPrade, R.F. Biomechanical evaluation of the transtibial pull-out technique for posterior medial meniscal root repairs using 1 and 2 transtibial bone tunnels. *Am. J. Sport. Med.* **2015**, *43*, 899–904. [CrossRef] [PubMed]
7. Oh, S.Y.; Jang, Y.H.; Chae, I.S.; Kim, S.H. Prevalence and Clinical Impact of Acromial Cupping after Arthroscopic Rotator Cuff Repair: Does Acromioplasty Matter? *Clin. Orthop. Surg.* **2021**, *13*, 520–528. [CrossRef] [PubMed]
8. Lee, Y.G.; Shim, J.C.; Choi, Y.S.; Kim, J.G.; Lee, G.J.; Kim, H.K. Magnetic resonance imaging findings of surgically proven medial meniscus root tear: Tear configuration and associated knee abnormalities. *J. Comput. Assist. Tomogr.* **2008**, *32*, 452–457. [CrossRef] [PubMed]
9. Chung, K.S.; Ha, J.K.; Ra, H.J.; Yu, W.J.; Kim, J.G. Root Repair Versus Partial Meniscectomy for Medial Meniscus Posterior Root Tears: Comparison of Long-term Survivorship and Clinical Outcomes at Minimum 10-Year Follow-up. *Am. J. Sport. Med.* **2020**, *48*, 1937–1944. [CrossRef] [PubMed]
10. LaPrade, C.M.; Jansson, K.S.; Dornan, G.; Smith, S.D.; Wijdicks, C.A.; LaPrade, R.F. Altered tibiofemoral contact mechanics due to lateral meniscus posterior horn root avulsions and radial tears can be restored with in situ pull-out suture repairs. *J. Bone Jt. Surg. Am.* **2014**, *96*, 471–479. [CrossRef] [PubMed]
11. Park, M.C.; Pirolo, J.M.; Park, C.J.; Tibone, J.E.; McGarry, M.H.; Lee, T.Q. The effect of abduction and rotation on footprint contact for single-row, double-row, and modified double-row rotator cuff repair techniques. *Am. J. Sport. Med.* **2009**, *37*, 1599–1608. [CrossRef] [PubMed]
12. Quigley, R.J.; Gupta, A.; Oh, J.H.; Chung, K.C.; McGarry, M.H.; Gupta, R.; Tibone, J.E.; Lee, T.Q. Biomechanical comparison of single-row, double-row, and transosseous-equivalent repair techniques after healing in an animal rotator cuff tear model. *J. Orthop. Res.* **2013**, *31*, 1254–1260. [CrossRef] [PubMed]
13. Lee, D.W.; Kim, M.K.; Jang, H.S.; Ha, J.K.; Kim, J.G. Clinical and radiologic evaluation of arthroscopic medial meniscus root tear refixation: Comparison of the modified Mason-Allen stitch and simple stitches. *Arthroscopy* **2014**, *30*, 1439–1446. [CrossRef] [PubMed]

medicina

MDPI

Review

Current Narrative Review—Application of Blood Flow Restriction Exercise in Clinical Knee Problems

Saehim Kwon [1], Ki-Cheor Bae [2], Chang-Jin Yon [2] and Du-Han Kim [2,*]

[1] Department of Orthopaedic Surgery, Konkuk University Medical Center, Konkuk University School of Medicine, Seoul 05030, Republic of Korea; kwonjamming@gmail.com
[2] Department of Orthopedic Surgery, Keimyung University Dongsan Hospital, Keimyung University School of Medicine, Daegu 42601, Republic of Korea; bkc@dsmc.or.kr (K.-C.B.); poweryon@dsmc.or.kr (C.-J.Y.)
* Correspondence: osmdkdh@gmail.com; Tel.: +82-2-53-258-4771

Abstract: Quadricep weakness is frequently observed in patients following anterior cruciate ligament (ACL) injury or in those with knee osteoarthritis, often contributing to functional impairments and persistent symptoms. While high-intensity resistance training has been shown to effectively improve muscle strength, its application may be limited in certain populations due to pain or the risk of surgical complications. In recent years, blood flow restriction (BFR) training has emerged as a promising alternative. Growing evidence indicates that low-load BFR exercise can significantly improve muscle strength, induce hypertrophy, and enhance knee function, with outcomes comparable to those of high-intensity resistance training. When implemented using appropriate protocols, BFR training appears to be a safe and efficacious rehabilitation strategy for individuals with knee pathology.

Keywords: blood flow restriction; exercise; quadriceps muscle; anterior cruciate ligament reconstruction; knee osteoarthritis

1. Introduction

Quadricep atrophy is commonly observed in patients undergoing knee surgery or those with knee osteoarthritis, often leading to long-term complications such as abnormal gait patterns, persistent pain, and even surgical failure [1–5]. Resistance training is a primary intervention to prevent or mitigate quadricep atrophy, with exercise intensity playing a critical role. It is generally accepted that loads exceeding 60–70% of one repetition maximum (1RM) are required to improve muscle strength, while 70–85% of 1RM is necessary to induce hypertrophy. However, high-intensity (HI) resistance training is often contraindicated in individuals with knee osteoarthritis or in post-operative patients due to pain, joint irritation, or the need to protect healing tissues [6–9]. Moreover, the mechanical load associated with HI training may surpass the joint's tolerable limits, making it unsuitable during the early phases of rehabilitation. To address these limitations, various alternative modalities—such as neuromuscular electrical stimulation, blood flow restriction (BFR) training, and biofeedback-guided exercise—have been explored [10,11]. Among these, BFR training has recently garnered attention as a viable and strategic rehabilitation approach.

BFR training, also referred to as occlusion training, was first developed by Dr. Sato in Japan in 2004 [12,13]. This technique involves the application of a pressure cuff or elastic band to the proximal portion of a limb, resulting in partial restriction of arterial inflow and complete occlusion of venous outflow during exercise. The typical equipment used for BFR training includes a tourniquet cuff, a manometer, and a manual or automatic pump (Figure 1) [6]. Despite growing interest in its potential benefits, there remains a lack of well-organized clinical research regarding the standardized application protocols and long-term outcomes of BFR training.

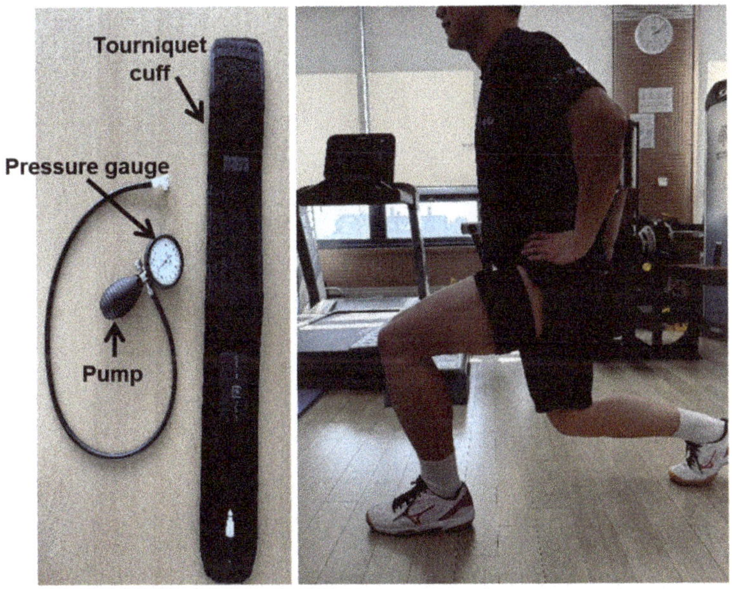

Figure 1. Blood flow restriction instruments consist of a tourniquet cuff, blood pressure gauge, and pump. The tourniquet cuff is used to partially restrict arterial inflow and fully restrict venous outflow during exercise. The blood pressure gauge is used to measure the pressure within the cuff. The pump is used to inflate the tourniquet cuff to the desired pressure.

This narrative review aims to summarize and elucidate recent advancements in BFR training, with a particular emphasis on its application in knee-related pathologies. The review is structured as follows: (1) an overview of the fundamental principles and application techniques of BFR training; (2) an evaluation of its safety profile; and (3) a discussion of its analgesic effects, which are critical for assessing clinical feasibility. Subsequently, we review clinical outcomes in two major patient populations—individuals with (4) anterior cruciate ligament (ACL) injuries and those with (5) knee osteoarthritis—where BFR training is being increasingly utilized. Based on the current body of evidence, we then outline (6) practical application strategies commonly employed in clinical settings and conclude with (7) a discussion of limitations and directions for future research.

2. Principle and Application Methods of Blood Flow Restriction Training

The principle of BFR devices is to restrict blood flow to the muscles, thereby creating a hypoxic environment within the tissues and inducing temporary ischemia in the exercised area [14]. This hypoxic condition generates metabolic stress, which activates the mammalian target of the rapamycin signaling pathway responsible for muscle protein synthesis and anabolism [15,16]. This process stimulates the production of several growth factors, such as insulin-like growth factor and growth hormone, which promote muscle fiber recruitment and muscle hypertrophy [17]. In addition, BFR training activates vasoactive metabolites and vascular endothelial growth factor, thereby stimulating angiogenesis and eventually increasing post-obstructive blood flow to the limb [18].

These effects are systemic, leading to strength gains and muscle hypertrophy not only in the proximal and distal musculature of the tourniquet site but also in the contralateral limb muscles [19]. The level of muscle protein synthesis and activation of the mammalian target of rapamycin pathway achieved through BFR training is comparable to that observed with HI resistance training [20]. Furthermore, signaling pathways involving protein tyrosine kinase may help inhibit mitochondrial permeability transition pores and reduce the overall concentration of reactive oxygen species, thereby minimizing cellular damage and supporting the metabolic demands of skeletal muscle, which in turn improves exercise performance capacity [15]. These mechanisms may also reduce pain and inflammation associated with HI training, thus enhancing the effectiveness of BFR training in functional recovery programs for postoperative patients or individuals with osteoarthritis [21] (Figure 2).

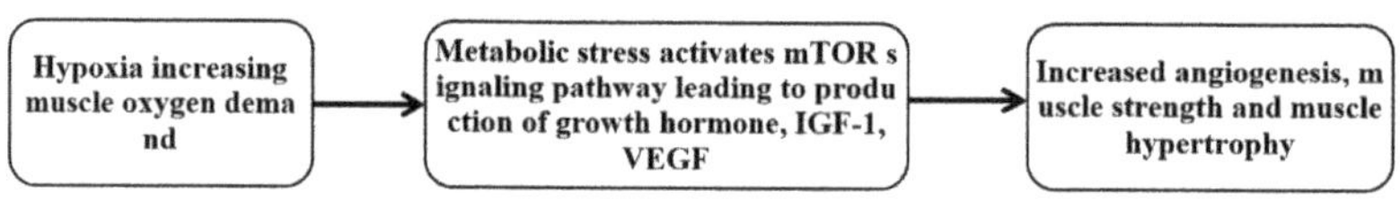

Figure 2. The physiological processes of the blood flow restriction exercise.

When implementing BFR training, specific parameters such as the degree of restriction pressure, cuff width, duration of restriction, and rest intervals vary across studies. The restriction pressure has been reported as either a fixed value of 160–200 mm Hg [9,22–25], or as a relative value set at approximately 60–80% of the arterial occlusion pressure measured using Doppler ultrasound [6,8,26–29]. Cuff widths have ranged from 6 to 20 cm [6,8,23–25,29], and rest intervals between sets have varied from 30 s to 1 min [6,8,23–29]. Some studies applied BFR only during exercise [7,22,25], whereas others maintained BFR continuously throughout the training session [8,9,23,24,26,27,29].

Due to these methodological variations, recent efforts have been made to establish standardized guidelines to enhance both the safety and efficacy of BFR training. Patterson et al. [6] proposed that, given individual differences in arterial occlusion pressure, applying restriction at 40% to 80% of the measured pressure is the safest and most appropriate approach. In a clinical trial, Mattocks et al. [30] divided participants into groups with occlusion pressures of 0%, 10%, 20%, 30%, 50%, and 90%, and found that while higher restriction pressure increased cardiovascular responses such as enhanced blood flow, it also elevated exercise intensity to a level that reduced total training volume and diminished hypertrophic adaptations.

Conversely, Hughes et al. [31] compared low-intensity (LI) exercise under low (40%) and high (80%) arterial occlusion pressures and found significantly greater pain reduction in the high-pressure group. Neto et al. [32] examined the effects of continuous versus intermittent BFR training on maximal voluntary strength (isometric and dynamic), muscle hypertrophy, and muscular endurance. While strength and hypertrophy outcomes were similar between groups, the continuous BFR group demonstrated superior gains in muscular endurance. Nielsen et al. [33] reported no muscle damage when BFR was applied at 100 mm Hg with high-frequency exercise to voluntary failure, using 30 s rest intervals and continuous restriction. Lastly, Mouser et al. [34] concluded that when restriction pressure is standardized based on arterial occlusion, variations in cuff width have minimal impact on training outcomes.

3. Safety of Blood Flow Restriction Training

Potential complications associated with BFR include cardiovascular responses, limb ischemia, and thrombosis [35]. Patterson et al. [18] reported that fluctuations in peripheral hemodynamics may occur following LI BFR exercise. However, Clark et al. [36] found no significant changes in pulse wave velocity or ankle-brachial index, both of which are indicators of arterial stiffness. Takano et al. [37] demonstrated that although systolic blood pressure and heart rate increased in BFR compared to non-BFR, there were no statistically significant changes in total peripheral resistance index or cardiac output, and stroke volume was significantly decreased in BFR due to reduced preload. These findings suggest that BFR does not impose a greater cardiovascular or hemodynamic risk compared to non-BFR exercise.

Furthermore, the degree of blood pressure elevation induced by LI BFR was comparable to that seen with HI non-BFR, indicating no additional risk [38]. Clark et al. [36] also conducted a study in 16 young adults who performed BFR training for four weeks, reporting no significant increases in D-dimer, high-sensitivity C-reactive protein (hs-CRP), or prothrombin time, thereby supporting the safety of BFR with respect to venous thromboembolism.

Tennent et al. [39] investigated 17 patients aged 18–65 years who underwent knee arthroscopy and were divided into BFR (80% arterial occlusion pressure) and non-BFR exercise groups. No thrombus formation was observed in either group. Calatayud et al. [40] studied eight patients with hemophilia and found that low-load resistance training with BFR at 40% of arterial occlusion pressure resulted in no adverse effects such as bleeding, and no significant differences in pain, rate of perceived exertion (RPE), or tolerability compared to the control group.

Madarame et al. [41] reported that in patients with stable ischemic heart disease who were not on anticoagulants, BFR led to significant increases in heart rate and plasma noradrenaline levels, but no significant changes were observed in D-dimer, fibrin degradation products, or hs-CRP, suggesting that BFR may be relatively safe in this population. However, due to the cardiac load it induces, caution is warranted, and the use of BFR is contraindicated in patients with unstable ischemic heart disease.

The application of BFR is not recommended for individuals with arterial calcification, sickle cell traits, severe hypertension, heart failure, unstable ischemic heart disease, or those taking procoagulant medications. Local complications may include subcutaneous hemorrhage and transient numbness due to peripheral nerve compression, though these symptoms typically resolve over time [42]. To minimize the risk of systemic or local complications, BFR should be applied under the supervision of trained professionals, following appropriate screening and individualized assessment.

4. Analgesic Effects of Blood Flow Restriction Training

The results of studies investigating the analgesic effects of BFR training have been variable. In patients who have undergone anterior cruciate ligament (ACL) reconstruction, research indicates that the initial perception of pain and exercise intensity, as measured by the rating of perceived exertion, in the LI BFR group is comparable to or even higher than that in the HI non-BFR group [38,43]. This heightened pain sensitivity is believed to result from the hypoxic environment within the muscle and the accumulation of lactic acid, which stimulate the release of algogenic substances such as substance P, bradykinin, histamine, and prostaglandins.

However, Martín-Hernández et al. [44] reported that although the perceived exercise intensity was similar between the LI BFR and HI non-BFR groups at the onset of training, it significantly decreased in the LI BFR group over the course of repeated sessions. In addition, anterior knee pain was found to be lower in the BFR group. Hughes et al. [31] compared four groups—low-intensity, high-intensity, low-intensity low BFR (40% arterial occlusion pressure, 30% of one-repetition maximum), and low-intensity high BFR (80% arterial occlusion pressure, 30% of one-repetition maximum)—and observed increased pressure pain thresholds and exercise-induced hypoalgesia in both BFR groups. Furthermore, the BFR groups maintained a reduced level of exercise-induced pain 24 h after the training session.

In studies by Segal et al. [23,24] involving patients with knee osteoarthritis, the LI BFR group demonstrated significantly greater reductions in pain following a 12-week exercise program compared to the non-BFR group.

5. Application and Clinical Outcomes of Blood Flow Restriction Training in Patients with Anterior Cruciate Ligament Injuries

Most patients who undergo ACL reconstruction exhibit quadricep weakness and muscle atrophy, which can persist for a significant period after surgery [45,46]. This condition has been associated with an increased risk of re-injury and residual instability [47]. To address this issue, BFR training after ACL reconstruction has demonstrated improvements in strength and hypertrophy of the quadriceps, hamstrings, and adductor muscles in most studies [6,22,25,28,48].

Research indicates that BFR applied for more than three months is clinically effective (Table 1). For instance, a study by Ohta et al. [22] evaluated 44 young men and women who underwent ACL reconstruction, comparing a BFR exercise group with a non-BFR exercise group over a three-month period. The results showed significant improvements in maximal strength during knee extension and flexion, as well as in the cross sectional area of the quadriceps, hamstrings, and adductor muscles in the BFR group. Muscle biopsies assessing type 1 and type 2 muscle fiber diameters in eight patients per group revealed an increase in fiber diameter in the BFR group, although the difference was not statistically significant. The Cochrane risk of bias for each study is summarized in Table 2.

Table 1. Outcomes of blood flow restriction exercise in anterior cruciate ligament reconstruction.

Author	Study Design	Population	Method	Outcomes
Ohta et al. [22] (2003) *	RCT	BFR (n = 22, mean age 30) -non BFR (n = 22, mean age 28)	180 mmHg, 16 weeks	-Knee extensor and flexor strength: BFR > Control CC60 86 ± 14: 84 ± 13 CC180 90 ± 9: 84 ± 14 IM60 94 ± 21: 92 ± 19 -CSA ratio of knee extensor: BFR (101 ± 11) > Control (92 ± 12)
Lambert et al. [28] † (2019)	RCT	BFR (n = 7) vs. non BFR (n = 7)	12 weeks, 20% 1RM	-Thigh lean muscle mass: BFR > Control -Similar improvements in single leg squat distance, Y-balance
Zargi et al. [25] † (2018)	RCT	BFR (n = 10) vs. non BFR (n = 10)	12 weeks, 150 mmHg, 14 cm, 30% 1RM	-Isometric endurance: BFR > control -Muscle blood flow: BFR > control
Hughes et al. [6] (2019) L	RCT	BFR (n = 12) vs. non BFR (n = 12)	8 weeks -BFR: 80% LOP 11.5 cm, 30% 1RM -non BFR: 70% 1RM	-10RM and Isokinetic strength: increased in both groups (104% and 106%) -Muscle thickness: increased in both groups (5.8% and 6.7%) -Self-reported function, Quality of life and Y-balance performance(18–59 > 18–33): BFR > HL-RT -Joint pain and effusion: HL-RT > BFR

Table 1. *Cont.*

Author	Study Design	Population	Method	Outcomes
Vieira de Melo et al. [29] (2022) [L]	RCT	BFR (n = 12) vs. non BFR (n = 12)	12 weeks -BFR: LOP 80% 30% 1RM -non BFR: 70% 1RM	-Isometric strength: BFR > control -Lysholm, IKDC and KOOS questionnaires: BFR > control -Quality of life improvement: BFR > control
Karampampa et al. [27] (2023) †	RCT	BFR (n = 8) vs. non BFR (n = 8)	12–18 w -BFR: LOP 60–80% 10–20% 1RM -non BFR: 10–20% 1RM	Thigh circumference: BFR > control Isokinetic strength: BFR (13.4) > control (9.6) No significant difference in quality of life
Robert A Jack 2nd et al. [26] (2023) [L]	RCT	BFR (n = 17) vs. non BFR (n = 15)	12 weeks -BFR: LOP 80% 20% 1RM -non BFR: 20% 1RM	LE-LM: BFR (−0.39) > control (−4.67) LE bone mass: BFR (−2.58) > control (−16.95) Similar improvement in single-leg squat, single-leg eccentric step-down, Y-balance Return to sports time: BFR group < control

RCT; randomized control study; BFR; blood flow restriction; CSA; cross sectional area; EMG; electromyography; LOP; limb occlusion pressure; HL-RT; heavy-load resistance training; IKDC; the international knee documentation committee; KOOS; the knee injury and osteoarthritis outcome; LE; lower extremity; LM; lean mass. Risk of bias: high risk *; some concern †; low risk [L].

Table 2. Cochrane risk of bias 2.

	Randomization Process	Deviations from Intended Interventions	Measurement of the Outcome	Missing Outcome Data	Selection of the Reported Result	Overall Risk of Bias
Ohta et al. [22] (2003)	Some concerns	High risk	High risk	Low risk	Low risk	High risk
Lambert et al. [28] (2019)	Low risk	Some concerns	Low risk	Low risk	Low risk	Some concerns
Zargi et al. [25] (2018)	Some concerns	High risk	Some concerns	Low risk	Low risk	Some concerns
Hughes et al. [6] (2019)	Low risk	Some concerns	Low risk	Low risk	Low risk	Low risk
Vieira de Melo et al. [29] (2022)	Low risk	Low risk	Low risk	Low risk	Low risk	Low risk
Karampampa et al. [27] (2023)	Low risk	Some concerns	Low risk	Low risk	Low risk	Some concerns
Robert A Jack 2nd et al. [26] (2023)	Low risk	Low risk	Low risk	Low risk	Low risk	Low risk

Additionally, Hughes et al. [6] investigated the effects of exercise following ACL reconstruction by dividing 24 young men and women into a LI BFR exercise group and a HI non-BFR exercise group. The authors compared outcomes including muscle strength, muscle mass, knee range of motion, physical function scores, and pain levels. The LI BFR group showed improvements in strength and muscle mass that were comparable to those observed in the HI non-BFR group. Moreover, the LI BFR group demonstrated greater gains in knee range of motion, higher physical function scores, and lower pain levels [6].

6. Application and Clinical Outcomes of Blood Flow Restriction Training in Patients with Knee Osteoarthritis

Quadriceps weakness and thigh muscle atrophy are recognized as significant contributors to the development and progression of knee osteoarthritis [1]. In particular, as the radiographic severity of osteoarthritis advances, quadricep strength has been shown to be closely associated with the performance of daily activities and overall functional capacity [49]. Numerous studies applying BFR training in patients with knee osteoarthritis have reported improvements in muscle strength and mass, as well as enhancements in functional performance and reductions in pain levels [7–9].

Key studies examining the effects of BFR training in individuals with knee osteoarthritis are summarized in Table 3. Some discrepancies have been noted regarding the short-term efficacy of BFR training based on gender. Segal et al. [23,24] conducted separate studies in men and women. In a study involving 41 men aged 45 years and older with knee osteoarthritis or risk factors for osteoarthritis, a four-week intervention comparing a BFR exercise group with a non-BFR group showed no significant differences in maximal strength. However, knee clinical pain scores were higher in the BFR group. In contrast, a similar four-week study in 40 women aged 45 to 65 years with osteoarthritis or osteoarthritis risk factors demonstrated significantly greater improvements in maximal strength in the BFR group, while no significant differences in knee clinical pain scores were observed between the groups.

Table 3. Outcomes of blood flow restriction exercise in osteoarthritis patients.

Author	Study Design	Population	Method	Outcomes
Segal et al. [23] (2015) [L]	RCT	BFR (n = 19, 58.4 years) vs. non BFR (n = 22, 56.1 years)	160–200 mmHg, 4 weeks 30% 1RM	-Bilateral leg press 1RM: Increased significantly in both groups -Isokinetic strength: BFR (3.1) < control (4.7) -KOOS scores: BFR (4.9) < control (14.2)
Segal et al. [24] (2015) [L]	RCT	BFR (n = 19) vs. non BFR (n = 21)	160–200 mmHg, 4 weeks 30% 1RM	-Bilateral leg press 1RM: BFR (28.3) > control (15.6) -Isokinetic strength: BFR (0.07) > control (−0.05) -Quadriceps volume: no significant group differences -Knee pain: no significant group differences
Bryk et al. [9] (2016) †	RCT	BFR (n = 17) vs. non BFR (n = 17)	6 weeks -BFR: 200 mmHg 30% 1RM -non BFR: Pressure not described; 70% 1RM	-Improved strength, function, pain in both groups -Anterior knee discomfort: BFR < control
Ferraz et al. [8] (2018) †	RCT	BFR with LIRT (n = 16, 60.7 years) non BFR HI-RT (n = 16, 59.9 years) non BFR LI-RT (n = 16, 60.3 years)	12 weeks -BFR with LIRT: LOP 70%, 20–30% 1RM -non BFR HI-RT: 50–80% 1RM -non BFR LI-RT: 20–30% 1RM	-Significant leg press (26% and 33%) and knee extension 1RM (23% and 22%) increase in BFR and HI-RT but not in LI-RT -Quadriceps CSA (7% and 8%) increase in BFR and HI-RT but not in LI-RT -TST improvement in HI-RT and BFR but not significant with TUG -WOMAC physical function (−42% and −49%) improved in HI-RT and BFRT -WOMAC pain (−49% and −42%) improved in BFRT and LI-RT -No difference in quality of life among the three groups

Table 3. *Cont.*

Author	Study Design	Population	Method	Outcomes
Harper et al. [7] (2019) ^{L}	RCT	BFR (n = 19) vs. non BFR (n = 16)	12 weeks -BFR: [Pressure = 0.5 × SBP + 2(thigh circumference) + 5] 20% 1RM -non BFR MI-RT: 60% 1RM	-Isokinetic strength: improvement in both groups -Function (400 m walk, SPPB, LLFDI) improvement in both groups -Pain (WOMAC and NPRS) improvement in both groups -No significant difference in Serum P3NP, TWEAK, IGF-1 levels

RCT; randomized control study; BFR; blood flow restriction; KOOS; the knee injury and osteoarthritis outcome; LI-RT; low-intensity resistance training; HI-RT; high-intensity resistance training; CSA; cross sectional area; TST; Timed stands test; TUG; timed up and go test; WOMAC; the Western Ontario and McMaster universities osteoarthritis index; MI-RT; moderate-intensity resistance training; SPPB; short physical performance battery; LLFDI; late life function and disability instrument; NPRS; numeric pain rating scale; P3NP; N-terminal peptide of procollagen type III; TWEAK; tumor necrosis-like weak inducer of apoptosis; IGF-1; insulin-like growth factor. Risk of bias: some concern †; low risk ^{L}.

In contrast, most studies involving BFR applied for more than six weeks have reported clinically meaningful outcomes. For example, Ferraz et al. [8] investigated 48 women with Kellgren and Lawrence grade 2 or 3 knee osteoarthritis, who were assigned to one of three groups, LI BFR, HI non-BFR, or LI non-BFR, over a twelve-week training period. The LI BFR group demonstrated increases in maximal strength and muscle mass comparable to those observed in the HI non-BFR group, whereas no significant improvements were noted in the LI non-BFR group. Both the LI BFR and HI non-BFR groups exhibited significant gains in functional performance, including improved results on the timed stands test and enhanced knee clinical scores. Notably, only the LI BFR group showed a significant reduction in clinical stiffness. Knee clinical pain scores decreased in both the LI BFR and LI non-BFR groups, while 25% of participants in the HI non-BFR group withdrew from the study due to pain experienced during exercise. Other studies have similarly reported that the LI BFR group achieved significant improvements in muscle strength, muscle mass, and functional performance compared to the LI non-BFR group. The Cochrane risk of bias for each study is summarized in Table 4.

Table 4. Cochrane risk of bias 2.

	Randomization Process	Deviations from Intended Interventions	Measurement of the Outcome	Missing Outcome Data	Selection of the Reported Result	Overall Risk of Bias
Segal et al. [23] (2015)	Low risk	Low risk	Low risk	Low risk	Low risk	Low risk
Segal et al. [24] (2015, Men)	Low risk	Low risk	Low risk	Low risk	Low risk	Low risk
Harper et al. [7] (2019)	Low risk	Some concerns	Low risk	Low risk	Low risk	Some concerns
Bryk et al. [9] (2016)	Low risk	Some concerns	Low risk	Low risk	Low risk	Some concerns
Ferraz et al. [8] (2018)	Low risk	Low risk	Low risk	Low risk	Low risk	Low risk

7. Current Methods and Recommendations of BFR Application Used by the Authors

In patients with ACL reconstruction or knee osteoarthritis, BFR training can be applied using a progressive algorithm (Figure 3), tailored to the individual's ambulatory capacity and tolerance to exercise intensity.

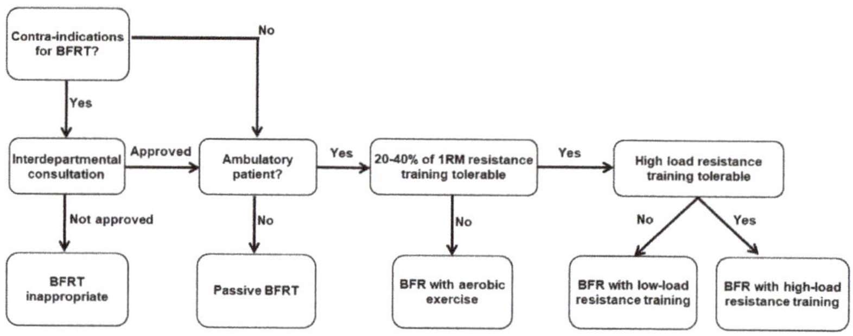

Figure 3. Algorithm for blood flow restriction training in a similar protocol as reported in the previous review article by Brendan R. Scott et al. [50].

Passive BFR is indicated for patients who have difficulty with weight-bearing exercise or walking. When ambulation is possible, aerobic exercises such as walking or cycling are typically performed in combination with BFR (Figure 4A). BFR resistance training is introduced when the patient is able to tolerate exercise at an intensity of 20–40% of 1RM (Figure 4B).

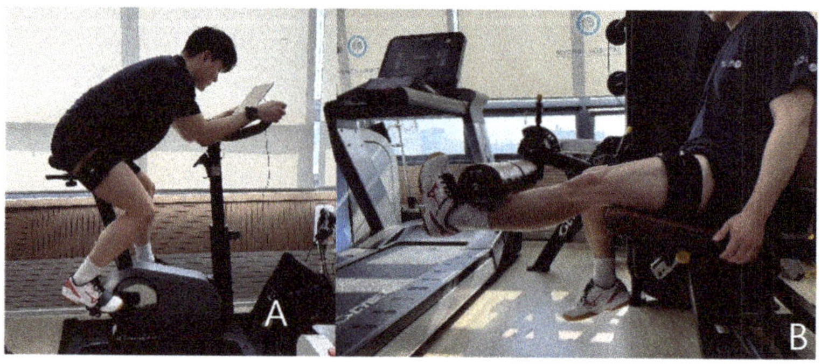

Figure 4. Blood flow restriction aerobic exercise (**A**) and blood flow restriction resistance training (**B**).

According to current safety guidelines, BFR training is considered contraindicated in individuals with severe cardiovascular disease, uncontrolled hypertension, active thromboembolic disorders, or sickle cell anemia, unless cleared through comprehensive interdepartmental consultation. In patients with relative risk factors—such as hemophilia or stable ischemic heart disease—BFR training may still be implemented under appropriate clinical supervision, with continuous monitoring of hemodynamic responses and neurovascular status to ensure safety.

8. Limitations

Most of the studies cited in this review are small-scale randomized controlled trials or pilot studies, which limits the overall strength and generalizability of the current evidence. Additionally, substantial variability in BFR protocols—such as cuff pressure, cuff width, duration, and training frequency—poses challenges in establishing standardized clinical recommendations. Many studies also lack long-term follow-up and fail to incorporate functional outcome measures that accurately reflect real-world improvements in patient function. To validate the clinical efficacy of BFR in the management of knee conditions, large-scale, prospective, multicenter randomized controlled trials are warranted.

9. Conclusions

BFR training may serve as an effective rehabilitation strategy for patients following knee surgery or those with knee osteoarthritis who are unable to perform HI exercise and are at risk of muscle disuse. Substantial evidence supports the efficacy of low-intensity BFR training in improving muscle strength, muscular endurance, quadriceps volume, and patient-reported functional outcomes. However, findings related to performance-based functional tests and pain relief remain inconsistent across studies, highlighting the need for further investigation. Nonetheless, when applied using evidence-based protocols and maintained for an adequate duration, BFR training can provide meaningful clinical benefits while minimizing the injury risk associated with HI non-BFR exercises. Moreover, adherence to established safety guidelines reduces the risk of adverse events, including cardiovascular stress, muscle damage, thrombosis, and embolism, thereby supporting the safety and utility of BFR as a rehabilitation modality.

Author Contributions: D.-H.K. contributed to the conceptualization of the approach, surgical procedures, data analysis, writing of article, and submission of article; D.-H.K. and S.K. to the writing of the article; K.-C.B. and C.-J.Y. to the data collection and critical review of the article. All authors have read and agreed to the published version of the manuscript.

Funding: This research received no external funding.

Institutional Review Board Statement: Not applicable.

Informed Consent Statement: Not applicable.

Data Availability Statement: Data sharing is not applicable. No new data were created or analyzed in this study.

Conflicts of Interest: The authors declare no conflicts of interest.

References

1. Segal, N.A.; Glass, N.A.; Felson, D.T.; Hurley, M.; Yang, M.; Nevitt, M.; Lewis, C.E.; Torner, J.C. Effect of quadriceps strength and proprioception on risk for knee osteoarthritis. *Med. Sci. Sports Exerc.* **2010**, 42, 2081–2088. [CrossRef] [PubMed]
2. Bi, Z.; Cai, Y.; Sun, C.; Shi, X.; Liao, S.; Liu, J. Different Radiological Indices of Patellar Height Predict Patients' Diverse Outcomes Following Total Knee Arthroplasty. *Clin. Orthop. Surg.* **2024**, 16, 741–750. [CrossRef] [PubMed]
3. Kim, S.E.; Ro, D.H.; Lee, M.C.; Han, H.S. Can individual functional improvements be predicted in osteoarthritic patients after total knee arthroplasty? *Knee Surg. Relat. Res.* **2024**, 36, 31. [CrossRef] [PubMed]
4. Lawrence, K.W.; Link, L.; Lavin, P.; Schwarzkopf, R.; Rozell, J.C. Characterizing patient factors, perioperative interventions, and outcomes associated with inpatients falls after total knee arthroplasty. *Knee Surg. Relat. Res.* **2024**, 36, 11. [CrossRef]
5. Londhe, S.B.; Shetty, S.; Shetty, V.; Desouza, C.; Banka, P.; Antao, N. Comparison of Time Taken in Conventional versus Active Robotic-Assisted Total Knee Arthroplasty. *Clin. Orthop. Surg.* **2024**, 16, 259–264. [CrossRef]
6. Hughes, L.; Rosenblatt, B.; Haddad, F.; Gissane, C.; McCarthy, D.; Clarke, T.; Ferris, G.; Dawes, J.; Paton, B.; Patterson, S.D. Comparing the Effectiveness of Blood Flow Restriction and Traditional Heavy Load Resistance Training in the Post-Surgery Rehabilitation of Anterior Cruciate Ligament Reconstruction Patients: A UK National Health Service Randomised Controlled Trial. *Sports Med.* **2019**, 49, 1787–1805. [CrossRef]
7. Harper, S.A.; Roberts, L.M.; Layne, A.S.; Jaeger, B.C.; Gardner, A.K.; Sibille, K.T.; Wu, S.S.; Vincent, K.R.; Fillingim, R.B.; Manini, T.M.; et al. Blood-Flow Restriction Resistance Exercise for Older Adults with Knee Osteoarthritis: A Pilot Randomized Clinical Trial. *J. Clin. Med.* **2019**, 8, 265. [CrossRef]

8. Ferraz, R.B.; Gualano, B.; Rodrigues, R.; Kurimori, C.O.; Fuller, R.; Lima, F.R.; DE Sá-Pinto, A.L.; Roschel, H. Benefits of Resistance Training with Blood Flow Restriction in Knee Osteoarthritis. *Med. Sci. Sports Exerc.* **2018**, *50*, 897–905. [CrossRef]
9. Bryk, F.F.; dos Reis, A.C.; Fingerhut, D.; Araujo, T.; Schutzer, M.; Cury, R.d.P.L.; Duarte, A.; Fukuda, T.Y. Exercises with partial vascular occlusion in patients with knee osteoarthritis: A randomized clinical trial. *Knee Surg. Sports Traumatol. Arthrosc.* **2016**, *24*, 1580–1586. [CrossRef]
10. Kong, D.H.; Jung, W.S.; Yang, S.J.; Kim, J.G.; Park, H.Y.; Kim, J. Effects of Neuromuscular Electrical Stimulation and Blood Flow Restriction in Rehabilitation after Anterior Cruciate Ligament Reconstruction. *Int. J. Environ. Res. Public Health* **2022**, *19*, 15041. [CrossRef]
11. Gabler, C.; Kitzman, P.H.; Mattacola, C.G. Targeting quadriceps inhibition with electromyographic biofeedback: A neuroplastic approach. *Crit. Rev. Biomed. Eng.* **2013**, *41*, 125–135. [CrossRef]
12. Sato, Y. The history and future of KAATSU Training. *Int. J. KAATSU Train. Res.* **2005**, *1*, 1–5. [CrossRef]
13. Abe, T.; Kearns, C.F.; Sato, Y. Muscle size and strength are increased following walk training with restricted venous blood flow from the leg muscle, Kaatsu-walk training. *J. Appl. Physiol.* **2006**, *100*, 1460–1466. [CrossRef] [PubMed]
14. Hughes, L.; Paton, B.; Rosenblatt, B.; Gissane, C.; Patterson, S.D. Blood flow restriction training in clinical musculoskeletal rehabilitation: A systematic review and meta-analysis. *Br. J. Sports Med.* **2017**, *51*, 1003–1011. [CrossRef] [PubMed]
15. Fry, C.S.; Glynn, E.L.; Drummond, M.J.; Timmerman, K.L.; Fujita, S.; Abe, T.; Dhanani, S.; Volpi, E.; Rasmussen, B.B. Blood flow restriction exercise stimulates mTORC1 signaling and muscle protein synthesis in older men. *J. Appl. Physiol.* **2010**, *108*, 1199–1209. [CrossRef] [PubMed]
16. Fujita, S.; Abe, T.; Drummond, M.J.; Cadenas, J.G.; Dreyer, H.C.; Sato, Y.; Volpi, E.; Rasmussen, B.B. Blood flow restriction during low-intensity resistance exercise increases S6K1 phosphorylation and muscle protein synthesis. *J. Appl. Physiol.* **2007**, *103*, 903–910. [CrossRef]
17. Hwang, P.S.; Willoughby, D.S. Mechanisms Behind Blood Flow-Restricted Training and its Effect Toward Muscle Growth. *J. Strength Cond. Res.* **2019**, *33* (Suppl. S1), S167–S179. [CrossRef]
18. Patterson, S.D.; Ferguson, R.A. Increase in calf post-occlusive blood flow and strength following short-term resistance exercise training with blood flow restriction in young women. *Eur. J. Appl. Physiol.* **2010**, *108*, 1025–1033. [CrossRef]
19. Bowman, E.N.; Elshaar, R.; Milligan, H.; Jue, G.; Mohr, K.; Brown, P.; Watanabe, D.M.; Limpisvasti, O. Proximal, Distal, and Contralateral Effects of Blood Flow Restriction Training on the Lower Extremities: A Randomized Controlled Trial. *Sports Health* **2019**, *11*, 149–156. [CrossRef]
20. Dreyer, H.C.; Fujita, S.; Cadenas, J.G.; Chinkes, D.L.; Volpi, E.; Rasmussen, B.B. Resistance exercise increases AMPK activity and reduces 4E-BP1 phosphorylation and protein synthesis in human skeletal muscle. *J. Physiol.* **2006**, *576*, 613–624. [CrossRef]
21. Bani Asadi, M.; Sharifi, H.; Abedi, B.; Fatolahi, H. Acute Inflammatory Response to a Single Bout of Resistance Exercise with or Without Blood Flow Restriction. *Int. J. Sport Stud. Health* **2020**, *3*, e110594. [CrossRef]
22. Ohta, H.; Kurosawa, H.; Ikeda, H.; Iwase, Y.; Satou, N.; Nakamura, S. Low-load resistance muscular training with moderate restriction of blood flow after anterior cruciate ligament reconstruction. *Acta Orthop. Scand.* **2003**, *74*, 62–68. [CrossRef]
23. Segal, N.; Davis, M.D.; Mikesky, A.E. Efficacy of Blood Flow-Restricted Low-Load Resistance Training For Quadriceps Strengthening in Men at Risk of Symptomatic Knee Osteoarthritis. *Geriatr. Orthop. Surg. Rehabil.* **2015**, *6*, 160–167. [CrossRef]
24. Segal, N.A.; Williams, G.N.; Davis, M.C.; Wallace, R.B.; Mikesky, A.E. Efficacy of blood flow-restricted, low-load resistance training in women with risk factors for symptomatic knee osteoarthritis. *PM&R* **2015**, *7*, 376–384.
25. Zargi, T.; Drobnic, M.; Strazar, K.; Kacin, A. Short-Term Preconditioning With Blood Flow Restricted Exercise Preserves Quadriceps Muscle Endurance in Patients After Anterior Cruciate Ligament Reconstruction. *Front. Physiol.* **2018**, *9*, 1150. [CrossRef] [PubMed]
26. Jack, R.A., 2nd; Lambert, B.S.; Hedt, C.A.; Delgado, D.; Goble, H.; McCulloch, P.C. Blood Flow Restriction Therapy Preserves Lower Extremity Bone and Muscle Mass After ACL Reconstruction. *Sports Health* **2023**, *15*, 361–371. [CrossRef] [PubMed]
27. Karampampa, C.; Papasoulis, E.; Hatzimanouil, D.; Koutras, G.; Totlis, T. The Effects of Exercise with Blood Flow Restriction (BFR) in the Post Operative Rehabilitation of Anterior Cruciate Ligament (ACL) Reconstruction Patients: A Case Series. *J. Orthop. Res. Ther.* **2023**, *8*, 1314. [CrossRef]
28. Lambert, B.; Hedt, C.A.; Jack, R.A.; Moreno, M.; Delgado, D.; Harris, J.D.; McCulloch, P.C. Blood Flow Restriction Therapy Preserves Whole Limb Bone and Muscle Following ACL Reconstruction. *Orthop. J. Sports Med.* **2019**, *7*, 2325967119S00196. [CrossRef]
29. Vieira de Melo, R.F.; Komatsu, W.R.; Freitas, M.S.; Vieira de Melo, M.E.; Cohen, M. Comparison of Quadriceps and Hamstring Muscle Strength after Exercises with and without Blood Flow Restriction following Anterior Cruciate Ligament Surgery: A Randomized Controlled Trial. *J. Rehabil. Med.* **2022**, *54*, 2550. [CrossRef]
30. Mattocks, K.T.; Jessee, M.B.; Counts, B.R.; Buckner, S.L.; Mouser, J.G.; Dankel, S.J.; Laurentino, G.C.; Loenneke, J.P. The effects of upper body exercise across different levels of blood flow restriction on arterial occlusion pressure and perceptual responses. *Physiol. Behav.* **2017**, *171*, 181–186. [CrossRef]

31. Hughes, L.; Patterson, S.D. The effect of blood flow restriction exercise on exercise-induced hypoalgesia and endogenous opioid and endocannabinoid mechanisms of pain modulation. *J. Appl. Physiol.* **2020**, *128*, 914–924. [CrossRef]
32. Neto, G.R.; Sousa, M.S.; Costa e Silva, G.V.; Gil, A.L.; Salles, B.F.; Novaes, J.S. Acute resistance exercise with blood flow restriction effects on heart rate, double product, oxygen saturation and perceived exertion. *Clin. Physiol. Funct. Imaging* **2016**, *36*, 53–59. [CrossRef]
33. Nielsen, J.L.; Aagaard, P.; Prokhorova, T.A.; Nygaard, T.; Bech, R.D.; Suetta, C.; Frandsen, U. Blood flow restricted training leads to myocellular macrophage infiltration and upregulation of heat shock proteins, but no apparent muscle damage. *J. Physiol.* **2017**, *595*, 4857–4873. [CrossRef]
34. Mouser, J.G.; Dankel, S.J.; Jessee, M.B.; Mattocks, K.T.; Buckner, S.L.; Counts, B.R.; Loenneke, J.P. A tale of three cuffs: The hemodynamics of blood flow restriction. *Eur. J. Appl. Physiol.* **2017**, *117*, 1493–1499. [CrossRef] [PubMed]
35. Manini, T.M.; Clark, B.C. Blood flow restricted exercise and skeletal muscle health. *Exerc. Sport Sci. Rev.* **2009**, *37*, 78–85. [CrossRef] [PubMed]
36. Clark, B.C.; Manini, T.M.; Hoffman, R.L.; Williams, P.S.; Guiler, M.K.; Knutson, M.J.; McGlynn, M.L.; Kushnick, M.R. Relative safety of 4 weeks of blood flow-restricted resistance exercise in young, healthy adults. *Scand. J. Med. Sci. Sports* **2011**, *21*, 653–662. [CrossRef] [PubMed]
37. Takano, H.; Morita, T.; Iida, H.; Asada, K.-I.; Kato, M.; Uno, K.; Hirose, K.; Matsumoto, A.; Takenaka, K.; Hirata, Y.; et al. Hemodynamic and hormonal responses to a short-term low-intensity resistance exercise with the reduction of muscle blood flow. *Eur. J. Appl. Physiol.* **2005**, *95*, 65–73. [CrossRef]
38. Hughes, L.; Paton, B.; Haddad, F.; Rosenblatt, B.; Gissane, C.; Patterson, S.D. Comparison of the acute perceptual and blood pressure response to heavy load and light load blood flow restriction resistance exercise in anterior cruciate ligament reconstruction patients and non-injured populations. *Phys. Ther. Sport* **2018**, *33*, 54–61. [CrossRef]
39. Tennent, D.J.; Hylden, C.M.; Johnson, A.E.; Burns, T.C.; Wilken, J.M.; Owens, J.G. Blood Flow Restriction Training After Knee Arthroscopy: A Randomized Controlled Pilot Study. *Clin. J. Sport Med.* **2017**, *27*, 245–252. [CrossRef]
40. Calatayud, J.; Ogrezeanu, D.C.; Carrasco, J.J.; Martinez-Valdes, E.; Pérez-Alenda, S.; Cruz-Montecinos, C.; Andersen, L.L.; Aagaard, P.; Suso-Martí, L.; Casaña, J. Safety, feasibility, and neuromuscular activity of acute low-load resistance exercise with or without blood flow restriction in patients with severe hemophilia. *Eur. J. Haematol.* **2023**, *111*, 47–56. [CrossRef]
41. Madarame, H.; Kurano, M.; Fukumura, K.; Fukuda, T.; Nakajima, T. Haemostatic and inflammatory responses to blood flow-restricted exercise in patients with ischaemic heart disease: A pilot study. *Clin. Physiol. Funct. Imaging* **2013**, *33*, 11–17. [CrossRef]
42. de Queiros, V.S.; Dantas, M.; Neto, G.R.; da Silva, L.F.; Assis, M.G.; Almeida-Neto, P.F.; Dantas, P.M.S.; Cabral, B.G.D.A.T. Application and side effects of blood flow restriction technique: A cross-sectional questionnaire survey of professionals. *Medicine* **2021**, *100*, e25794. [CrossRef] [PubMed]
43. Hollander, D.B.; Reeves, G.V.; Clavier, J.D.; Francois, M.R.; Thomas, C.; Kraemer, R.R. Partial occlusion during resistance exercise alters effort sense and pain. *J. Strength Cond. Res.* **2010**, *24*, 235–243. [CrossRef] [PubMed]
44. Martín-Hernández, J.; Ruiz-Aguado, J.; Herrero, A.J.; Loenneke, J.P.; Aagaard, P.; Cristi-Montero, C.; Menéndez, H.; Marín, P.J. Adaptation of Perceptual Responses to Low-Load Blood Flow Restriction Training. *J. Strength Cond. Res.* **2017**, *31*, 765–772. [CrossRef] [PubMed]
45. Sinsurin, K.; Kiratisin, P.; Irawan, D.S.; Vachalathiti, R.; Richards, J. Residual deficits of knee and hip joint coordination and clinical performance after return to sports in athletes with anterior cruciate ligament reconstruction. *Knee Surg. Relat. Res.* **2024**, *36*, 22. [CrossRef]
46. Yoon, K.H.; Lee, S.M.; Park, J.Y.; Lee, H.S.; Hwang, S.H. A Comparison of Results in Older, Middle-aged, and Younger Patients after Primary Anterior Cruciate Ligament Reconstruction: Minimum 10-Year Follow-up. *Clin. Orthop. Surg.* **2024**, *16*, 57–65. [CrossRef]
47. Gupta, R.; Singhal, A.; Malhotra, A.; Soni, A.; Masih, G.D.; Raghav, M. Predictors for Anterior Cruciate Ligament (ACL) Re-injury after Successful Primary ACL Reconstruction (ACLR). *Malays. Orthop. J.* **2020**, *14*, 50–56. [CrossRef]
48. Takarada, Y.; Takazawa, H.; Ishii, N. Applications of vascular occlusion diminish disuse atrophy of knee extensor muscles. *Med. Sci. Sports Exerc.* **2000**, *32*, 2035–2039. [CrossRef]
49. McAlindon, T.E.; Cooper, C.; Kirwan, J.R.; Dieppe, P.A. Determinants of disability in osteoarthritis of the knee. *Ann. Rheum. Dis.* **1993**, *52*, 258–262. [CrossRef]
50. Scott, B.R.; Loenneke, J.P.; Slattery, K.M.; Dascombe, B.J. Exercise with blood flow restriction: An updated evidence-based approach for enhanced muscular development. *Sports Med.* **2015**, *45*, 313–325. [CrossRef]

MDPI AG
Grosspeteranlage 5
4052 Basel
Switzerland
Tel.: +41 61 683 77 34

Medicina Editorial Office
E-mail: medicina@mdpi.com
www.mdpi.com/journal/medicina

MDPI

www.ingramcontent.com/pod-product-compliance
Lightning Source LLC
Chambersburg PA
CBHW062039220926
51850CB00010B/2605
* 9 7 8 3 7 2 5 8 6 5 6 4 2 *